A Handbook for Action Research in Health and Social Care

A Handbook for Action Research in Health and Social Care

Richard Winter and
Carol Munn-Giddings

with contributions by

Cathy Aymer, Peter Beresford, Jane Bradburn,
Valerie Childs, Brenda Dennett, Philip Ingram,
Philip Kemp, Noreen Kennedy, Richard Lawrence,
Cherry Mackie, Vicky Nicholls, Fergal Searson,
Michael Turner and Yan Weaver

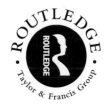

London and New York

First published 2001
by Routledge
11 New Fetter Lane, London EC4P 4EE

Simultaneously published in the USA and Canada
by Routledge
29 West 35th Street, New York, NY 10001

Routledge is an imprint of the Taylor & Francis Group

Typeset in Times by Keystroke, Jacaranda Lodge, Wolverhampton
Printed and bound in Great Britain by Biddles Ltd, Guildford
and King's Lynn

British Library Cataloguing in Publication Data
A catalogue record for this book is available
from the British Library

Library of Congress Cataloging in Publication Data
Winter, Richard, 1943–
    A handbook for action research in health and social care /
    Richard Winter and Carol Munn-Giddings.
        p. cm.
    Includes bibliographical references and index.
    1. Human services—Research. 2. Action research.
    3. Action research—Case studies. I. Munn-Giddings, Carol,
    1961–   II. Title.

HV11 .W597 2001
362'.07'2—dc21   00–047058

ISBN 0–415–22484–5 (pbk)
        0–415–22483–7 (hbk)

To Ella and Anenti

Contents

PART III
Undertaking an action research project: a practical guide

205

PART IV
Action research as a form of social inquiry: a 'theoretical' justification

253

Contributors

Cathy Aymer is a Senior Lecturer in the Department of Social Work and Director of the Centre for Black Professional Practice at Brunel University. Her main areas of work are anti-discriminatory practice and race and gender diversity in organisations. Her other interests are the ways in which welfare services respond to the needs of African refugees and of young black men.

Peter Beresford was convener of the Citizens' Commission on the Future of the Welfare State. He is Professor of Social Policy at Brunel University and works with the 'Open Services Project' and the Brunel University Centre for Citizen Participation. He is a long-term user of mental health services and is actively involved in the psychiatric system survivors' movement.

Jane Bradburn is a Research Associate at the College of Health, London. She carried out this research with cancer self-help groups at the Mount Vernon Hospital as part of a doctorate funded by the UK Economic and Social Research Council. She has since developed the 'Cancer Voices' project with the national charity Cancerlink.

Valerie Childs wrote this report when she was a social worker with Essex Social Services Department, where she is now a senior social work practitioner. She has worked with children and their families since 1976, in residential and fieldwork settings. She currently contributes to Diploma in Social Work training at Anglia Polytechnic University and offers consultation to colleagues undertaking complex casework and group work.

Brenda Dennett qualified as a social worker in 1983 and obtained a post-qualifying Honours Degree in Social Work in 1995. She undertook the piece of work reported here when she was working for Essex Social Services Department as the manager of a day-care centre for people with profound learning disabilities and complex needs often leading to behaviour which challenges service provision. She is now working as respite care manager for South Essex.

Philip Ingram is an engineer by training but retired prematurely to care for his wife during her early-onset dementia. He is now a freelance trainer and writes on dementia and on service-users' and carers' issues. He has been active in promoting user involvement in service design and monitoring, has set up a number of carers' groups and helped to establish a branch of the Alzheimer's Society in Ipswich, Suffolk.

Philip Kemp has many years of experience in the mental health field and has a particular interest in supported housing. The work reported here was undertaken when he was working for the London borough of Barking and Dagenham Social Services Department. He is now a Senior Lecturer in the Faculty of Health at South Bank University, London.

Noreen Kennedy undertook the work reported while she was working as a ward sister at the Middlesex Hospital in central London, where she is now Senior Nurse in Practice Development for General Surgery, Trauma and Orthopaedics. She has also facilitated action research projects in other clinical areas and takes a lead role in developing evidence-based practice.

Richard Lawrence undertook the work reported when he was working as a community development officer with Carlisle City Council. He is now a community development project officer with Warwickshire County Council, supporting a multi-agency partnership team in the development of a community strategy for Stratford-upon-Avon district.

Cherry Mackie is a long-term survivor of breast cancer and works as co-ordinator of the cancer service-user support groups at the Lynda Jackson Macmillan Centre, Mount Vernon Hospital, London.

Vicky Nicholls is a research support worker at the Mental Health Foundation, London. She previously worked at the Greater London Association of Community Health Councils and has completed an MA in Health and Social Policy, including research into community involvement in health needs assessments.

Fergal Searson is a Senior Lecturer in the Department of Acute and Critical Care Nursing, University of Central Lancashire, Preston, with a specific focus on coronary care nursing. He has a particular interest in involving patients in their experience of illness.

Michael Turner was the lead worker with the Citizens' Commission on the Future of the Welfare State and also with the 'Shaping Our Lives' and 'Our Voice in Our Future' projects, based in the National Institute of Social Work, London.

Yan Weaver initiated and co-ordinated the service-user-led 'Making Choices' project in Camden, London, and the 'Alternative Choices in Mental Health' research project (with support from the Mental Health Foundation) and produced a mental health handbook/directory for the borough of Camden. He has experience of receiving mental health services of various kinds, including in-patient psychiatric treatment. He also has several years' training and experience in psychotherapy and counselling, and has worked as a mental health residential and community support worker. He currently co-ordinates the work of a telephone information and advice service for 'Lambeth Mind', a user-led mental health charity in South London.

Acknowledgements

Richard Winter's work on the book was funded by the award of a Research Fellowship by the Leverhulme Trust.

Carol Munn-Giddings' contribution was partly funded by a grant from the HEFC RAE funding to the Social Work and Social Policy Division of the University.

Many thanks for the careful work of our panel of 'critical readers' – nurses, social workers, professional educators and service-users: Jane Arnett, Mary Barrett, Leo Bishop, Paul Chidgey, Jill Clark, Jayne Crow, Susan Hart, Lindsay Hill, Brenda Landgrebe, Rollanda Law, Liz Morris, Fungai Nhiwatiwa, Vivien Nice, Tony Porter, Jane Scoggins and Jan Thurlow. Chapters 1, 2 and 3 were substantially revised in the light of their suggestions.

Particular thanks, also, for helpful advice on the sections concerning service-user research and anti-racist research in Chapter 3, to: Jill Aylott, School of Health and Community Studies, Sheffield Hallam University; Cathy Aymer, Brunel University Department of Social Work; Peter Beresford, Professor of Social Work at Brunel University; Sharon Dennis, Nurse Adviser at Lewisham University Hospital.

Chapters 5 and 6 are reprinted by permission of the editors of the journal *Educational Action Research*.

Chapter 14 is published with the agreement of the Royal College of Psychiatrists: an earlier abridged version was published in R. Ramsay (ed.) *Light at the End of the Tunnel* (London: Gaskell, 2000).

Preface

The title *Handbook* is intended to indicate the varied nature of the contents and the different ways in which the book may be used or approached. In Part I there is a sequence of chapters giving a general theory of action research, first as a simple outline, then in more detail – comparing action research with other forms of social research – and finally emphasising its range and variety. Some may wish to start with this material, but others may prefer to begin by looking at the series of practical examples from different contexts presented in Part II and then go on afterwards to compare them with the theoretical discussions. The most abstract presentation of a 'theory' for action research is postponed to the end of the volume, to signal that although it may be of key importance for some readers, others may not find it necessary, and that in any case it is not essential for an understanding of the rest of the book. There is also a 'Practical guide' (Part III) which is intended specifically for groups wishing to use the *Handbook* to support them in undertaking their own practical developmental work, either independently or as part of a tutor-led course. For such readers, Part III may be their starting point for approaching the other material.

The book is a joint enterprise arising from a longstanding commitment on the part of both authors to the democratisation of social research. The themes and structure of the book were the outcome of lengthy discussions in which we combined our different but complementary approaches. Thus, Carol Munn-Giddings contributes experience and knowledge of service-user movements, service-user research, the community development tradition, and feminist research; and Richard Winter has particular expertise concerning practitioner action research, theories of management, and research methodologies based on collaborative developmental reflection.

Most of Parts I and IV of the book were initially drafted by Richard Winter, and revised in response to commentary and additions by Carol Munn-Giddings. Chapter 3 was written jointly, and represents a synthesis of our differing perspectives on action research. The same is true of the series of practice examples in Part II, for which we were jointly involved in identifying the contributors. Part III consists of material devised over many years for Richard Winter's courses on action research at Anglia Polytechnic University for social workers, nurses, managers, lecturers and school teachers. The final editorial work was undertaken by Richard Winter.

Carol Munn-Giddings worked for many years as a social researcher in various health and social services settings, including the voluntary sector, undertaking, facilitating and managing projects relating to service-users' perspectives. In her current post at Anglia Polytechnic University she is Reader in Participative Inquiry and Director of Research in the School of Community Health and Social Studies. Her work includes teaching research and innovation to practitioners and supporting staff in developing their own research.

Richard Winter has been involved with action research for most of his professional career. He is Professor of Education at Anglia Polytechnic University, where he leads an action research course providing support for practitioners and managers in a variety of professions, including health, social services and education. He is also Co-ordinator of the international action research group Collaborative Action Research Network, and co-editor of the journal *Educational Action Research*.

Email addresses
r.j.winter@anglia.ac.uk
c.munn-giddings@anglia.ac.uk

The nature of action research

Chapter 1

Introduction

Prologue

This book is about the use of action research as a strategy for inquiry and development. It proposes a form of social research which is not a separate, specialised, technical activity but one which is closely linked to practice and which can be undertaken by practitioners and service-users. It presents a general theoretical explanation, a series of specific examples illustrating a variety of approaches and contexts, and detailed practical guidance for those wishing to undertake an action research project.

The book is particularly addressed to managers, service-users, staff workers and educators involved in social and health care and community development but those concerned with teaching and with management more generally will also find almost all the arguments and examples applicable to their own contexts. We have in mind several rather different forms of inquiry, and the following list gives an idea of the range of contexts and people we hope to address:

- efforts on the part of staff in caring organisations (hospitals, social services departments, voluntary agencies, residential facilities, day centres, etc.) to develop their care work with patients/clients/ service-users;
- efforts on the part of service-user groups to develop their own services and/or improve the quality of services provided, either by gathering the views of service-users or by working in partnership with staff;
- efforts on the part of professional educators/trainers/tutors to facilitate the development of community, health and social care practices and to foster 'professional' learning;
- efforts on the part of managers to improve the quality of services through developing managerial processes and relationships;
- efforts on the part of community-based staff in mobilising efforts to develop and promote community action and support facilities such as advice and drop-in centres.

This variety means that it is sometimes difficult to find words which will seem exactly appropriate for all our anticipated readers. In particular, such words as 'work' and 'practice' are intended to refer to *all* the activities listed above, whether undertaken by managers, educators, service-users or social and health care staff and community workers (with or without professional qualifications). Similarly, the term 'practice context' is intended to refer to service-user group meetings, hospitals, care agencies and educational/training processes. If sometimes our phrasing seems to be excluding some of these activities, we apologise: our arguments about action research and our examples of practical work are fully intended to be relevant for the whole variety of readers and contexts indicated above.

Outline structure of the book

As indicated in the Preface, the book may be used in different ways by readers with different purposes. As a handbook, it is not necessarily intended to be read straight through.

The next section of this chapter introduces the concept of action research through discussion of a specific example, and ends with a preliminary 'definition'.

Chapter 2 explores further how action research is different from other forms of research, arguing that it is an extension of 'reflective practice' in professional work and showing how it is different from (but related to) conventional quantitative research and conventional qualitative research. It shows how action research transforms key aspects of the inquiry process and ends with an account of 'cultures of inquiry' in the workplace.

Chapter 3 presents the range and variety of action research, discussing key themes of power, validity, collaboration, and reflection on personal experience, drawn from:

>   service-user research
>   community development
>   theories of management and organisational change
>   theories of critical reflection and evaluation
>   educational action research
>   feminist research
>   anti-racist research

Part II (Chapters 4–14) illustrates further the variety of action research, comprising a series of contrasting reports of practical projects from differing contexts: nursing, social work, community development, professional education and service-user research. Each report is complete and self-explanatory, and provides for those interested in undertaking an action research project a possible way of focusing, planning and carrying out a useful piece of work. Together, these chapters demonstrate in practical detail action research's range of purposes, research relationships, results, methods, and styles of reporting.

Part II provides comprehensive step-by-step guidance on planning and undertaking an action research project. It contains detailed discussion documents, developed for action research courses over many years, to support each stage of work: clarifying the nature of the project, practical planning, consideration of ethical issues, data gathering, data analysis and writing a research report. It is particularly intended for readers who are about to undertake a research project, and includes advice on how to use the other sections of the book to inform their work at different stages.

Finally, Part IV provides a brief 'theoretical' justification for action research to reassure those who are concerned that it may lack the rigour and objectivity of 'proper research'. This part of the book may be of particular interest to senior managers and those responsible for allocating research funding, in contexts where action research often finds difficulty in gaining recognition and support. The argument of Part IV complements earlier arguments derived from the action research literature (in Part I) to provide a more general grounding for action research's intellectual and professional rationale.

What is 'action research'?

In discussions of methods for social research, professional development and organisational change, the term 'action research' is both appealing and yet somewhat mysterious. Its ambiguity is easy to see: 'action research' suggests a single activity which is simultaneously a form of inquiry and a form of practical action. Clearly, any 'research' process involves some form of 'action' (interviewing, distributing questionnaires, etc.), but 'action research' refers to something rather different. It suggests the possibility of a form of social research which involves people in a process of change, which is based in professional, organisational or community action, and which is thus no longer beset by the age-old problem of the gap between 'theory' and 'practice'. (We all know jokes about, for example, professors of physics who can't change a fuse and psychologists who can't manage their own personal relationships.) At the same time, it proclaims an ideal of practical work which is also a form of *learning* for those involved (action *as* research). Hence its appeal.

Putting these ideas together, then, 'action research' refers to a process which alternates continuously between inquiry and action, between practice and 'innovative thinking' (Hart, 2000) – a developmental spiral of practical decision-making and evaluative reflection. It is both reflective practice and practice-based research. A nice idea, perhaps (you say), but what does it really involve? Is it feasible, and if so what does it achieve? Is it really 'research'? If so, in what sense? In what sense are its outcomes 'valid' and/or generalisable? Is it a worthwhile use of precious time? It sounds like hard work: is it worth it? Who benefits? Does it have a sound basis, or is it just a wishy-washy ideal? These are some of the questions we hope to answer in this book.

An introductory example/practical exercise

In order to get some feel for the processes of an action research project and how they differ from other sorts of research, imagine the following scenario. Your organisation has had a windfall: suddenly the sum of £4,000 is available; this will pay for, say, seventy hours of someone's time to investigate an aspect of the work that you are engaged in; and it is up to you to say what the focus of the inquiry should be.

> *(Before you read any further, make a note of such a topic – something that strongly affects your current work and which you really wish you understood better than you currently do.)*

Having decided on your topic, now imagine that you have received the money on condition that the inquiry is carried out by a professional research worker from the organisation's research department or from a university or other external body. What would you ask the researcher to do, and what sort of outcomes would you expect by the end of the inquiry process? And now, in contrast, imagine a slightly different scenario: it is stipulated that you must carry out the inquiry yourself, with the £4,000 being used to 'cover' the work you usually do. (Again the time available is seventy hours, to be structured as you wish – perhaps two weeks full time or three hours a week for about four months.) What activities would you engage in, and what outcomes would you expect? Finally, consider the probable differences between these two contrasting situations: what differences might there be in the way you and the outside researcher set about conducting the inquiry, what different conclusions might emerge, and how might the two inquiry processes have a different impact on the work situation?

Let us now consider a concrete example, which reveals, in a preliminary way, some important clues to the nature of action research. Barbara Stansell, a social worker, was, in 1997, responsible for a small team of staff working in a centre for people with learning difficulties. She was worried by what seemed to be an unacceptably high rate of staff absence due to sickness (Stansell, 1997). If resources had been available she could have commissioned an outside researcher to interview the staff and collect their explanations for their absences, together with their proposals for any changes which might improve matters. She might also have asked the researcher to collect comparative data on rates of absence in other, similar teams, in the hope that some useful patterns might emerge, indicating the factors influencing staff absence rates – the size of the team, the profile of its members in terms of age, gender and family situation, the type of client, type of neighbourhood served, level of service-user involvement, etc. At the end of the work, Barbara would have received a report containing a collection of different possible 'reasons' for staff absence (some offered by the staff, some in the form of suggested contextual influences) and some positive proposals. This would have been, let us say, a piece of 'conventional' social research.

But, in this case, Barbara undertook the inquiry herself, as an 'action research' project. And as soon as she began to consider how to approach her staff interviews, she realised that to focus directly on staff absence and sickness might seem so threatening as to be merely counterproductive for all concerned. Instead she needed to focus, positively, on how to improve staff morale, and that decision eventually resulted in her project being very largely concerned with her own management style, and especially with the contradictions in her attempts to be 'democratic'. (She thought of herself as leaving her staff plenty of scope for their own decisions, but found that in many ways she was much more 'directive' than she had thought.) So part of her work involved, for example, discussions with her staff as to how the arrangements for group meetings might be used to increase a sense of participation and achievement. What had started out as a proposal on the part of a manager to 'interview' individuals thus became a much more long-term project which was collaborative, focused on the staff group as a whole, and self-evaluative.

Commentary

This example is drawn from an organisational context: it happened to be a day-centre staff team, but it could easily have been a hospital ward or a service-user group. And one can also see how a similar set of alternatives might arise in the context of community work or service-user research, if one was worried about, let us say, the apparent under-utilisation of an Advice and Support Centre. So what general conclusions can we draw?

To begin with, we may note that action research is an approach to *social* research – understanding how human beings interact with one another, and how we respond to events and situations. Next, it is clear that action research is concerned just as much with the *process* of inquiry as with its 'findings': any research process creates relationships, and action research is concerned that its long-term impact on relationships should be positive as well as illuminating. Even more importantly, action research emphasises the value of insights derived from practical involvement in a situation, rather than the contribution of supposedly 'objective' methods applied by outsiders. An outsider acting on Barbara's original formulation of the problem could have done considerable damage to what were already fragile relationships: it was Barbara's concern for her team that led her to realise that the project needed to be refocused. And it is doubtful whether the comparative data would have offered Barbara as much guidance on the nature of her 'problem', and what to do about it, as the collaborative process she set up with her staff.

Action research seeks to bridge the ever-present gap between 'theory' and practice. It does so in two ways. It places value on the *experiential* basis for knowledge and it emphasises the *practical* motive for developing one's understanding:

> Action researchers . . . are inclined to see the development of theory or under-standing as a by-product of the improvement of real situations, rather than [seeing] application as a by-product of advances in 'pure' theory.
>
> (Carr and Kemmis, 1986: 28)

> Action research might be defined as: the study of a social situation with a view to improving the quality of action within it.
>
> (Elliott, 1991: 69)

In other words, action research is based on the assumption that increased understanding will flow from our commitment to try to bring about practical changes.

Finally, it is important to notice the 'political' ideal underlying action research. Action research starts from the belief that knowledge about human situations can be generated from our commitment to practical situations, and that our practical involvement can in itself create the understanding which our circumstances require. So we do not need to be dependent on outside experts on social science theory and methodology in order to be able to formulate issues or to determine appropriate methods. Action research is therefore about establishing inquiry processes which are specifically designed to be 'empowering' for the subjects of the inquiry. There is a danger of this becoming mere rhetoric: for many of us, encounters with the reality of power are both depressing and distressing, and 'action research' doesn't magically change this. But the concept of empowerment *is* of central importance. It embodies action research's fundamental optimism concerning people's ability and willingness to work together constructively, and also an ideal of democratic participation and responsible citizenship. Action research envisages a process whereby our understanding of ourselves and of the social world in which we are engaged can be developed and deepened as a direct consequence of our practical commitments. For action research, hierarchies of power and status (between academic and practical knowledge, between researchers and practitioners, between professionals and their clients, between experts and laypersons) are seen as inhibiting and impoverishing the creation and distribution of knowledge.

A definition?

Some of the statements already presented could be taken as 'definitions' of action research. And by the time you have read further you will probably want to construct your own definition. But at this stage, as a start, we might suggest the following.

Action research is the study of a social situation carried out by those involved in that situation in order to improve both their practice and the quality of their understanding.

Chapter 2

Action research as an approach to inquiry and development

The cycle of action and reflection as a model of 'work'

We have already noted that action research can be seen as a model of 'work' as well as a model of 'research' (see Chapter 1, p. 5). This chapter presents a general outline of action research from each of these perspectives in turn and concludes with a brief discussion of how we might try to bring the two together by attempting to create a 'culture of inquiry' in practice settings. This first main section presents action research in terms of a model of work, involving a continuous cycle of action and reflection. However, the term 'action research' immediately brings us face to face with the word 'research'. So we need to start by showing how 'research' can be reinterpreted in a way which brings out its potential link with the tasks and processes of 'work', i.e. practical interactions between colleagues, between staff and service-users, between staff and managers, and between service-users in group meetings, etc.

What does 'research' mean?

Dictionaries are useful here, as a starting point. They remind us that 'research' means to search 'again' or repeatedly, and that 'search' is connected with the Latin *circare*, to go round. So we can suggest that to research means to look at something 'from all sides' or from several different points of view. It is in this sense that we can understand 'research' as examining something 'carefully', 'intensively', 'closely', 'critically' in order to 'discover' something we did not know before (*Shorter Oxford English Dictionary*; *Concise Oxford Dictionary of English Etymology*).

Also, we live in a culture where research is conventionally seen as a *specialised* role, whose particular task is to describe and report upon the work of others. In contrast, in the light of what was said in the previous chapter it is clear that action research aims to be a form of inquiry which can be undertaken by those who are *not* specialist 'researchers'. So the 'research' aspect of 'action research' needs to be defined in such a way that it is free from this 'specialist' connotation.

Finally, we need to be careful how we interpret the suggestion that 'research' means *systematic* inquiry (Stenhouse, 1985a: 8). We can easily slip into thinking that in order to be systematic, research needs a rigid plan which predetermines both the issues and the forms of evidence to be sought. But if research is to be an activity which can arise from practical experience, then it needs to be systematic *only* in the general sense of being planned and carried out in accordance with 'general principles', e.g. that hunches should always be checked out and differing opinions compared. *Practice-based* research, therefore, needs not only to be systematic but to be *responsive* to the shifts in perspective and focus as the process unfolds; it needs to be flexible enough to accompany the complex and developing interactions arising from practice, without interrupting or distorting them.

Work and action research as a 'spiral' between action and reflection

In order to achieve the delicate balance between being systematic and being flexible, most action researchers have tended to adopt some version of Kurt Lewin's formulation of the process. Action research, he suggests, 'proceeds in a spiral of steps, each of which is composed of a circle of planning, action and fact-finding about the result of the action' (Lewin, 1946: 38). Kemmis and McTaggart elaborate this slightly in their *Action Research Planner*: action research proceeds in a series of 'cycles', in each of which we plan, act, observe, reflect and then draw up a revised plan (Kemmis and McTaggart, 1988: 11).

This is a necessary starting point, but it has certain weaknesses. First, it can be interpreted as an oversimplification, and as suggesting that the overall focus has to remain fixed; it does not allow for discovering that our concerns may need to shift and become more complex as our actions, observations and reflections deepen our understanding of the situation (McNiff, 1988: 43–6). Second (and more importantly), the emphasis on repeated cycles seems to suggest that even the basic process necessarily requires a long period of time to complete, and may be difficult to sustain in many work settings. For example, staff may be short of time even for reflection (Palmer *et al.*, 1994: 1), the long-term commitment of management to an inquiry process may be doubtful (Fuller and Petch, 1995: 5), and there may be a very high rate of turnover among participants (Meyer, 1993: 1071). We therefore need to look for an interpretation of the action research cycle which can be implemented over a relatively short period of time, i.e. weeks or months rather than years.

But if we emphasise that the action research cycle of 'plan, act, observe, reflect, re-plan' can refer to quite a small scale of events, we meet a third difficulty. Action research described in this way may seem to be so general as to refer to any moderately complex activity. For example, every time we conduct a significant conversation with peers, colleagues or clients, we first consider what to say, then we say it, then we note the response and decide on our next comment accordingly. Surely, action research must be distinguishable from such everyday interactions.

Before agreeing with this, let us nevertheless note that there is indeed an important overlap between action research and the familiar patterns of practical interaction. And this is why action research can, in principle, be accommodated within the collaborative, reflective and developmental process which most people (managers, practitioners and service-users) would accept as the appropriate ideal for workplace activity.

Let us then return to the central question of this section: is there a sense in which practical experience itself offers an opportunity for those involved to undertake the 'intensive, critical and careful' examination of their activities characteristic of 'research'? To reply 'Yes' to this, albeit tentatively, does not seem too controversial. Admittedly, pressures of time often threaten to reduce workplace interactions (between colleagues, between managers and staff, between professional workers and service-users) to a mere routine, but this is not *always* the case. On the contrary, work settings, organisational relationships and service-user needs are so *individualised* that general procedures can never prescribe *exactly* what needs to be done on particular occasions (Marks-Maran and Rose, 1997: 122): 'reflection' is always part of the process.

The significance of this last point is made clear when we examine the details of the UK 'Research in Practice' initiative, which attempts to introduce 'evidence-based practice' in the social work profession. Its aims are described as follows:

> to provide a link between social work professionals and the best research knowledge available . . . to assemble and assess findings about good practice . . . and make them available in a variety of forms to practitioners, senior managers, elected members and consumers . . . to assist all those working in social services departments who want *to build an evidence base for their practice*.
>
> (Dartington Social Research Unit, 1997 [italics added])

So here we have a managerial initiative (the project was initiated by the Association of Directors of Social Services) which assembles research findings provided by universities as a 'base' for practice, in a volume containing summaries and findings from twenty research studies carried out in universities on behalf of the government (Department of Health, 1995). But how exactly does research 'evidence' provide a 'base' for practice decisions? The brief answer is: only through further interpretive work on the part of those directly concerned. In the Foreword, by the Parliamentary Under-Secretary of State (no less), we read, 'This document is not intended as a practice text-book. . . . Professionals must be experienced, knowledgeable and skilled and no amount of central or local guidance can substitute for this.' The Introduction repeats the message: 'This publication . . . is not a text book or practice guide which tells professionals what to do with individual cases' (ibid.: 8). And the rest of the document demonstrates why such a non-prescriptive emphasis is inevitable. Most of the text consists of discussion and argument, rather than rules to be followed, and the research 'findings' are presented in general evaluative terms ('appropriate', 'sensitive', 'wrong') which beg the question as to how we interpret them in a particular case, whether 'we' are care staff or service-users:

> Five features of best practice have been identified: sensitive and informed professional/client relationships; an appropriate balance of power between the key parties; a wide perspective on child abuse; effective supervision and training of social workers; and a determination to enhance the quality of children's lives.
>
> Clients suffered whenever professionals became preoccupied with a specific event, ignored the wider context, chose the wrong 'career avenue' for the child, or excluded the family from the enquiry.
>
> Protection is best achieved by building on the existing strengths of the child's living situation.
>
> (ibid.: 52)

The conclusion, then, is that in the context of social interaction (which is the context both for action research and for social and healthcare work) 'evidence' in the form of generalisations does not build up into a *prescriptive* basis for action, even though perhaps organisational policy directors and government ministers might wish that it did. Of course, we have a responsibility to 'know about' research evidence, and we are held accountable by policy guidelines. But research evidence and policies are necessarily general in nature, and what exactly we need to do here and now, 'for the best', requires us (always) to *interpret* and *evaluate* evidence and policy for specific cases, in particular contexts. Moreover, working with people always involves working with uncertainties, conflicts and dilemmas. 'Work', therefore, always offers scope for 'research', in the sense of subjecting our decisions, our relationships, our knowledge base and our interpretations of 'the evidence' to *more than usually sustained examination* (looking at matters 'critically', i.e. from more than one point of view). So research (and action research in particular) does not need to be thought of as an *interruption* of work, but as a means for *furthering and developing* the work we are already engaged in. 'Action research is simply a form of self-reflective inquiry undertaken by participants in social situations' (Carr and Kemmis, 1986: 162). (The relationship between action research and evidence-based practice is examined further in Chapter 3, Section 5.)

Action research as reflective decision-making

So how does this actually work? How can we try to ensure that an action research inquiry is both substantial (leading to valuable learning and practice development) and yet not so unwieldy as to be a distraction from the actual work process?

To begin with, let us remember that one of the most important aspects of action research involves negotiating 'collaborative' ways of working (based on principles of partnership, mutual respect and equality) among people who usually interact within a set of hierarchical power relations. This may still be true even if you are wishing to set up a joint project with a group of peers (professional colleagues, service-users, community members, etc.). For example, the project may have started off as the initiative of one member of the group, who thus may be perceived as personally having the 'backing' of management or sponsoring fund-holders; in any case, there are always informal differences in status between members of a group. This negotiation of collaborative roles, then, is not something which occurs *before* undertaking an action research project: it is a complex and continuing dimension of the project itself, requiring plans, actions, observations and reflections.

Another important point is that the value of action research arises just as much from the quality of the reflection it stimulates as from the comprehensiveness of the data collected. In other words, one does not have to collect a vast amount of data; new and useful insights can be generated from critical reflection on a few carefully selected incidents or responses (Winter, 1989: 25, 32–3). 'Critical reflection' is easier said than done, of course. Even when we are trying out something new, many aspects of the situation will remain familiar, and so many of our tried and trusted interpretations will spring to mind. We need to work carefully and systematically to permit alternative perspectives to emerge. A useful indication of what might be involved is provided by the work of Susan Hart on 'innovative thinking'. She suggests that the way we think about practical situations frequently includes a number of 'questioning moves' in response to one's first interpretation of an event, as follows:

- 'Making connections': what contextual influences are at work here?
- 'Contradicting': is there a contrasting way in which this might be understood?
- 'Taking the other's view': what might be the logic and purpose of the other person's response from within their own frame of reference?
- 'Noting the impact of feelings': how do I feel about this, and what do these feelings tell me about what is going on here?
- 'Suspending judgement': what else do I need to find out about before making a judgement about this?

(Summarised and adapted from Hart, 1995: 224)

Further discussion of 'critical reflection' is presented later (see Chapter 3, Section 6 and the 'Practical guide' (Part III), Section 3). At this stage the important point to note is that it involves a more sustained and elaborate application of ways of thinking that we all engage in (in a more condensed and rapid form) as part of our workplace decision-making. The action research 'cycle' is therefore fully under way as soon as a group of people with different roles in a 'work' situation *plan* to *observe* and record their practice, *reflect* critically on the observations they have made, meet to *compare and evaluate* these reflections and draw up a further *plan* for future work, based on the conclusions drawn from what they have *learned* from one another so far.

We can understand the action research cycle, then, in a way which is both simple and flexible, as a process consisting of just two continuously interacting aspects. On the one hand, there is our immediate practical experience of a situation (either a longstanding practice or a current attempt at innovation); and on the other hand there are our attempts (individual and collective) to consider other ways of understanding this experience and (consequently) to imagine practical alternatives. This alternating movement to and fro between practical experience and critical yet constructive reflection may be thought of as embracing and including the conventional action research sequence previously indicated.

Conclusion

In conclusion, then, action research tries to foster not only a model of research which arises naturally out of our practical experience of work, but a model of work which in itself presents opportunities for critical, constructive reflection. In one sense, at one level, we engage in critical reflection all the time (as we try to formulate effective responses to complex and rapidly shifting situations). But in another sense we don't. Work is arduous, hours are long, external forces seem to exert a dis-empowering constraint, and gradually, in order to survive, we slip into routines – comfortably familiar ways of doing things and of thinking about what we do. We have good reasons for our routines, of course, but we know that, at the very best, they do not represent the summit of what is possible or desirable. Undertaking an action research project, then, is a way of remembering the complex problems and possibilities inherent in the work we are engaged in. We also know that although our current expertise may be considerable, it is also tiny: only God would not benefit from undertaking an action research project from time to time.

Action research and other models of social research

In this section we examine how action research relates to other conceptions of research. It is important to consider this carefully, because the often heard suggestion that our practical decision-making must be based on 'research' or 'evidence' usually refers to conceptions of research and evidence which are in many ways not appropriate for action research. Action research does indeed emphasise that practice should be based on research and evidence, but it interprets the key terms in different ways, with important practical consequences. There are two forms of social research which are commonly contrasted with each other and whose relationship with action research needs to be examined, namely *quantitative*, survey-based research and *qualitative*, case-study research – the former based on numerical data and the latter (mainly) on linguistic data such as transcripts or notes from discussions, observations, etc.

Quantitative research – 'positivism'

In some respects, the gathering of numerical data might seem to be straight-forward, valuable and obviously necessary: for example, statistics showing the low proportion of black or female managers relative to the proportion of female or black staff in an organisation or nationally; the high proportion of young males committing certain types of offence; or the correlation between one-parent families and poverty. Such social statistics can reveal patterns, confirm the existence of problems and suggest directions for further inquiry.

However, although it is essential to be aware of such data it is equally important to be aware of their limitations. Statistical patterns are always open to different interpretations because theories and values always influence which statistics we choose to collect: statistics are *created*, not discovered. Moreover, human action is so complex and varied that there will always be individual cases which contravene even the most 'significant' statistical correlation. So statistics in themselves can never tell us exactly what to do in response to a specific situation. Consequently, statistics can never demonstrate causal links, since any measured correlation could always be due to other ('intervening') factors not included in the selected variables.

If quantitative research consisted merely of gathering very general data, providing background awareness as a *prelude* to detailed inquiry, it might not have become the focus of heated controversy about how social research should be conducted. However, quantitative social research usually aspires to go beyond the collection of routinely available surface data, and constitute a complete method of inquiry which makes claims to provide both understanding of, and guidance for, practical situations. In this guise, it is usually termed 'positivism', although this is in many ways a somewhat old-fashioned term. The word 'positivism' was coined early in the nineteenth century by Auguste Comte to sum up and popularise his hope and belief that knowledge of human affairs must be (and could be) given the same sort of 'positive' (purely factual and law-like) structure as Newtonian physics. He hoped that social *science* could become the basis for a universal consensus, free from dependence on political values and religious or metaphysical beliefs, which would finally end the disruptive conflicts between rival ideologies which characterised the society in which he was writing (just before the second French Revolution of 1830) (Comte, 1974 [1830–42]: 210–11, 24, 37–8, 129). Our own society, of course, like any other, continues to be torn by rival ideologies, and it is easy to see the enduring appeal of Comte's vision of a 'positive' social science, which claims to use the impersonal measurement of objective data to place our knowledge of human affairs beyond opinion, beyond value conflicts, beyond doubt and dispute. It is a vision which yearns for a social world finally at peace with itself, where the awkward idiosyncrasies of individuals and the disruptive antagonisms between sub-cultures have been brought under rational control through technical methods similar to those which have successfully tamed the forces of the physical world. Thus, many social scientists continue to assume that by using carefully constructed questionnaire forms the varieties of human experience and opinion can be coded, categorised and counted; and that by controlling the variables in setting up sample populations to receive and respond to questionnaire forms social science can imitate the physicists' control of experimental conditions. (Comte initially called his new social science 'social physics' (ibid.: 124).)

However, modern theories of knowledge are no longer based on Comte's vision of absolute certainty founded on incontrovertible and unambiguous 'facts'. This is true for the natural as well as the social sciences. 'Theories are . . . *never* empirically verifiable'; they can only be falsified (Popper, 1959: 40). The knowledge created by scientific inquiry exists as a set of 'conjectures', always awaiting possible refutation by future events. The authority of science is not its certainty but its 'rationality', i.e. our willingness to engage in critical debate about interpretations – a process of continuous learning from our current mistakes (Popper, 1963: Preface). Consequently, many would argue that Comte's vision of a purely factual, consensual social science is not only politically objectionable but also methodologically implausible.

The *political* problem is that if the data from the people being researched are to be collected and analysed numerically, they must be reduced to a set of prior categories; people's interpretations of their own experiences are thus enclosed within the definitions of the researcher. The ideas of the researched only 'count' (as relevant) if they can be 'counted' (numerically) as instances within the researcher's theoretical framework. Positivist research, then, involves the exercise of social power: it includes people as countable 'subjects', but it excludes them as definers of meaning. Indeed, by seeking general laws positivism implies that human behaviour is determined, and this assumption, in itself, tends to undermine any emphasis on human autonomy and creativity.

There are also a number of reasons why the positivist model of social research is rejected as *methodologically implausible*.

1   If human behaviour is generally determined by factors identifiable by researchers (e.g. by motives and ideologies), the activity of the researcher must also be determined by identifiable factors (e.g. by motives and ideologies), so that the research cannot then claim to be an impersonal, 'objective' process.

2   In the formulation of a set of categories in which to 'code' people's responses or behaviour, the values and purposes of the researcher and the organisation commissioning the research can never be excluded. Again, the apparent objectivity of the process is an illusion.

3   Reducing respondents' answers to a unified set of pre-coded categories does not *remove* individual differences of meaning; it merely conceals them. Consequently, although positivist research findings have the form of generalisations they give no clue as to how they relate to actual situations as people experience them, and do not, therefore, provide an adequate *understanding* of human experience. Moreover, since individual varieties of meaning are merely concealed, it is by no means clear that positivist research findings are replicable, even though that is their main claim.

4   By focusing on only one or two variables in a situation, the positivist model of research assumes that the complex interlocking systems of social reality can be understood as a series of abstracted fragments. But this fragmented conception of human reality is highly artificial, and the results of any research which depends on such a conception are unconvincing.

If the methodological problems of quantitative research, as outlined above, are borne in mind, then its outcomes will be properly recognised as being no more than modest conjectures, open to refutation (see above references to Popper). But, unfortunately, the results of quantitative research are still frequently treated (by politicians and organisational managers, for example) as though they actually do provide 'objective facts' about a situation, and thus constitute the basis for prescription and control. Thus, the Comtean vision of 'positivism' remains influential, even though its inadequacies have been frequently noted (e.g. Giddens, 1976; Habermas, 1978).

Qualitative research

To proponents of *qualitative* social research, the positivist attempt to bring the human world under scientific control through the measurement of quantities misses out the essential 'qualities' of human experience. And in the light of the criticisms of positivist research outlined above, *qualitative* researchers propose a very different model of inquiry. There are several different traditions of qualitative research and the following description is only intended to sum up the general perspective which they all share. It is loosely based on an influential account of what the authors call 'naturalistic inquiry' – a revealing term, as we shall see (Lincoln and Guba, 1985: especially 36–43). Qualitative researchers argue that human beings don't 'naturally' *experience* the world in numerical terms, as a series of quantities. We quantify experiences only in those special circumstances where we wish to exert a sort of *control* over social situations (Fay, 1975), for example where we wish to 'specify targets' or 'measure performances'. 'Control', here, usually means the exercise of social power and authority, but since the objectivity of the process is, as we have seen, always open to question, such attempts at authoritative objectivity are frequently contested, e.g. in controversies about performance 'indicators', 'performance-related pay' or organisational 'league tables'.

In contrast, qualitative research rejects the 'scientific' aspiration of controlling social affairs by producing general laws or 'measuring' behaviour; instead, the emphasis is on *understanding* social situations. Through intensive interviewing, open-ended observation and exhaustively descriptive case studies, researchers aim to create an interpretation which is sufficiently complex in its recognition of differences to be agreed as acceptable by all concerned. In this way, qualitative research seeks to avoid the politically 'disempowering' effects of quantitative research. Instead of trying to achieve 'objectivity' by using 'impersonal' procedures to create quantitative results, *qualitative* research aims to achieve a *consensus* as to the meaning of a situation, through respectful negotiation of interpretations between the researchers and those being researched. Its plausibility rests on a claim to represent the full, 'natural' complexity of social realities, including an explicit account of the 'credentials' of the researchers (Lincoln and Guba, 1985: 362–3). It also recognises that generalisations about social realities does not produce *laws* but tentative 'working hypotheses' (ibid.: 38), derived from a full understanding of an individual case which may potentially illuminate other cases. (Stake distinguishes between the generalisations of positivism (from a sample to a total 'population') and 'naturalistic' generalisation, i.e. generalisation from one situation to another situation in which we are interested (Stake, 1980: 70–1).)

What is different about action research?

Although quantitative and qualitative research may be clearly differentiated, they normally tend to share the following characteristics which, in principle, set them both apart from action research.

1   In both cases the purpose of the inquiry is to analyse a supposedly static situation; this is accomplished from a position of detachment, either through the experimental manipulation of variables or through exhaustive observation.
2   In both cases it is hoped that the process of the inquiry can avoid having any impact on the situation being investigated. Otherwise, the situation will no longer be in its 'naturally occurring' state but will have been changed by the 'distorting' impact of the inquiry process.
3   In both cases the researcher is clearly distinct from the people being researched: the researcher is in the role of the observer, gathering and analysing data provided by others.

In contrast, action research, as a form of inquiry, is clearly different with respect to the three points noted above. (The argument concerning feminist, anti-racist and service-user controlled research is slightly more complex – see Chapter 3.)

1   The purpose of action research is to work towards change, not merely to describe a current situation 'as it is'.
2   The process of an action research inquiry aims to be *constructive* rather than invisible – in many ways a more plausible ambition, since no social research process can actually avoid changing the situation it investigates: human beings will always *respond* (in one way or another) when research in any form appears on their scene.
3   Action researchers need to investigate their own practice as well as the practice of others, since they are participating members of the situation being investigated. Where the action researcher is in the role of facilitator the purpose is to encourage participants to examine their own practices, and the inquiry should always include an explicit evaluation of the facilitation process. In

principle, therefore, action research should involve *all* participants in *self*-questioning and *self*-evaluation, although it is not hard to find examples where this is not the case.

To sum up this stage of the argument: the debate about the nature of action research is quite distinct from the debate about the rival claims of quantitative and qualitative research methods. Action research always uses qualitative methods (interviews, observations, documents, etc.), and can quite easily also incorporate quantitative data, as a starting point for critical/self-critical reflection or as a preliminary form of evaluation. (A group of action researchers might even, at some stage, try to agree some quantitative 'targets' for the next phase of their work: 'control' does not have to be external; it can be an expression of autonomy – 'taking control'.) What is distinctive about action research is, as we have already noted, that it is a form of research which is organised around a process of action rather than a process of description. The main contrast, then, is between action research and 'descriptive research', including both quantitative methods and the case-study approach of 'naturalistic inquiry'. The main purpose and process of 'descriptive research' is to create an 'accurate account' of a situation from a stance of detachment, assuming that it remains static while the researcher observes it and writes up the report. The main purpose of action researchers, on the other hand, is not only to improve their understanding of a situation with which they are already intensively involved, but also to engage in an attempt to change things (even if only on a small scale) and to describe what is learned from the change process as it occurs.

How action research transforms some key aspects of social inquiry

With these distinctions in mind, then, let us look briefly at some of the key terms common to any form of social inquiry and notice how they are transformed when they refer to the dynamic, practice-oriented, self-reflective and collaborative processes of an action research project.

Data-gathering

In an action research project all participants are researchers. Data-gathering is thus a *joint* enterprise, undertaken by all participants in order to give a 'voice' to differing perspectives. Hence, gathering data needs to go beyond simply 'asking questions' and to include processes which encourage all participants to present the details of their experience and their conceptions of desirable changes in practice, so that their ideas and perceptions become available for comparison and exploration. Data-gathering sessions are therefore likely to resemble developmental workshops just as much as conventional 'interviews'. Furthermore, deciding which data to collect is not settled in advance but is negotiated between participants as the inquiry progresses. For example, agreeing the structure and content of a questionnaire form will require intensive collaborative work, and this is just as significant a part of the inquiry as analysing the eventual responses. Everyone's early thoughts and interpretations of events need to become 'data' at later stages of the inquiry; this is why it is often helpful for all participants to keep an on-going reflective diary from the outset of the project. In this way, individual insights can be compared and revised as part of the collaborative learning process.

Data analysis

The problem for data analysis is: how can we push beyond familiar interpretations of events which do not tell us anything new? With large samples or exhaustive and comprehensive details this can sometimes be achieved through a simple process of 'coding' all data under general headings. But the relatively small scale of an action research inquiry often means that merely 'coding' our data is unlikely to be very revealing. During an action research project, therefore, although quantitative data may be coded at some point in the work, 'analysis' will more usually take the form of open-ended critical reflection. This involves, above all, *questioning* our spontaneous interpretations of events, and then sharing and comparing our interpretations and questions, in order to create the maximum opportunity for challenge, surprise and mutual learning. Any eventual framework of categories for 'coding' data will gradually emerge as a negotiated *outcome* of the inquiry (see 'Data-gathering' above). More importantly, the form of analysis we choose needs to be appropriate for 'feeding back' into the developmental process, as an agenda for the discussion of possible action.

Theory

For an action research process, 'theory' is not a fixed, authoritative body of general propositions which determine in advance either what the inquiry must be about or how our findings are to be explained. Instead, 'theory' needs to be interpreted as 'a varied collection of possible general explanations or implications', which can be 'brought into play' as the inquiry progresses. Theory is to be found stored in libraries, to be sure, but it is also to be found activating our thoughts and feelings as we go about our business. Negotiating an action research project among participants thus always involves, among other things, an interchange of theoretical perspectives. Making these theoretical perspectives explicit, questioning one perspective in the light of another, and suggesting possible sources of ideas which might be illuminating and might help to carry the inquiry forward: this is the 'theorising' dimension of action research. Thus, although an action research project is always *focused* on practice, it always has a theoretical *scope* – a specific but shifting horizon of general ideas and general possibilities and implications, arising both from the outcomes of the work (as they emerge) and from the process itself. This means that action research can also 'generate' theory, not by establishing links between variables or by supporting a hypothesis but by portraying a specific sequence of events in such a way (in such complexity of detail, in such 'depth') that others can perceive its implications for different situations (see Winter, 1998).

Validity

We have already noted that modern theories of knowledge emphasise that our knowledge exists as a set of 'conjectures' always awaiting possible refutation by future events, and that 'rationality' is a matter of our willingness to engage in a process of continuous learning. Action research has this principle at the centre of its processes. The inquiry proceeds through continuously negotiating between differences of perspective, and its validity resides in the carefulness and rigour of this process, not merely in a claim to have made an accurate *representation* of reality (the main claim of both positivism and naturalistic inquiry). Certainly, action research *does* attempt to portray practical developments accurately and to evaluate them soundly, but it also seeks validity in a further dimension – the openness of its communicative processes. Thus an action research project must show that differing views have been fully expressed and that the judgements which make up the inquiry have been open to scrutiny and debate. Thus, part of the 'validity' of an action research project depends on how far it seriously addresses the crucial issues of organisational and professional power.

Generalisability

We have already noted that action contexts are so complex and individualised that the relevance of general statistical trends and of detailed evidence from other contexts is always a matter of interpretation. With this in mind, we can suggest that the lessons from an action research project based on the experience of a single situation are just as likely to be illuminating and interesting for colleagues elsewhere as the outcomes of other forms of research. An action research project has its own in-built safeguards against 'purely subjective' interpretations – namely, its focus on evaluating practical change and its emphasis on the negotiation of meaning between different participants. In other words, through co-operative negotiation and evaluation of practice developments an action research inquiry can uncover significant underlying structures in the situation (conflicts of values, difference of motive, power relations, etc.), which will 'resonate' strongly with a wide variety of other situations. Moreover, the account of the *process* of the inquiry (the sequences of negotiations, the strategies adopted in response to methodological problems) provides a further dimension in which an action research report can offer significant insights to people involved in other situations. We can therefore suggest that not only are action research reports, like other research, 'generalisable' (in the restricted and tentative sense we must always keep in mind), but that, like other research, it *needs* to be made 'public' (Stenhouse, 1985a). By being shared in a public forum (team and group meetings, newsletters, journals, the Internet), the report of an action research project contributes to the critique and refinement of knowledge (ibid.: 9, 17–18).

Organisational politics

Action research always aims at creating a constructive practical *effect* on the work of an organisation. And since it is a collaborative process involving various people in different roles, it cannot help recognising that it has an organisational/political dimension. Thus, even if an action research project is on a very small scale, initially involving a very few people, it can never be private or covert. On the contrary, it needs always to be explicitly negotiated, from the outset, with key managers, relevant committees and all who may (even potentially) be concerned. In this way, an action research inquiry must become (as quickly as possible) a *shared* project, the intersection of different people's interests. This is equally true whether the inquiry is undertaken within a single organisation or involves a number of community agencies or when a service-user group is developing an evaluation of service provision. In an important sense, then, an action research project needs to start with a political analysis of possible alliances and potential opposition in the practical context, to ensure that proposals can eventually be effectively implemented. To create and maintain this aspect of the work is not just a background concern but a crucial part of the project itself. Otherwise the inquiry risks failing to have a practical impact and ending up as merely another survey of opinion.

Research ethics

Action researchers explore situations to which they 'belong', and in which they therefore already have ethical responsibilities towards others – as colleagues (or group members) towards each other and as care workers towards service-users. In undertaking action research one does not step aside from the ethical relations of a work role in order to 'do research'; on the contrary, action research is an extension and an intensification of those same ethical relations. In other words, such principles as the duty of care for others' well-being, the prevention of harm, respecting rights, facilitating autonomy and preserving confidentiality can easily be reasserted for the research process, since they are, as it were, already 'in place'. Indeed, since action research is a process in which (typically) practical developments are introduced by those most directly involved and responsible, it can be both 'experimental' and yet at the same time guided by the ethics of practice itself, in a way which resolves some of the moral dilemmas otherwise faced by 'outside' researchers. Of course, this still leaves in place the *challenges* posed by the ideal of consistently ethical practice, the ethical *dilemmas* of practice (e.g. the potential conflict between organisational policy and the needs of service-users), and the question of how to resolve the conflicts which are inherent in professional decision-making (e.g. disagreements between practitioners' and service-users' interpretations of 'need'). This is a reminder that action research needs to specify ways in which its principles and ideals can be safeguarded against the various forms of 'malpractice' (oppression, concealment, etc.) which are, alas, not unknown, either in professional work or in research activity. (See also the section 'Ethical issues and principles of procedure' in Part III, Section 5.)

Creating a 'culture of inquiry' in practice settings

In many ways, action research suggests that 'inquiry' can be (indeed needs to be) part of the culture of the contexts in which we work – whether these are large organisations and agencies or small support/self-help groups. Admittedly, many of us probably feel that our own work setting, far from resembling a 'culture of inquiry', is dominated by (for example) 'getting the job done on time', or staying within cost limits, or even (crudely) 'not stepping out of line'. So, in the final section of this chapter we consider the development of a culture of inquiry in terms of practical opportunities and strategies. (A number of the ideas are taken up in more detail in Chapter 3.)

To begin with, let us consider some organisational/managerial perspectives which seem to offer opportunities or (in general terms at least) grounds for optimism. Optimism is important here, since we know that life in organisations can be harsh – competitive, highly pressured and under-resourced, with high levels of stress and low levels of support leading to low morale and high rates of staff turnover and illness. On the other hand, organisational managers know as well as anyone else that this state of affairs is inefficient and wasteful. They are increasingly aware that they need to care for the morale and well-being of staff not simply as an expression of humanity but as a hard-headed calculation – as prudent management of an expensive resource. Moreover, managers know that an organisation needs to keep *changing*, in order to adapt to changing political and economic circumstances and the changing needs and demands of clients. And for this they need staff to be prepared to commit their creativity to learning from and learning about their work. Hence the popularity among senior managers (of all types of organisations) of the 'Investors in People' movement – a government-sponsored initiative focusing on strategies to encourage staff 'commitment', 'initiative', 'problem-solving' and 'learning' in order to achieve higher 'productivity' and 'quality' (Investors in People, 1994: 4).

The managerial argument for a culture of inquiry in the workplace can be put in another way. For an organisation to be effectively 'responsive' to external demands, it needs to be engaged in regular, even continuous *evaluation* of its activities (see Chapter 3, Section 3). This requires a culture in which criticism is not suppressed (as a threat or an act of blaming) but is welcomed as part of a process of learning. Evaluation, therefore, needs to be, above all, *self*-evaluation, based in a mutually supportive group process and involving client responses as a resource for the improvement of practice. And if evaluation is to be genuinely of value, it must lead directly to action. So management systems need to *delegate* to *all* staff the responsibility for practical initiatives concerning their own work, thereby reassuring them that they are *trusted* to exercise autonomy (Fox, 1974). Otherwise, systems of accountability merely achieve a semblance of 'control' at the cost of stifling staff commitment and initiative (Deming, 1986: 23–4, 60). For a variety of reasons, then, some senior managers (at least) are beginning to define their 'leadership' role in terms of creating and supporting, quite specifically, a 'culture of inquiry', with a responsibility to create *confidence*, among their staff, to take the risks that innovation requires.

Further arguments for an inquiry-oriented work culture are provided by professional bodies' attempts to create more widely accessible post-qualifying qualifications, which increasingly focus on portfolios of evidence demonstrating work-based learning rather than attendance at formally taught courses. In social work, for example, staff need to present evidence demonstrating analysis and evaluation of their own work and the ability to 'empower' others (Central Council for Education and Training in Social Work, 1992: 14–15). A broadly similar emphasis is to be found in the 'Framework' document for post-qualifying profes- sional development published by the English National Board for Nursing, Midwifery and Health Visiting (1990). The 'Framework' is designed 'to meet the needs of the majority of practitioners who work and will continue to work . . . closely with patients and clients . . . in practice settings', and presents 'Ten Key Characteristics' of the work to be demonstrated, including 'using research to plan, implement and evaluate strategies to improve care', 'team working', and 'facilitating and assessing development in others'. More broadly, even the much criticised checklists of work-based 'competences' which make up the vocational qualifications recently developed in the UK, Australia and New Zealand *can* be adapted and interpreted so that they stimulate critical evaluation, practice development and action research-like inquiry, involving clients (Yelloly and Henkel, 1995: 62–3; Winter and Maisch, 1996: 138; Brown Lee, 1997: 231–5).

The various service-user research movements are also beginning to influence both practitioners and managers in healthcare and community organisations at every level, leading to an emphasis on involving service-users in defining good practice (see Chapter 3, Section 1).

The thesis so far, then, is that, in arguing for a 'culture of inquiry' in work settings, practitioners concerned to improve their qualifications and to create the conditions for work satisfaction can make common cause with service-users wishing to make their voices 'heard' and with senior managers concerned simply with organisational effectiveness. In principle, the apparent conflicts of interest are, in the end, sur- mountable, because all have a vested interest in evaluating and developing services. Admittedly, when we are actually experiencing a state of demoralisation we are all tempted to 'block' the possibilities for developmental inquiry, blaming others for 'the fact' that 'nothing can be changed' and seeking emotional refuge by stressing our powerlessness. But at least all concerned (from senior managers to service-users) would admit that this is a pathological and counterproductive state of affairs, urgently needing remedy. So let us turn to some practical suggestions.

- Groups of staff at every level can be encouraged to develop and evaluate innovative practice 'standards' – as exemplified in the *RCN Standards of Care Project* (Royal College of Nursing, 1990).
- Staff meetings at every level can regularly include an agenda item for the sharing of inquiry-focused developments.

- Organisations concerned with the delivery of health and social care can demonstrate their commitment to a 'partnership' with service-users by setting up consultation processes which involve them in the planning and evaluation of their services (see Essex County Council Social Services, 1997: 90–1). There are examples of care organisations which have issued policy statements committing them to a wide variety of methods for service-user participation, including workshops, individual interviews, staff attendance at user-group meetings, opportunities to make written comments from home, use of Email/Internet links, use of a variety of languages, etc.
- Organisational newsletters can include brief accounts of developmental work initiated by staff and/or service users, together with details of where fuller reports can be obtained.
- Local 'conferences' can be arranged (by large employers or by groups of local employers, with or without the contribution of local educational institutions) at which staff can gain support and advice through sharing accounts of their developmental work.
- Appraisal criteria for staff at every level can include reference to their involvement in developmental work and to their involvement of service-users in such work.
- Appraisal criteria for managers can include reference to the involvement in creative developmental work on the part of the staff in their team or section.
- Organisations can make specific allocations of *time* for staff to engage in developmental activities built into budgets and given a high level of priority – not as an optional luxury but as an operational necessity. Similarly, staff need to be encouraged to 'give themselves permission' to see their time spent on developmental work (with colleagues and with service-users) as a requirement, not an indulgence.

So far we have concentrated on organisational arrangements. But cultures of inquiry (and their opposite: cultures of stress, fear and resistance to innovation) are created not only by formal processes but by the 'emotional climate' of relationships and interactions. From this perspective even a small working group (e.g. a local staff group or a group of service-users meeting in a community support centre) may either succeed or fail in generating a culture of inquiry. At this level most of us have much to learn about what Goleman calls 'emotional intelligence' – the arts of *supportive* criticism, emotional self-awareness, respecting diversity of opinion (as a resource rather than a personal threat), listening to and learning from one another, and maintaining the harmony of a group as a precondition of its productivity (Goleman, 1996: Chapter 10). We need to recognise when our defensive/aggressive emotions have been 'hooked', when we have been sucked into a group interaction which is 'going wrong' (closing off the inquiry process) and to feel able to step back and ask the group to consider what is 'going on' at the emotional level. Goleman's work has obvious parallels with Nancy Kline's suggestions about the 'feminine' skills required by 'the thinking environment'.

Like Goleman, she emphasises that creative, productive thinking takes place more effectively in groups where members listen carefully and empathetically to one another, as equal partners, and explicitly express appreciation of each other's contributions; where diversity of opinion is clearly valued and feelings are recognised as part of the thinking process (Kline, 1993: Chapter 3). In other words, we must not forget that 'inquiry' carries a real 'emotional risk', as we expose our experiences, our interpretations and our value judgements to challenge. These are especially important lessons to learn for those of us who have become used to 'macho' styles of debate, where the process of inquiry is supposed to arise from competition and confrontation.

Conclusion

To sum up: action research requires (and fosters) a working environment which encourages collaboration and reflection, evaluation and exploration – and a culture which is innovative because it is supportive. This has implications for the way we manage organisations and for the way we interact as individuals with others. At both levels, the concept of a culture of inquiry draws upon familiar but challenging ideas of what we know to be generally desirable and effective – conceptions of what makes for a responsive, 'learning' organisation, and what makes for productive, creative group processes. Of course, it is important to acknowledge that what goes on in organisations and group meetings often fails miserably with respect to the ideas we have outlined here, indicating the real difficulties involved, but it is also important to recognise that these ideas *are* both well known and widely accepted. In attempting to implement them, therefore, we can try to proceed with some degree of real hope while not expecting immediate or complete success.

Chapter 3

Action research

Contexts and dimensions

Introduction

So far we have presented action research in terms of a single, fairly general definition. In this chapter we examine more closely the *variety* of action research. This variety is sometimes presented as a set of different 'types', e.g. 'diagnostic', 'participant', 'empirical', 'experimental' (Chein *et al.*, 1948; Adelman, 1993). But these terms seem less than helpful, since any given action research project would in some sense contain (almost by definition, as we have seen) all of these aspects. Hart and Bond use a slightly different set of distinctions: 'empowering'/ 'experimental'/'organisational'/'professionalising' (Hart and Bond, 1995: 43–4). But here again one might argue that in some sense all of these are essential components of a coherent model. In this chapter, in contrast, we do not present the variety of action research as a set of different types (between which we may have to choose) but as a set of contributory traditions, developed in different contexts, but overlapping and displaying many common themes.

Section 1 looks at issues of power and partnership in the context of service-user research. Section 2 considers the problem of 'collaboration' in the context of action research for community development. Section 3 considers the long tradition of work in organisational management, and contrasts the notion of action research as a process of expert consultancy with the newer management theory which has arisen around the concept of the learning organisation. Section 4 reviews the role of facilitation in action research and suggests that all participants, including facilitators, need to be creatively involved as researchers into their own practice, including the practice of facilitation. Section 5 considers the evaluation dimension of action research in the light of the tension between 'science' and 'empowerment'. Section 6 considers the nature of 'critical reflection' as a process common to action research and professional practice. Finally, Sections 7 and 8 focus on the *politics* of action research, through analogies with feminist and anti-racist research traditions.

The purpose of this chapter is to illustrate key themes, not to present a comprehensive review of the whole action research literature. Thus, for example, the influential work of Peter Reason and John Rowan (Reason and Rowan 1981;

Reason, 1988) presents a conception of 'new paradigm research' and 'co-operative inquiry' which may be thought of as a general methodology implicit in our conception of 'collaborative' action research, but which is too broad-ranging to be accommodated in this chapter as either a specific 'tradition' or a particular 'context'. It is also important to note that our presentation of many of the issues is not intended to 'resolve' them. In many cases the key concepts are inherently vague (e.g. 'empowerment', 'collaboration'), and they merely serve to point a direction and to indicate problems that need to be addressed through the *practice* of inquiry.

In this chapter, then, we try to present the variety of action research, to provide pointers to further reading, and to illustrate the different ways in which the ideas outlined so far have been, and can be, realised in practice. This seems important: each practice context contains certain unique features and it is helpful to see action research as a repertoire of possibilities, so that we can better interpret the breadth of the general principles we have outlined.

I Service-user research

One of the most important aspects of action research is that it sets up processes which *question* conventional hierarchies of expertise, by recognising and involving forms and sources of knowledge and understanding which other modes of research have neglected or dismissed. Action research thus raises issues of power and authority, both within the research process and also in the definition and provision of services. The involvement of service-users in researching and contributing to the development of social and healthcare services thus needs to be a central theme in any comprehensive conception of action research.

The history of the relationship between service-users and research, in the health and social services, parallels in many ways that of women and members of ethnic minority groups: research was conducted on them and theory was made about them, with little, if any, reference to their views or the details of their own perceptions of their experience. However, the 1980s and 1990s witnessed a variety of movements by service-users and by carers' groups (particularly in the fields of mental health, learning disability and physical disability) demanding that their perspectives should be taken into consideration in the formulation of policy and practice. And, increasingly, there has been a demand by service-user movements (and by those sympathetic to them) that service-users should pose the questions for inquiry about their own condition and treatment, and should be active in undertaking the research. Otherwise, it is argued, service provision will lack a crucial dimension of understanding, which only service-users can make available (see Beresford, 1999). And unless service-users take the lead in defining the issues and in carrying out the research, there is a risk of collusion with existing models of practice, many of which are discriminatory and oppressive (Oliver, 1996). From the early 1990s UK government legislation and policy documents began to emphasise the importance of the service-user's view in service development and related education, for example the NHS and Community Care Act, 1992, and the 1997 document

The New NHS, where we read: 'The Government will take special steps to ensure that the experience of users and carers is central to the work of the NHS' (Department of Health, 1997: 66). Service-users and their carers can therefore be seen to have a particular interest in 'action research', i.e. in research where the purpose of inquiry is to make *changes* in the relationships and procedures which permit professionals and organisations to intervene in their lives.

The early accounts of service-users' perceptions and opinions were practitioner research (e.g. Mayer and Timms, 1970) but in a more traditional mould than that advocated by action researchers. Practitioners were indeed 'inquiring' into their own practice but not in a way that fully or equally involved service-users in developing either the area for study or lines of inquiry. Instead, they were assigned the passive role of answering the questions that practitioners or their managers had set (although the novelty, at the time, of hearing the clients' voices and raising their profile should not be underestimated). Such forms of inquiry had clear limitations. There was a tendency for users to evaluate their own practitioner's work rather than the quality of the service in general, and it was particularly difficult for clients (many of whom were 'captive' – i.e. obliged to accept a service) to criticise the work of an agency on which they were dependent. It was therefore suggested that researchers should be independent of direct service provision, so that service-users would feel more comfortable in giving their honest opinions (Fisher, 1983), leading to involvement in service-user research on the part of academics and the research departments of service organisations. This, of course, risks reproducing another sort of expertise hierarchy and the dependence of service-users on the independent researcher, so researchers involved in such work increasingly advocated the use of more participatory research methods, seeing the researcher as a facilitator of research rather than as an 'expert'.

Examples, methods

However, the need for service-users and carers themselves to undertake research has been increasingly advocated (Oliver, 1996; Beresford, 1999). For example, the Patients' Council of the Royal Edinburgh Hospital has developed a 'Quality Assurance Framework' derived from a survey of patients' views (MacFarlane, 1998), and a service-user group attached to the West Yorkshire National Health Trust undertook a revision of the official documentation, which was found to be too technical and to have too high a reading age to be an effective information source (Barton-Wright, 1998). On a larger scale, the Sainsbury Centre for Mental Health has developed a 'user-focused monitoring' procedure, involving service-users as interviewers and using a framework of questions derived from the experiences of an initial 'pilot group' of service-users. The findings of the first series of interviews included: service-users felt that their treatment did not draw on their strengths, did not offer the opportunity for discussion and did not involve them in the drawing up of their care plan (Rose, 1999). A survey of the experiences of over 400 users of mental health services (Faulkner, 1997) involved service-users in managing the project, designing the questionnaire and analysing the results; they concluded that service-users were dissatisfied with purely medical treatments, and recommended wider use of 'holistic' and 'talk-based' therapies (ibid.: 9, 18).

Some would argue that the ideal of collaborative action research aims, as far as possible, to merge the roles of researcher and researched, whereas the methods adopted in the work referred to above (reporting findings from interviews and questionnaires) retain a clear distinction between these two roles. There are sound political reasons for this: service-user research has an uphill battle to achieve credibility in the contexts where this is crucial (i.e. where funds are allocated and where policy is made), and so it seemed more prudent to adopt a conventional methodology. Nevertheless, the danger that service-user researchers could recreate another conventional expertise hierarchy needs to be recognised: the 'democratic' or 'participatory' quality of a research process obviously depends not simply on the *identities* of those involved, but also, crucially, on how the process itself is designed (see Section 8, below).

On the other hand, there is one research 'method' which does seem to be particularly appropriate for service-users, namely the telling and discussion of 'stories'. Telling one's 'story' is a way of 'bearing witness to' one's experience, and it is precisely by presenting the detail of their experience and structuring it in their own way, through 'stories' and critical analysis, that service-users can contribute to a better understanding of what these services actually 'feel like' (see Borkman, 1999). Again, there is a parallel with methodological traditions in feminist research, which (as with service-user research) highlights the specific value of a form of knowledge, 'experiential knowledge', gained only through living with or in specific health and social conditions. Such knowledge is itself a form of 'expertise', based on both individual and collective experience, and when shared in self-help/mutual aid groups has the potential to challenge, and thus help to improve, professional conceptions and treatment in health and social care (Ramon, 1997; Munn-Giddings, 1998).

'Partnership'?

After the acceptance of the value of research carried out by self-help groups of service-users, the next question arises: can service-users work *with* practitioners and service-providers without losing control of the research process, and if so, how? This leads us back to the problems indicated earlier. Oliver's work illustrates the importance of this issue by showing that both the starting point and the outcomes of research can be quite different if they are defined and conducted by service-users. He notes, for example, how social services at both a policy and a practice level concern themselves almost exclusively with counting the numbers of disabled people and ascertaining their needs, thereby reinforcing a 'dependent' relationship between service-providers and those labelled 'disabled'. Disabled researchers, in contrast, have advocated that local authorities should construct indicators of *disabling environments*, addressing this as an issue for the community as a whole

(Oliver, 1990). This example also indicates how adopting the agenda of service-users raises issues which are much broader than the 'needs' of particular individuals or groups stigmatised as 'having problems'. It also shows how such work raises the issue of the power relation between practitioner and user, and indicates potential differences in their concerns. At some level practitioners who engage in inquiry to develop their practice are probably (and understandably) making a prior assumption that their practice (in some form or another) is required and beneficial, whereas that may be precisely what service-users wish to question.

All this alerts us to the real difficulties in a 'partnership' model, in which service-users and practitioner-researchers work constructively together to improve services. Nevertheless, much of the action research tradition presupposes that it is possible, as much of the argument in the previous chapters indicates. Elliott and Adelman, for example, reviewing their work as directors of one of the most influential large-scale action projects in an education context, suggest that it was based on the 'hypothesis' that 'the best means' that teachers have for 'diagnosing' important problems in their classroom practice is the process of 'monitoring *pupils' accounts of teaching*' (Elliott and Adelman, 1996: 17). Beresford (1992) addresses the issue in a social services context. He describes two main approaches to involving service-users and carers in research, namely 'consumerist' research and 'democratic' research. In the first model users are simply 'consulted': they participate, but only insofar as they respond to the agenda set by the service-providers. The researchers (whether independent outsiders or practitioners) are instrumental in initiating the research, defining the area for study, and persuading service-users to become involved. In the second model users are involved from the beginning, initiating the area for study, defining the research area, conducting the research and interpreting the data. But the issue need not be defined quite so sharply. Holman (1987) presents a series of examples from community development projects, showing a range of solutions to the problem of how practitioners and service-users might work together. These included: (1) the views of service-users gathered by an independent researcher; (2) a tenants' association 'commissioning' a team of researchers to gather data documenting their concerns; (3) a community worker helping a tenants' association to design and carry out their own data collection exercise; and (4) a 'steering group' of local residents with two community workers planning and carrying out an investigation for which the report was 'put together and typed by the residents' (ibid.: 679).

More recently, Bond *et al.* (1998) provide an interesting example of what Beresford might call 'democratic' research undertaken collaboratively by prac-titioners and service-users. The jointly written account describes how a practitioner studying for a higher degree worked with her academic supervisor and with a group of mothers whose children had been sexually abused, in order to inquire into and develop support services for the mothers' group and, more generally, for mothers in families where sexual abuse has taken place. The work resulted in changes in local services, the development of a dynamic service-user group ('For Mothers by Mothers'), and the production by this group of an information service for other service-users. Perhaps a key element here was that the service-users involved consciously formed themselves as 'a group' and have since successfully developed what was originally a self-help group into an agency that provides training for those involved in child protection. This report illustrates both the mutual learning and the organisational change that can take place when academics, practitioners and service-users collaborate in ways which draw fully and creatively on their different forms of knowledge.

Summary

Is there a general perspective within which we can view the relationship between service-user involvement, research and the development of professional practice, in a way which contributes to our conception of action research? Mullender *et al.* (1993/4) provide a useful starting point. They suggest that professional practice and research into professional practice share the same value base, namely 'empowerment' (ibid.: 17) (i.e. a concern with individual dignity and autonomy) – 'seeing people as people, not as labels ['cases', 'problems', disabilities'] or as research "subjects"' (ibid.: 12).

> Participatory forms of research are needed, then, which can encompass not just the subjective experience of those whose circumstances or behaviour are to be studied but their *active* contribution. Research needs to see them as the experts on the direct experience involved. . . . Workers and researchers who attempt to pursue empowering principles will wish to facilitate service users to make decisions for themselves and to control whatever outcome ensues – such as deciding whether to release findings and to whom. Though special skills and knowledge are employed, these do not accord privilege and are not solely the province of professionals. . . . People who lack power and who would be nervous of engaging in anything bearing the grand name of 'research' can gain it through working together in well facilitated groups.
>
> (ibid.: 12, 14)

Although we need to remember that 'empowerment' can easily lapse into an empty, simplistic or even patronising buzz-word, this quotation evokes quite clearly some key aspects of action research as outlined in earlier chapters, for example the emphasis on questioning the expertise embodied in our current knowledge through attempting to work collaboratively with others. Other issues raised by service-user research (e.g. the process of 'facilitation', the link between the value base of research and the value base of practice, and the power relations of research and service provision) are discussed further in later sections of this chapter.

2 Action research and community development

The politics of community development

The idea of a 'community' is central to action research. Frequent references have already been made to the 'collaborative' principle (including participants as 'co-researchers'; treating the researcher as a 'member' of the inquiry ather than as an 'outside' expert) and the action research literature is full of references to *group* processes, e.g. 'co-operation' (Heron, 1996), 'participation' (Reason, 1994). The emphasis in action research methodology on 'empowerment' refers not only to encouraging individual 'reflection' but including individuals within a mutually supportive collective endeavour, what Carr and Kemmis call a 'self-reflective community' (Carr and Kemmis, 1986: Chapter 7).

There is also a long tradition of community-based action research and, indeed, some of the earliest influential examples of action research are set within a community development context. Thus, in Lewin's article 'Action research and minority problems'– often seen as the founding text of action research – the main example describes a workshop for community workers seeking to improve 'race relations', that is to remove 'economic and social discrimination' against 'minority groups' (Lewin, 1946: 40). Then there is the work of John Collier, also frequently cited by writers on action research, including Lewin himself (ibid.: 46). Between 1933 and 1945 Collier was the civil servant responsible for the United States government policy on native Americans. He describes his department's attempts to counteract centuries of racist policies which had refused to recognise the diversity of native American cultures (Collier, 1945: 268) and destroyed their coherence, 'atomising' these people into isolated individuals without land, family or belief systems (ibid.: 272). Collier emphasises that local cultures need to be given 'status, responsibility and power' through fostering education and local organisation (ibid.: 274) and that the process through which this is to be accomplished is 'action research' (ibid.: 294), i. e. research which is 'evoked by needs of action . . . [and which] feed[s] itself into action' (ibid.: 300). For Collier, action research is a form of research which must be *jointly* created and implemented by administrators and community members (ibid.: 276, 300) and in which administrators, in order to be 'faithful to . . . the spirit of that knowledge which [they have] not yet mastered' (ibid.: 300), must see themselves above all as *learners*.

These examples show the essentially political and critical dimension to the community development version of action research. We live in a society where, many would argue, the human values of 'community' – social responsibility, mutual caring – have been (and are still being) destroyed by two key features of modernisation: (1) hierarchical bureaucracies, in which power is exercised at the top and those at the bottom lack control over their lives, which limits the capacity of community members to exercise autonomy; (2) competitive individualism – the supposed motivating ideology of capitalism – which 'atomises' (Collier's term) community life into aggregates of self-interested individuals. Community development through action research, then (as envisaged by Collier and Lewin), seeks to empower the disempowered and is thus an attempt to redress structural problems at the heart of modern societies.

An important methodological point arises here: the political dimension of community development means that there is an important sense in which researchers and facilitators do *not* see themselves as adopting a 'neutral' stance, since the idea of community *development* represents a critical perspective on some of the key features of current social structure. Consequently, community/research workers may well feel that an important part of their role is that they share an identity with community members (e.g. identities of class, gender or ethnicity), so that they see their task as *advocacy* or *representation* as well as analysis (cf. service-user research, feminist research and anti-racist research, discussed elsewhere in this chapter).

There is a further key question about action research *as* community development (arising from this political analysis). Can small-scale projects 'build up to' structural change, or are they always destined to be 'defeated' by the surrounding political structure (massive bureaucratic organisations seeking profits for shareholders) and the dominant culture (self-oriented individualism)? From this perspective, small-scale projects producing merely local 'adaptations' may even be seen as counterproductive from the point of view of more radical structural change.

Examples

However, contemporary society is not simply and exclusively dominated by the forces of bureaucracy and competition, though sometimes it does take some effort to remember this. There are other, contrasting political ideologies at work, which offer support to the community ideal. First, the managers of formerly 'bureaucratic' organisations are beginning to recognise that they can only be effective if they succeed in fostering teamwork (see Section 3, below). Second, community participation is increasingly being recognised as a necessary general strategy for addressing problems of poverty and cultural deprivation. Early examples are the community development projects of the 1960s and 1970s in the UK (Lees and Smith, 1975) and the anti-poverty and family advice services projects in the USA. More recent examples include the comprehensive collection of processes and procedures for creating community participation reported by the New Economics Foundation (1997) and the rapidly spreading 'micro-credit' Grameen Bank movement originally initiated by Muhammad Yunus in Bangladesh (see Yunus, 1998). Third, one may find theoretical encouragement in Kropotkin's classic argument that mutuality and collective support are just as crucial to survival as competitive individualism, and are just as firmly embedded in 'human nature' (Kropotkin, 1987 [1902]). He cites examples ranging from individual acts of dramatic self-sacrifice – e.g. an escaped prisoner who emerged from his hiding place to save a child from a burning house knowing that as a consequence he would be rearrested (ibid.: 219) – to spontaneous economic arrangements in which a whole village joins forces to harvest the crop of communal plots of land so that the poor benefit from the superior resources of the rich (ibid.: 203).

The political impetus behind community development work perhaps explains why it is the strongest tradition of action research in Third World countries, where the political forces undermining 'the community' have had their most obviously destructive impact. The original figure here, frequently cited in action research writing in both community development and educational contexts, is Paolo Freire. For Freire, education must be a process of cultural consciousness-raising rather than direct instruction, a process of giving a voice to communities which have been 'silenced', as a step towards cultural and political emancipation (Freire, 1972: 16). In Freire's work, as in the work of John Collier mentioned earlier, the process of inquiry starts with the researcher in the role of learner: the educator must first learn what it is that the community needs to learn; educational 'texts' must be developed from the words of community members (ibid.: 46). Similarly, for Fals-Borda, 'participatory action research' is a combination of research, adult education and sociopolitical action, an 'experiential methodology' for the construction of 'power or countervailing power, for the poor, oppressed and exploited groups and social classes' (Fals-Borda and Rahman, 1991: 3). Research is a 'collective' process, involving the researcher in dialogue and discussion through public meetings with villagers, to 'recover' their awareness of their own history and its political lessons (ibid.: 8).

Problems and 'solutions'

Valla (1994), writing about community health research in Brazil, raises a key question about the nature of 'participation' in such approaches. How can professional workers or researchers avoid dominating the interpretive process, even when their intention is to create a 'new space' outside the professional delivery of services so that professional judgement can be questioned? 'There is a great possibility that professionals may unconsciously assume responsibility for the choice of criteria and categories' (ibid.: 406–7). To address this problem he suggests that professional workers, in order not to 'miss' key aspects of community members' experience, need to adopt an informal approach to 'data gathering', including listening to community talk and reading community newsletters, rather than insisting always on formal interviews, which may in some situations be regarded with suspicion (ibid.: 410).

Valla's emphasis on the difficulties involved in 'facilitating' developmental work returns us to the work of Lees and Smith (1975) in the UK, mentioned earlier; they also emphasise the internal tensions in community development work which may threaten its effectiveness. Lees, for example, notes the conflicts between researchers demanding rigorous evaluation strategies (based on before-and-after measures) and community workers whose professional emphasis is on involving community members in clarifying their own needs and making their own decisions as to courses of action. An 'emergent' self-help group cannot have its objectives spelt out for it in advance by a project director under pressure to 'prove' statistically the success of a particular programme (Lees, 1975: 61–2). Also, neighbourhood groups may well be critical of official provision, and when encouraged to express these views and to organise themselves to improve services the stage is set for outcomes which will not be welcomed by all parties (ibid.: 64). Consequently, as Smith (1975) suggests, the situations in which community development action research are attempted are always so 'turbulent' and 'messy' (ibid.: 193, 198) that no clear-cut findings as to the 'success' or 'failure' of specific programmes are likely to emerge. Community development work should therefore (modestly) content itself with 'open[ing] up possibilities by presenting the range of effects from any change and bringing forward the attitudes of otherwise unrepresented groups' (ibid.: 197).

In general, then, Lees and Smith present a somewhat pessimistic review of the problems inherent in community development programmes, focusing on the permanent tension between the objectives of 'researchers' and those of community members and local politicians. But this may be in part due to the fact that the work they report is not based on any clearly formulated methods for 'action research' as opposed to conventional social science. In contrast, Stringer's more recent account of 'community-based action research' (Stringer, 1996) – which presents a fairly positive view – is explicitly based on Guba and Lincoln's model of 'responsive evaluation', i.e. a set of procedures for evaluation which is 'responsive' to the various interest groups within a community (see Section 5, below). Stringer rejects in principle the 'power and control' dimension of positivist social science (ibid.: 144–150) with which Lees and Smith are struggling and which always presents a problem for community development since it always installs the researcher in the roles of outsider and 'expert'. Stringer's model of inquiry emphasises that knowledge of social affairs is always created locally and its 'authenticity' is therefore always 'multiple' and varied (ibid.: 156). 'Community based action research', he says, 'works on the assumption that all stakeholders – those whose lives are affected by the problem under study – should be involved in the processes of investigation' (ibid.: 10). It is a form of 'collaborative exploration' in which community members develop 'more constructive analyses of their situation', 'create solutions to their problems', and 'improve the quality of their community life' (ibid.: 10). Its 'working principles' include: relationships of equality among all participants, acceptance, co-operation, attentive listening, maximum inclusion of individuals and representative groups, and ensuring that all participants benefit from the project activities (ibid.: 38). And Stringer also echoes John Collier's emphasis on the researcher as learner, ending the section in which he criticises the claims to 'legitimacy' of conventional social science by quoting the words of the Aboriginal social worker Lillie Watson: 'If you've come to help me you're wasting your time. But if you've come because your liberation is bound up with mine, then let us work together' (ibid.: 148).

Summary

These words are a reminder that the community development model of action research must always be seen as an attempt to intervene in the *politics* of knowledge: the *power* of the researcher's expertise always threatens to 'disempower' community members and thus to undermine the researcher's desire to 'help'. A coherent model of community-oriented action research thus requires facilitators to recognise the wider political structures which devalue community members' own self-understanding, in relation to the interpretations of academics and politicians. From this point of view Stringer may perhaps place too much reliance on Guba and Lincoln's model of evaluation, where the central criterion of success is the achievement of consensus among the various stakeholders. The obvious interface between community development work and the structural politics of the wider society reminds us that any local consensus may be both incomplete and short-lived. Thus, in community development and in action research generally it is important to recognise the political limits of one's work and to welcome and appreciate the significance of even small improvements.

3 Action research as management: consultancy or organisational learning?

Expert consultants, learning organisations and teamwork

At first sight there seem to be key features of large organisations which suggest that they are not fertile places for the development of action research as we have described it. We tend to think of organisations as 'bureaucratic' structures, i.e. as a hierarchical system of roles in which staff at each level prescribe the rules to be followed and the objectives to be achieved by the level below (Weber, 1947). However, the bureaucratic model of organisational life clearly leaves out much of the reality of what goes on. Alongside 'formal' lines of authority and accountability there are always 'informal' patterns of behaviour which redefine goals and relationships in unpredictable ways (Selznick, 1964). And an organisation can also be understood as a political system where interest groups compete or as a system of 'self-organising' groups capable of changing functions and substituting for one another (Morgan, 1986: Chapters 6, 4).

Bearing all this in mind, it is not surprising that although there *is* a long tradition of action research involving organisational managers, it is rather ambiguous in terms of some key action research principles. Thus, both Rapoport (1970) and Foster (1972) chart the continuing and expanding work of the Tavistock Institute, from the 1940s to the present, in developing action research work in commercial and governmental organisations (Tavistock Institute, 1993). Similar work has been undertaken over many years by William Foote Whyte (Whyte, 1991). However, most of this work describes not organisational managers actually carrying out action research themselves, but social science experts working in a consultancy role with managers to solve problems or to initiate change. Chisholm and Elden (1993) refer to 'early action research', in which 'researchers remained in control of key aspects of the process, [and] the nature of meaning within the organisation or system came from the outside expert, not members of the organisation'. And they go on to recommend a more 'participative' model in which the contributions of outside researcher and organisational members are combined, but which still preserves a clear differentiation between the roles of researcher and practitioner. This general problem was recognised by Sanford as early as 1970 in a paper with the eloquent title 'Whatever happened to action research?'. What happened was that action research became a process in which an expert in a 'social science' discipline (such as 'social dynamics', psychotherapy or operational research) acts as a 'change agent', revealing to managers the short-comings of the group processes within their organisation (see Foster, 1972).

Detailed discussions of the 'expert change agent' model of action research are provided by Elden (1981) and Hart and Bond (1995: Chapters 5, 6). Elden was employed as a social science-qualified expert to help management set up a 'participative' approach to the installation of a new computer system. He describes how difficult he found it to learn not to impose his own agenda or 'pre-packaged' methods, but to work with staff in developing their own priorities and their own language for analysing their situation (Elden, 1981: 265). This required new role relationships, which were difficult for staff (conscious of being short of time and pressured by events), for managers (who needed to let go of some of their power prerogatives) and, in particular, for Elden himself, who found that he needed to discard much of the expertise which he had originally thought of as his main qualification for his role. Hart and Bond's account brings out even more clearly the conflictual position of the external consultant called in by senior management to work within an 'autocratic organisational culture' in order to achieve 'empower-ment among groups lower down the hierarchy' (Hart and Bond, 1995: 104). They show the major political problems this generates, even including the rejection of the research report (ibid.: 109).

Given the inherent conflict between action research and the bureaucratic model of organisational management, the recent emergence of the notion of the 'learning organisation' is potentially both significant and helpful. It is a model of organ-isational learning which is concerned not with formulating a socially relevant role for social scientists but with the roles and purposes of managers themselves, as practitioners. In describing this 'new' model it is appropriate to start with the work of W.E. Deming. In the late 1940s Deming achieved fame through his introduction of statistical performance data to enable managers to control the quality of the operations for which they were responsible (Hutchins, 1988: 146). But in 1986 Deming published a deeply worried account of the 'crisis' of organisational life to which his own ideas had led. Pre-specified standards, statistical outcome measures, and hierarchical appraisals of staff performance were creating a climate of distrust which inhibited innovation, team-work, critical thinking and effective long-term planning, and were leading to simplistic decision-making based on what was easily measured rather than what was important (Deming, 1986: 54, 60, 97, 123).

This is a crisis not just of morale but of effectiveness. The argument originally underlying the work on learning organisations was that the renewed intensity of global competition meant that organisational survival required increased responsiveness to client demand in a rapidly changing market, and this in turn required the creativity and continuous learning fostered above all by collaborative teamwork (Senge, 1990: 4; Peters, 1987: Chapter 1). Thus, as early as 1982 Peters and Waterman's popular best-seller argued that in order to survive commercially an effective organisation needed to focus on creating autonomy for small, fluid, experimental task forces (Peters and Waterman, 1982: Chapters 5, 6), and Peters' follow-up text (1987) is even more explicit. Organisational survival requires 'constant change and constant improvement' (ibid.: 4), so managers should see themselves as 'facilitators' of 'self-managed teams', each responsible for evaluating the quality of its own work and for continuous innovation through listening carefully to clients' responses (ibid.: 43, 75, 58, 145ff.). Similarly, Hakes (1991: 14–16) emphasises that each organisational operation must be fully 'owned' by those who are involved in it and can influence it on a 'minute-by-minute' basis, so that staff can offer criticism of, and suggest improvements for, their own work, as part of a culture of free and open discussion. Senge's book, subtitled *The Art and Practice of the Learning Organisation*, summarises and elaborates these various themes. In order to survive, all organisations must become learning organisations (Senge, 1990: 4). And in order to do so, organisations must transcend defensive interdepartmental politics, create an open exchange of ideas (ibid.: Chapter 13), delegate decision-making down to 'local' contexts (ibid.: Chapter 14), and (above all) develop 'team learning' (ibid.: Chapter 12), i.e. encourage the sharing of different perspectives, using a 'systems' analysis of how perspectives influence one another (ibid.: Chapters 5–8).

As yet, of course, the learning organisation is not so much an observable reality as a remote ideal or even merely a political buzz-word, often masking a deceptive ideology: for many of us, life in organisations feels *increasingly* bureaucratic, as computerised information systems create new forms of hierarchical control (Huws, 1999: 51). However, it is arguable that the new responsive, interactive model of management is part of a real historical change (Heckscher, 1994: 43–4) and two of the historical factors tending to encourage this development have already been referred to: (1) the intensification of competition for markets; and (2) the increasing recognition, by writers on organisations and on education, of the crucial importance of team working (Dixon, 1994; Heckscher, 1994; Gibbons *et al.*, 1994).

Management and the unpredictability of social events

Another factor tending to push management theory in the direction of action research is the increasingly widespread acceptance of the fundamental unpredictability of social events (Omerod, 1994; Aspden, 1994). This argument is at the heart of Stacey's elaborate account of how management theory must be rethought to take into account the *theoretical* (as well as practical) uncertainties of organisational processes (Stacey, 1996). His argument is largely based on systems theory (ibid.: 250ff.) and chaos theory (ibid.: 319ff.), both of which emphasise the continuous feedback mechanisms operating over time between social events, leading to patterns which are so complex that they cannot be predicted except in very general terms. Hence, the 'technical rationality' model of management (the collection and processing of all relevant information followed by prescriptive decision-making *by* managers *for* staff) is usually ineffective, since the amount of relevant data is too enormous to be fully analysed in the time available. Stacey's argument is thus based on a much broader set of considerations than the unpredictability of markets, and helps to emphasise that the notion of the learning organisation is equally applicable to management in organisations such as social services departments, hospitals, medical centres and schools, where the role of purely commercial markets is less clear-cut. His point is quite general: except in very rare circumstances, *effective* management must recognise the *lack of certainty* in its field of operations and allow maximum *flexibility* and *discretion* (ibid.: 33–5). In other words, organisations need to encourage 'states of instability, contradiction, contention and creative tension in order to provoke to new perspectives and continuous learning' (ibid.: xx).

Feminist theory and workplace learning cultures

A number of gender-based differences have been proposed which would be highly significant for the establishment of the sort of workplace 'learning culture' which action research requires. For example, Tannen suggests that men tend to approach conversational interactions as a negotiation for status and independence, as a 'contest . . . to achieve and maintain the upper hand if they can', whereas women treat conversation as a negotiation for 'connection' in which 'people try to seek and give confirmation and support and to reach consensus' (1992: 24–5). From this point of view it is interesting to note the difference between Nancy Kline's description of the 'thinking environment', with its emphasis on listening, expression of appreciation, encouragement, and recognition of feelings (Kline, 1993: Chapter 2) and the competitive, antagonistic version of 'dialectical' discussion proposed by Mike Pedler and his (male) colleagues in their evocation of 'the learning company' (Pedler *et al.*, 1991: 62). That there may be a gender-based cultural difference between 'adversarial' and 'empathetic' modes of collaborative understanding is also suggested by Belenky *et al.*, (1986: 96, 100–22). 'Explanations' of gender-based differences are notoriously contentious: our argument here is merely that the increasing participation of women in managerial roles may perhaps bring into organisational life a significantly new range of abilities, from which organisational staff in general (including men) will be able to benefit. Perhaps a more 'feminised' organisational culture might find it easier to follow Deming's urgent advice that 'leadership' must be reconstructed to mean acting not as 'a judge' of one's staff, but instead as a colleague and counsellor, 'learning from them and with them' (Deming, 1986: 117).

Summary: an example of the manager as learner

Thus there are various grounds for taking seriously an emerging school of thought which seems to suggest that effective management needs, above all, the qualities we have associated with action research. What might this look like in practice? This section concludes with a summary of a project based explicitly on a model of management practice *as* an action research process and specifically intended to foster the ideal of a learning organisation (Bishop, 1995). When Leo Bishop undertook this piece of work he was Senior Manager of Inspection Services for Essex Social Services Department. This meant that he had managerial responsibility for staff carrying out inspections of residential and day-care centres for children, elderly people and people with physical and learning disabilities. The problem he wished to address was as follows. The UK government had recently introduced a policy change which affected the work of inspection staff and had issued a policy statement concerning the new practices required. This statement, however, was of a very general nature. So how could Leo Bishop, as manager, oversee the creation of a more detailed document containing guidelines on the actual practice of inspection? He recognised that although he had management *responsibility* for the inspection work he did not know *how* (exactly) it should be carried out. He also recognised that a document which staff could fully 'own' (because they had created it themselves) would be much more effective than a prescriptive document 'issued' by management (ibid.: 19). In other words, Leo Bishop suggests that the task required his staff to learn from each other and required him to learn from and with them (see Deming, 1986: 117). In this way the document would be used more intensively, and creating it would enhance morale.

Leo Bishop explicitly places his approach within the Peters and Waterman (1982) conception of the learning organisation (Bishop, 1995: 18) and, more particularly, the 'learning local authority' (Stewart and Sutherland, 1992). His model is one in which 'The role of the manager becomes . . . action research into the actual work of inspection and the manager's own work of communicating with his/her staff' (Bishop, 1995: 3). His method was in many ways quite simple. He conducted a series of workshops where staff 'brainstormed' a list of the key features of their work as inspectors, which entailed recognising, and learning from, the tensions between their different perspectives. He then edited the list (organising it and removing repetitions) and circulated it to the participating staff for amendment. The staff amendments were then incorporated into a final 'Draft statement of practice principles'. Finally, staff were sent a questionnaire on which they could register (confidentially and anonymously) how they had experienced the project. Almost all said they were 'pleased' with the outcome, and that their views had been 'genuinely sought', and approximately 50% said they had felt the process to be 'empowering' (ibid.: 56).

Of course, an organisational culture is not transformed overnight or by a single project, and 50% of Leo Bishop's staff did *not* report that they had experienced the 'empowerment' intended. But the project does represent an attempt to make use of the professional 'space' which remains even when governments are prescribing policy guidelines, given that *actual* practice (the 'how') always remains a matter for individual discretion even after 'guidelines' have been published. It also demonstrates that a senior manager can consciously adopt an action research model of her/his role in order to initiate a process which accomplishes an obvious management task (generating practice guidelines) in a way which involves the staff concerned as creators rather than as recipients, and which involves the manager also in a process of learning.

4 'Facilitation': issues of power and learning

It was helpful, as a starting point, to think of action research as, typically, an 'insider' process in which those involved in a situation work together to develop their own practices (see Chapter 1). But this is in some respects an oversimplification: action research traditionally does also formulate an important role for an 'outsider' contribution to the research process. In management and community development contexts this role has often been presented in terms of a social scientist acting as a 'consultant' (see Sections 2 and 3, above). More generally, action research projects are often initiated from within universities, organisational research units or public funding bodies, so that the project initiator becomes the 'facilitator' of action research, often co-ordinating work in a number of different contexts. This is obviously likely to be the case with large-scale initiatives, and these large projects have of course played a significant part in raising the profile of action research as an approach to social inquiry. Not surprisingly, therefore, 'facilitation' has played a key role in some of the most widely influential action research projects, especially in the contexts of nursing, community work and school teaching; indeed, Webb treats the facilitative process as the key relationship in the action research model of inquiry (Webb, 1991: 156). In this section, therefore, we consider the meaning of 'facilitation', and how it relates to the general action research principles already outlined.

An early example of an extended action research project in a nursing context (Towell and Harries, 1979) is built around what might be called the institutional-isation of the facilitator role. It describes how Towell (working in conjunction with the Tavistock Institute) and Harries (originally appointed as Senior Nursing Officer) developed their roles as 'social research advisers' in a large mental hospital. 'This role was intended to provide a service in the hospital such that any group of staff could seek help in identifying, investigating and tackling problems arising in their day-to-day work' (ibid.: 14). An important feature of the book is that ward nurses co-author the various accounts of the different projects, along with the research advisers. Although the funding for this arrangement was relatively short-lived, the project provides a valuable model of how a care organ-isation can institutionalise action research in such a way that support for staff is made permanently available, thereby blurring the distinction between insider and outsider research.

However, there are tensions implicit in the role of action research facilitator, as Towell himself admits (ibid.: 34), and an insight into the origin of these tensions, as well as a full statement on the nature of the facilitator role in general, may be found in the account provided by Brown *et al.* (1982). For Brown and his colleagues, the role of facilitator arises directly from the action research principle of collaboration: a *group* of participants always needs to be co-ordinated, group processes need to be organised, group assumptions need to be challenged, and there will be gaps in the group's collective expertise which need to be filled (ibid.: 4). The facilitator thus provides an outsider perspective, a focus for activity, emotional support, practical assistance and resources. The facilitator acts as critic, recorder and methodological teacher (ibid.: 5–7). The problem, however, is that the 'objective' of the facilitator is 'the enhancement of the autonomy' of the participants and 'the reduction of their dependency on others' (ibid.: 11). There is thus an inherent danger that all the well-intentioned work of the facilitator may become counterproductive, merely substituting another form of authoritative expertise within yet another hierarchical power relationship.

Facilitation and power

It is this issue – the implicit power relation within the facilitator role – which has provided the impetus for much of the writing by action researchers on facilitation. Posch, for example, writing about his work on a Europe-wide action research project on environmental education, notes the 'temptation' for facilitators to 'dominate' the interpretation of events with their own understandings, which, he says, may well seem 'clearer' than those of the participating school teachers, even to the teachers themselves (Posch, 1993: 454). Losito and Pozzo (1997) – also writing from within an international project, 'Management for Organisational and Human Development' – describe the facilitator role through two contrasting images, both of which allude to his/her power and authority over other participants: (1) the facilitator as an 'experienced sailor' advising the crew of a ship navigating without a captain (ibid.: 290); and (2) the facilitator as the weaver of a tapestry from the multicoloured threads provided by participants (ibid.: 291–2). Messner and Rauch address the power issue in terms of three 'dilemmas'. How does the facilitator provide 'support' without 'taking control' (Messner and Rauch, 1995: 45)? How does the facilitator both provide a critical outsider perspective *and* encourage participants to have confidence in their own experience (ibid.: 50)? How can the 'pressure' provided by the facilitator's presence be 'stimulating' rather than 'inhibiting' (ibid.: 51–2)?

Somekh (1994) attempts to point a way forward from such dilemmas. Her argument is that a fruitful division of labour operates within large-scale action research projects. *All* participants are 'researchers', and indeed they define and publish their own work (ibid.: 359), but they are researchers with a differing final emphasis: individual participants are largely concerned with developing and understanding the practical detail of their own work contexts, whereas project facilitators are more concerned with generalisations across the many contexts covered by the overall project (ibid.: 376–7). This addresses the issue of whether facilitators necessarily 'take over'. By working in partnership with each other, the members of an action research project (facilitators and 'other participants') can, together, create knowledge which is both locally effective and has some degree of generalisability. However, Somekh's implied distinction between the local and the general does not sit easily with action research's claim that there is potential general significance even in the individual case (see above, Chapter 2, p. 21, 'Generalisability'); this evokes the danger (for action research) that the role of the facilitator will somehow reinstate the outsider's expertise as 'superior' to that of the 'insider' participants.

Another response to the issue of the facilitator's 'superiority' is Elliott's influential proposal that facilitators always have a double task. They must support the 'first order' action research of participants working within their own individual contexts, but, in addition, they must also engage in a separate, 'second order' action research study of their own work of facilitating the work of the other participants (Elliott, 1991: 27, 30; Elliott and Adelman, 1996: 17). In this way facilitators are faced with the same task as any other participant: they are challenged to investigate and develop their own practice and understanding of their practice as facilitators. In other words, the tendency of the facilitator role to foster a sense of superiority is, partly at least, counteracted by a requirement to adopt a *critical* stance towards their own work. This idea that facilitators must place themselves, methodologically, 'alongside' other project participants by systematically subjecting themselves to the risks and challenges of investigating their own work as facilitators represents one way of attempting to reduce the status and power differentials within the research process.

Action research as facilitation

In some ways, *all* participants in an action research process may be thought of as engaged in a process of facilitation, in the sense of providing mutual support within a developmental process (see Losito *et al.*, 1998). The work of Titchen, in the context of nursing, provides a clear example. Titchen acted as facilitator for a ward sister who was in turn acting as facilitator for the nursing staff on her ward, to help them develop a more 'patient-centred' conception of their role (Titchen, 2000). Titchen's model of facilitation involves mutuality, reciprocity, attention to particulars, and 'care'. The key processes include 'observing, listening and questioning', 'feedback', and combining challenge and support within a 'critical dialogue'. Her model has at its centre not 'expertise' but the reflexive and 'accepting' awareness of the human relationships at work in the inquiry. Titchen calls this relationship 'critical companionship', and what is most important to note is that it describes the ideal underlying *all* the relationships of the action research process: the relationship between project facilitator and ward sister, between ward sister and staff nurses, *and* between nurses and their patients.

Summary

To sum up, action research's central principles of collaboration and empowerment mean that the relationships it seeks to establish in work contexts are the same as the relationships of the inquiry process itself. And these relationships can be thought of as 'facilitation' – as opposed to those of authoritative or expert 'instruction'. The initiators/co-ordinators of action research projects (whether large or small in scale) are not privileged by their experience or their expertise to simply 'get others to engage in' action research: they themselves are also always 'participants'. As such, their stance towards their own practice within the action research inquiry process must be no different from that of other participants. Their assumptions are available to be questioned by others, their strategies will change through the course of the inquiry, their aim is to *learn*. Even though facilitators *initially* provide support and advice, their work must, in the end, 'model' the collaborative relationships and principles of action research. Otherwise 'facilitation' will become self-contradictory, tending to recreate the relationships of authority and dependency which an action research project is always attempting to overcome.

5 Action research as 'responsive' evaluation

Two models of evaluation

The cyclic pattern of action research – its repeated alternation between practical action and reflection (see Chapter 2, p. 14) – suggests immediately its close links with the activity we call 'evaluation'. An action research project may or may not *start* by evaluating current practice (whether long established or recently introduced) but there will always be an explicitly evaluative *phase* at some point in the work. The essence of evaluation is the making of judgements: does this practice 'need' changing? has this attempt at improving practice been 'effective'? Evaluation focuses our understanding of experience by setting data and analysis against values and criteria. And, as with action research in general, the key questions are: what sorts of data are to be collected? who devises the criteria? and who makes the judgements?

The general shape of the debate about evaluation is indicated by the influential paper 'Evaluation as illumination' by Parlett and Hamilton (1977) in which they begin by presenting two contrasting models of the evaluation process. The first is based on the quantitative measurement of outcomes in relation to pre-specified criteria. In the pure form of this model evaluation takes the form of comparing 'before-and-after' measurements of the effects of a given 'intervention' and measuring the differences between experimental and control situations or groups. Parlett and Hamilton call this the 'agricultural-botany' model, since they see it as most appropriate for evaluating the yields of crops or plants. They also call it the 'traditional' model, because of its longstanding influence in experimental psychology (as well as in the testing of *medical* procedures – see below). Their argument is that this model is generally *not* appropriate for evaluating *human* situations, for a number of reasons. First, variables can never be wholly controlled, and even partial attempts to do so are 'artificial' (i.e. they have a distorting effect on the situation), unrealistically expensive and ethically dubious. Second, the attempt to control variables discourages flexibility and improvisation. Third, focusing on purely quantitative measures restricts the scope of the data considered. Fourth, local variations are ignored. Fifth, the differing concerns of the various interest groups are ignored (ibid.: 8–9). In the light of these criticisms of the 'traditional' model, the authors propose their alternative, namely 'illuminative evaluation':

> The aims of illuminative evaluation are to study the innovatory programme: how it operates; how it is influenced by the various [institutional] situations in which it is applied; what those directly concerned regard as its advantages and disadvantages. . . . It aims to discover what it is like to be participating. . . . In short it seeks to address and to illuminate a complex array of questions.
>
> (ibid.: 10)

The two models of evaluation obviously echo the distinction between 'positivist' and 'naturalistic' inquiry presented in Chapter 2, and also the difference between what Simons calls 'product' and 'process' evaluation (Simons, 1982a). The continued relevance of Parlett and Hamilton's distinction is illustrated in more recent writings. Oakley (1996) – acutely aware of the public pressure to 'guarantee' the effectiveness of social work interventions – argues that decisive evaluation must take the form of randomised controlled trials (RCTs), involving quantitative measurement of outcomes and comparing an 'experimental' group which receive the innovatory 'treatment' with a 'control' group which do not. The two groups are supposed to be established by purely statistical techniques in an attempt to ensure that they do not differ in any way which might 'bias' the results. MacDonald (1999) echoes the demand for RCTs in social work, but Taylor and Thornicroft (1996), writing in the context of mental health service provision, analyse in detail the difficulties involved and show that, in practice, neither treatment conditions nor the motivation and awareness of participants can be fully controlled (ibid.: 144–8). Fuller also argues that the random allocation of participants to experimental and control groups is often impractical, and that evaluation therefore usually involves comparisons carried out on a more informal basis, i.e. by comparing 'cases' (Fuller, 1996: 62). Fuller also points out that evaluating 'effectiveness' is not a straightforward matter, since the *intentions* of service managers and professionals may be at variance with the *concerns* of service-users (ibid.: 56), and statements of objectives often involve ambiguous and contested concepts, e.g. 'interests', 'needs' and 'well-being' (ibid.: 58). Fuller's emphasis therefore has much in common with that of Parlett and Hamilton: evaluation evidence can rarely be scientifically controlled; instead (in order to be usefully 'illuminating') it needs to be *varied*, so that it reflects the *complexity* of actual situations (ibid.: 59, 63).

Two models of 'evidence'

In many ways the key questions for evaluation are: what sort of judgements are to be made and what sort of evidence is therefore appropriate? Stenhouse, one of the central figures in the recent development of action research, provides a clear-cut reply in favour of the illuminative model. Illuminative evaluation, he says, seeks judgements not simply in the sense of 'verdicts' but ones which may provide a basis for future developmental work (Stenhouse, 1985b: 31). Moreover, since developmental work is located in a particular context, evaluative judgements need to be based on a 'dossier' of evidence, representing 'the case' as a whole and in depth (ibid.: 31–2), not the abstract, fragmented statistical 'results' generated by experimental 'trials'. The term 'trial' is suggestive here, reminding us that it is *lawyers* who have the most explicit concern with making judgements based on 'the evidence'. And *legal* 'trials' are based on accumulating a *mass* of evidence in the form of different 'stories' and interpretations from a variety of witnesses and competing advocates. Moreover, writers on legal theories of evidence emphasise that a legal judgement is always a matter of interpretation and discretion (Elliott and Phipson, 1987: 41) involving simultaneously many different types of decision (Twining, 1990: 362) and a recognition that 'reality' is elusive and complex since it is differently constructed by each of us (ibid.: 367–8).

It is thus highly misleading when the advocates of so-called 'evidence-based practice' attempt to hi-jack the term 'evidence' to mean, exclusively, *statistical* evidence of the sort generated by randomised control trials (Evidence-Based Medicine Working Group, 1992). The authors of this article suggest that the use of such evidence will provide 'superior patient care' (ibid.: 2421), although the example they give is hardly convincing. We are assured that a (male) patient informed simply that there is 'a high risk' that his acute condition might recur will be left 'in a state of vague trepidation' and fear. In contrast, if he is told (using the 'evidence-based' approach) that the risk is between 43% and 51% after one year, and between 51% and 60% after three years, and that if he has had no recurrence after eighteen months the risk will be 20%, then he will have 'a clear idea of his likely prognosis' (ibid.: 2420). But such statistics do *not* provide a full basis for judgements in individual cases, since they refer to large samples (cf. Stenhouse's argument above), so even according to statistical theory in this case the patient would hardly have been given 'a clear idea' of his individual 'prognosis', even if the statistics in this case were less obviously confusing. Of course, professional judgements must be (and always are) based on 'evidence', but statistical evidence of this sort, though clearly important, is necessarily only part of the picture, as the Evidence-Based Medicine Working Group themselves admit (ibid.: 2423). This argument of course applies all the more strongly to judgements outside a purely medical context, such as the likelihood of a recurrence of abusive behaviour in the context of social work with families.

The politics of evaluation

So far the discussion has focused mainly on methods and forms of data, but there is also the question of audience and purpose. MacDonald (1977) poses this issue succinctly. He argues that evaluation is necessarily and by definition concerned with making *value* judgements, and since social situations always involve 'competing interest groups' an evaluation process is always inherently *political* (ibid.: 224). To illustrate this, MacDonald presents three contrasting possibilities. First, an evaluation may adopt the objectives of the powerful agencies which control resources and dictate policy ('Bureaucratic Evaluation'). Second, an evaluator may adopt her/his own 'independent' objectives ('Autocratic Evaluation'). Third, an evaluation may be constructed as a process which 'recognises value pluralism and seeks to represent a range of interests in its issue formulation [with the evaluator acting as] a broker in exchanges of information between different interest groups' ('Democratic Evaluation') (ibid.: 226).

From what has been said so far, it is clear that it is the 'illuminative'/'democratic' model of evaluation which aligns with the action research principles outlined in Chapter 2. Further elaboration of this model is provided by the work of Guba and Lincoln. Their starting point is the concept of 'responsive evaluation' first proposed by Stake (1967). In responsive evaluation the process 'responds to' (a) the values and concerns of different individuals and interest groups, as 'stakeholders', and (b) the emergent issues as the inquiry proceeds (Guba and Lincoln, 1981: 33–6). In their later work Guba and Lincoln (1989: 43–4) also call their model 'con-structivist' – in that it rests on the philosophical argument that, since we have no direct access to any 'objective' reality existing independently of our interpretations, we necessarily 'construct' the reality of our experience. For evaluation, therefore, the 'key dynamic' is negotiation between the differing 'realities' of the various participants – a 'dialectical' process of discussion and mutual learning (ibid.: 44, 56), in which the aim is clarification (ibid.: 56) and, eventually, consensus (ibid.: 45). They also note that evaluation always threatens to place participating stakeholders 'at risk' (ibid.: 51), so that care must be taken to ensure that the impact of the evaluation is not oppressive but 'educational' and 'empowering' (ibid.: 149). In responsive/constructivist evaluation, therefore: 'All parties' . . . initial constructions are given full consideration and . . . each individual has an opportunity to provide a critique, to correct, to amend, or to extend all the other parties' constructions' (ibid.).

Practical problems

So far we have been concerned with a theoretical ideal of evaluation, seen as a democratic, responsive, illuminative process which shares many of the principles and ideals of action research. But practice never coincides exactly with theoretical ideals. One obvious problem is that of time. The process of negotiating and checking accounts needs to be completed within the time scale of a developing programme of action, which means that it can never be wholly comprehensive or exhaustive; and this in turn poses a question about the 'credibility' of the evaluation (ibid.: 236–7). Similarly, most evaluation work in small-scale localised projects will suffer from a shortage of resources, leading to the same problem. There is also always the tension between different audiences. An evaluation report may be both a means for self-evaluation within an institutional community (Simons, 1982b) and also part of the mechanism of accountability to a wider public. In theory these two functions can be made to coincide (ibid.: 287) but the potential conflicts (of motive, for example) are obvious.

Summary: some contrasting examples

In the light of these various general arguments, let us end this section by briefly considering a few specific examples of evaluation reports. Ovretveit (1986) began his evaluation of a new format for social work record-keeping by creating, in conjunction with a group of social workers, a set of general statements concerning practice values. From these statements a set of 'objectives' was devised which Ovretveit then used, in stage 2 of the project, as criteria for assessing whether or not various other groups of workers had made proper use of the new record-keeping forms. Although this work is described as both an evaluation and an action research project, it is clear that stage 2 participants were simply *subjected* to the assessment procedure, and were not involved either as 'stakeholders' or as 'co-researchers'. In contrast, Ward's (1996) evaluation of assessment procedures in child-care also began with a small 'working party' devising a set of assessment procedures, but the second stage of the work was used as an opportunity for refinement and revision by *broadening* the range of stakeholders, as Guba and Lincoln might have wished:

> The social workers, carers and children who completed these assessments have made numerous suggestions as to how the materials might be improved, and their comments will be taken into account as the materials are revised. . . . Feedback from users has led us to look more closely at issues such as the relative roles to be played by health professionals, social workers and educators in undertaking assessments, and to question whether the assumptions on which the materials are based are appropriate to the upbringing of children from a variety of cultures.
>
> (Ward, 1996: 84)

Loveland (1998) gives a further example of evaluation carried out by a social worker with the specific aim of consulting service-users and involving them in the development of service provision.

Turning now to examples from the health professions, Batteson (1997) describes the development of a training programme designed to improve communication and collaboration between nurses and occupational therapists. Like Ward's, Batteson's evaluation phase is a process of continued refinement of the programme, rather than (as with Ovretveit) a process of *assessment* against previously established criteria. In this context it is worth noting Elliott's observation that one of the 'criteria for good action research' is that it should involve participants in discussing and *defining* 'quality indicators', rather than taking for granted the relevance and adequacy of a pre-defined checklist (Elliott, 1995: 11). The Royal College of Nursing (1990) 'dynamic standard setting system' is a clear example of this process at work. Groups of nurses were involved in defining 'standards' of patient care to which they themselves wished to subscribe and which they judged to be feasible. They then monitored their own practice in the light of the criteria they had specified: a schematic approach, emphasising quantitative measures rather than illuminative documentation, but very obviously *self*-evaluation, even within a set of procedures for institutional accountability.

Finally, an example which allows us to consider the *form* of an evaluation report. MacVicar's evaluation of a respite care unit is interesting in that his report consists very largely of quotations from service-users describing their experiences and perspectives, even though it begins with a series of very closed questions, e.g. 'Is the project meeting the aims and objectives which have been set?' (MacVicar, 1995: 151). In this case, then, the evaluation report can be seen as 'empowering' clients simply by providing them with an officially audible (i.e. published) 'voice'. This example shows how an evaluation can be 'responsive', even when it is conducted within the general framework of a purely administrative decision as to whether or not a facility should continue to be funded.

6 Action research and 'critical reflection'

One of the central principles of action research is that the initiator of the research *learns* about her/his own practice (see Sections 3 and 4 in this chapter). Consequently, action research has become popular as a form of *education* for professional staff, in which learning arises from the process of engaging in practice-based *inquiry*. Two important points follow from this. First, a significant dimension of action research is its link with the concept of 'reflective practice', based on Schon's emphasis on the continuous reflection required by the complexities and uncertainties of professional practice (Schon, 1983). Second, one of the most significant contexts in which action research has been influential over the last twenty years is education, i.e. teaching. If action research is itself a form of education, it means that, for teachers, engaging in an action research inquiry has a direct similarity with their own professional practice. Thus, 'teachers-as-researchers' (Bartholomew, 1972; Stenhouse, 1975) are also 'teachers-as-learners' – learning *with* their students about the processes and structures of learning in which they are *jointly* engaged: teaching is itself a *research* process (ibid.: 141–3). In this section, therefore, expanding upon the first part of Chapter 2, we generalise this linkage (between action research and professional work) from teaching to other professions, using the concept of 'critical reflection' as a bridge between the two.

Action research and the 'reflective' professional practitioner

Schon's model of the reflective practitioner has a number of links with the rationale for action research. For example, he argues that professional decision-making is too complex to take the form of simply 'applying' general rules to specific situations, i.e. 'technical rationality' (Schon, 1983: 29). Instead, the reality of social inter-actions (including professional decision-making) has to be '*constructed*' by those involved (Schon, 1987: 36) as a process of 'reframing' experience and of 'experi-menting' with possible interpretations (Schon, 1983: 132, 141). The importance of Schon's ideas has been widely acknowledged. Palmer's introduction to *Reflective Practice in Nursing*, for example, emphasises the role of reflection in developing self-awareness and personal knowledge, combining patient care with learning from professional experience, and improving practice through critical self-questioning (Palmer *et al.*, 1994). Yelloly and Henkel (1995: 8–9) make a similar argument for social work. It is important to note that for all these writers reflection is conceived as a 'critical' process – a process of change and transformation. We need to consider, therefore, how action research contributes to *critical* reflection.

Writing in an educational context, Elliott draws an explicit parallel between Schon's 'reflective practice' and action research, arguing that collaborative action research, as a form of practitioner-based 'evaluation and development', is 'a unified conception of reflective educational practice' (1991: 50, 56, 54). For Elliott, a further important link is that professional *values* play a central part in defining both reflective practice and action research. Consequently, 'improving' practice (either within reflective practice or within an action research project) is never merely a technical matter of, for example, efficiency or productivity.

> The improvement of a practice consists of realising those values which constitute its ends. . . . [Thus] improving practice . . . necessarily involves a continuing process of reflection on the part of practitioners. This is partly because . . . what constitutes an appropriate realisation of values is ultimately a matter of personal judgement in particular circumstances.
>
> (ibid.: 49–50)

Action research, says Elliott, thus involves a 'reflective critique' of the 'value interpretations embedded in practice' because values are 'infinitely contestable . . . infinitely open to reinterpretation' (ibid.: 51, 50).

Two potential problems in this sort of argument need to be addressed. First, it might be interpreted as emphasising the discretion of professionals at the expense of their clients, and thus to reinforce their power *over* clients. But this would be to misread the significance of the 'values' at issue – which are always about the *rights* of clients (to justice, care, health, education, etc.) and the *responsibilities* of workers to 'realise' these rights *with* and *on behalf of* clients. And a continuous theme of educational action research is the transformation of authoritarian relationships between teachers and pupils into a relationship based on mutual respect and dialogue, involving teachers in *questioning* their own decisions (see, for example, Schindler, 1993). Second, there is also a danger that instead of saying that action research involves asking the always difficult question, 'How shall we *best* put our professional values into practice on *this* occasion?' (Elliott's argument), we ask, 'What is the *contradiction* between my professional values and my current practice, and how shall I resolve it?' (Whitehead, 1989).

What is being 'critical'?

This latter question, as presented by Whitehead, provides one interpretation of what might be meant by 'being critical' but it does so in a way which is unhelpful in several ways (in spite of its simplicity and thus its appeal). First, values represent ideals, and ideals are by definition never fully realisable in practice; so the relationship between values and practice is not simply a 'contradiction' which can be 'resolved'. Second, real contradictions exist *between competing values* in a given situation (e.g. the potential conflict between responding 'equitably' to different clients and responding fully to the 'unique individuality' of each client's circumstances); so 'practice' is a matter of 'working with' dilemmas or trying to 're-frame' them in order to find a constructive way forward. Third, real contradictions exist between the practices, interests and aims of different parties in a situation; so 'improving' a situation is often about negotiating new patterns of communication. In other words, the 'critical' dimension of action research cannot simply rest on an initial 'confession' of one's own 'failure' to enact professional values, still less on an invitation to others to do so; nor should it ever end with self-righteous claims to have 'removed a contradiction between' values and practice. The first makes action research seem unduly threatening, and the second renders action researchers' conclusions both implausible and suspiciously self-righteous.

The work of Carr and Kemmis is organised around a more complex conception of critical reflection, namely a process of 'emancipation' from cultural and institutional constraints (1986: 192). For Carr and Kemmis, the critical thrust for both reflection and action research arises from a socio-political ideal:

> The criteria of rationality (in communication), justice (in decision-making) and access to an interesting and satisfying life (in relation to work) provide benchmarks against which practices of communication, decision-making and work can be evaluated. . . . Educational action research . . . allows . . . teachers and others . . . to identify those institutional patterns of practice which limit the achievement of more rational communication, more just and democratic decision-making and access to an interesting and satisfying life for all.
>
> (ibid.: 193–4)

These criteria of rationality, justice and self-fulfilment are derived from the work of Habermas (see Carr and Kemmis, 1986: Chapter 5), and his conception of rationality is particularly significant for a theory of action research. The 'collaborative' principle of action research has as its ideal a form of discussion in which any hierarchical differences of power, status or authority between the various participants in a situation are temporarily 'suspended' (see Chapter 2 above), so that, in Habermas' terms, 'no force except the better argument is used', only genuinely common interests will be agreed and any attempts at deception will be exposed through critical scrutiny (Habermas, 1976: 108; Winter, 1987: 82).

But it is important to note that Habermas presents this explicitly as an *ideal* (Habermas, 1978: 314) and, again, the problem is: how can action research be 'critical' without simply pointing to the obvious and inevitable gap between a messy, contradictory reality and a pure but unrealisable ideal? On this point, Carr and Kemmis seem ambiguous. For example, at several points their analysis depends on a distinction between 'distorted' and 'non-distorted' (i.e. 'critical', 'emancipated') patterns of communication (e.g. 1986: 192, 194), and they identify participants' 'ideology' with 'erroneous self-understanding' (ibid.: 193). But if this is interpreted crudely it can easily seem as if the initiator of action research is claiming to be already in possession of a rational, emancipated perspective and inviting prospective participants to confess that they are as yet languishing in a state of error – not a good start for establishing *collaborative* work, fully owned by all concerned.

Carr and Kemmis are aware of this danger (1986: 149, 201, 203–5) and an important part of their argument is that action research must be founded upon 'the meanings and interpretations of practitioners' (ibid.: 149). In order to reinforce this emphasis, the definition of 'critique' proposed by Winter (1989, 1996) shifts the focus of 'critique' so that it more obviously starts from participants' own analysis of their situation and is less dependent on a pre-existing set of ideals. From this perspective, critical reflection has two major dimensions: 'reflexivity' (i.e. *self*-questioning, taking one's own interpretations of events as 'data' to be subjected to examination) and 'dialectics' (i.e. focusing on the contradictions, tensions and dilemmas inherent in a situation) (Winter, 1989: 39–55; 1996: 18–21). Within this perspective, 'ideology' is not a 'distorted' perspective but a not-yet-questioned perspective, and 'critique' is not the embracing of an 'emancipated' point of view but simply the *process* of *questioning* any point of view (Winter, 1989: 186–91).

It is important to emphasise that both these strategies (reflexive critique and dialectical critique) arise from forms of awareness that we *already* possess. They arise from our spontaneous recognition of the complexities of our experience. And they arise directly from the collaborative process of an action research inquiry, in which participants representing different roles (and thus different interests) *share* their differing perspectives on the same events. This sharing process enables us to recognise the existence of alternative rationalities, the limitations of our immediate interpretations, and, consequently, possibilities for change.

The ideal of learning through dialogue

Hence the important link in meaning between 'dialectics' and 'dialogue', and the significance of Schon's emphasis that the 'reflective' model of professional work requires a professional–client relationship based on 'conversation':

> [The professional worker] attributes to his [*sic*] clients, as well as to himself, a capacity to mean, know and plan. He recognises that his actions may have different meanings for his client than he intends them to have, and he gives himself the task of discovering what these are. He recognises an obligation to make his own understandings accessible to his client, which means that he needs often to reflect anew on what he knows. . . . The reflective practitioner tries to discover the limits of his expertise through reflective conversation with the client.
>
> (Schon, 1983: 295–6)

Hence, the professional is 'accountable to' the client, and by 'reflect[ing] publicly on his knowledge-in-practice [makes] himself confrontable by his clients' (ibid.: 297, 299). All this, of course, links with the suggestion in Chapter 1 that action research is a process of *mutual learning*, between colleagues, between group members, between practitioners and managers, and between staff and clients. It also serves to emphasise that action research as a learning process for professional workers is closely linked with action research as the involvement of service-users as full participants in (and frequently initiators of) the inquiry process.

Action research and learning through practice

This brings us back to the analogy between the relationships of action research and the relationships of professional practice. In education the analogy centres on the curriculum process (Carr and Kemmis, 1986: 7; Elliott, 1991: Chapter 2). Through the dialogue of inquiry teachers-as-action-researchers reconstruct and develop their understanding of their practice in the same way as pupils and teachers (through the dialogue of the teaching–learning process) reconstruct and develop their knowledge of, say, maths or geography. In nursing, Titchen (2000) uses the concept of 'skilled companionship' to describe both the 'helping relationship' between action research facilitator and practitioner and between nurse and patient. More elaborately, Heasman and Adams (1998: 341) trace the parallel between the 'helping cycle' of social work and the 'research cycle', neatly showing how both can be described in terms of a similar spiralling sequence: assessment – planning – implementation – evaluation – further assessment. Munn-Giddings (1993: 275, 284) draws the parallel slightly differently, arguing that social care practice and the practice of action research share the *values* of empathy and empowerment and, consequently, a critical stance towards the power relationships in which both are inevitably situated. And Hart's work (already referred to – see Chapter 2) makes the general point explicitly: practitioners' strategies for making professional decisions provide a guide to the strategies of reflection required by 'practitioner research' (Hart, 1995).

Summary

To sum up: the impetus towards critical reflection is already implicitly present in the complexities of 'professional' situations, i.e. those in which we struggle for such always elusive values as 'health', 'well-being', 'care', 'justice', 'equity' or 'education'. 'Critique', in other words, does not depend on 'importing' the criteria of a theoretical ideal but on realising our inherent potential for imagining people and situations in different ways, which effective work in these areas (i.e. health, social care, education, etc.) always requires. Thus, action research, from this perspective, is an activity which reinforces those forms of relationship and reflexivity to which professional work, almost by definition, aspires. To be 'critical' is not (simply or necessarily) to be 'oppositional', but to recognise that in order to realise values in each different practice situation we must be ready to *learn* from those whose perspective is different from our own.

7 Action research and feminist research

Although most feminist research would not explicitly be identified as action research, the two traditions share a number of key themes. For example, in both action research and in feminist research (in its many forms) there is an emphasis on 'experiential knowledge' (i.e. direct, personal knowledge, gained from 'living with' a situation or condition) as the basis for constructing research questions. In both cases there is also always a political purpose for 'knowing', since the pursuit of knowledge is explicitly dedicated to bringing about change and improvement in the lives of participants. Rose argues that 'empathy' and 'caring' need to be seen as inherent aspects of rationality itself (1994: Chapter 2), and Hammersley draws attention to the fact that both feminist research and action research are concerned to develop a 'collaborative' form of inquiry, i.e. 'involving the people studied in the research process' (1992: 95). In other words, like action research, feminist research emphasises inquiry undertaken *with* and *by* participants, rather than investigation *of* people, 'from the outside'. Hollingsworth elaborates the parallel in more detail, describing her own action research work as a 'feminist approach', while using terms which echo the general model of action research. In contrast to 'traditional research', her method, she says, involves: conversation, beginning with observations of one's own experience, clarifying differences, coding data by listening to and using personal theories, emphasising the social and political context, presenting results as tentative, and aiming for personal transformation (1994: 63).

Interviews, power, 'study groups'

Let us, then, consider some of the ways in which feminist writers on research have made specific suggestions which are particularly relevant for action research. An early example is Ann Oakley's work on interviewing (Oakley, 1981). She argues that the traditional approach to interviewing is 'a masculine paradigm' (ibid.: 31) with its emphasis on avoiding self-disclosure by the interviewer, avoiding any expression of feelings, and treating interviewees as merely sources of data whose role is simply to answer questions, not to pose their own. The social relationship of the conventional social science 'interview', therefore, is an expression of a hierarchical power relationship. For example, if the interviewees are, say, 'housewives' or 'single mothers' or 'rape victims' and the interviewer is male, then the interview process echoes and may even subtly reinforce the very societal power relations which are the topic of the interview. For feminist researchers, interviewing women in the 'detached' manner required by conventional social science textbooks is not only inappropriate but contradictory: a feminist researcher recognises that she *shares* a crucial part of her identity with the interviewees, and that 'personal involvement [rather than impersonal detachment] is the condition under which people come to know each other' (ibid.: 58). For feminist research, therefore, as for action research, 'interviews' are an opportunity for mutual education, not simply the gathering of objective data. Thus, there is a similarity between the collaborative learning that occurs in action research and the processes involved in women's self-study or 'consciousness-raising' groups (Wadsworth and Hargreaves, 1993). Both have a similar model of people gathering to discuss the matters that trouble them, taking responsibility for sharing personal views about these concerns and discussing critically what others have said, undertaking some form of action (personally and collectively) and reviewing these actions to decide on where to go next. All this is very similar to the 'evaluative cycle' of action research, outlined in Chapter 2.

Feminist research also places a general emphasis on the political and practical purposes of inquiry. Acker *et al.* include as one of the 'principles of feminist research', that it should 'contribute to women's liberation through producing knowledge that can be used by women themselves' (1991: 137). This echoes the familiar argument that the knowledge created by an action research inquiry should enable all participants to critique and develop the practical work with which they are concerned. As an example, Lather (1988) describes a research project set up in South Carolina, which involved a group of low-income and under-employed women working as researchers on a study of the lives of the low-income women in their community. The project was constructed to ensure that all the women involved in the project (the 'researchers' and the community members) raised their awareness, through discussion with each other, of the sources of their economic circumstances. The project examined the structure of community-based leadership and developed a self-help network for low-income women.

The importance of personal experience

The feminist emphasis on personal experience has particularly important consequences for research methods. Griffiths suggests that the single 'thread' underlying the many varieties of feminist thought is that 'they all emphasise the subjective consciousness or the self of an individual [as opposed to] the "objective" "view from nowhere"' (1994: 74). She goes on to describe her use of autobiography as a key method in her action research with school children, presenting extracts from her research journal which show how it is based on detailed accounts of her personal experience. But, she continues, autobiographical accounts also need to move on to include reflections on issues of power and to generalise from individual experience to collective or group experience – two further key 'connecting threads' in feminist thinking (ibid.: 75). In more general terms, Marshall argues that researchers need to be aware of the ways in which their own life themes contribute to the purposes and motives with which research is undertaken: an inquiry is not simply a search for 'objective truth', but involves one's emotions and values, one's 'personal and political biography' (1992: 289).

Research from a 'standpoint'

One important way in which feminist writers on research sum up the various ideas we have been considering is by emphasising that research is always conducted from a particular 'standpoint' (Harding, 1990). What is taken to be the 'objective' methodology of conventional social research is an expression of the particular standpoint (the values, the culture, the priorities and concerns) of male academics and administrators (ibid.: 92). And since the lives of men and women in our society are dramatically different in so many ways, the exclusion of the female standpoint from the conduct of social research is (even) more than a problem of political and cultural exclusion. It also means that research is impoverished and, indeed, 'distorted' (ibid.: 93) by the absence of crucial forms of experience and thus by the absence of crucial dimensions of understanding. Clearly, this is of particular importance where we are concerned with research into social and health care and education, where so many of the staff and service-users are women but so many of those who determine policy are men. In this context, the arguments of feminist 'standpoint theory' point in exactly the same direction as those of collaborative action research. Inquiry must begin with the experiences, perspectives and agendas for inquiry of those whose personal experience is at the centre of the enterprise (e.g. Ungerson's policy research on caring, which stems from her own experience as a carer (Ungerson, 1987)).

Including the standpoint of those whose standpoint has been ignored is a way of noting the *critical* thrust of both feminist theory and of action research. Dorney and Flood (1997) combine both perspectives in their account of an action research project aimed at 'breaking gender silences'. This work focused on developing strategies to enable female teachers and students to break their silence concerning their experience of anger and to enable male teachers and students to do likewise with the experience of tenderness. Clearly, as this example suggests, including ignored standpoints begins by including the emotional detail of personal experience in the 'data' of research; and by including men as well as women in their project the authors suggest a further general point. Women are not the only group whose voices are diminished by the oppressive qualities of the dominant culture; the same is true of people who are (for example) black, working class, disabled, disfigured, ill, impoverished, old or children. And, indeed, the sexism which directly oppresses women also demeans and impoverishes men. However, 'white middle class males are always tempted to ignore or repress such knowledge because the way is clear for us to regain our voices fairly rapidly simply by joining the chorus of the powerful' (Winter, 1994: 425). The strength of the feminist work on research methods is that it reminds *all of us* that our experience of oppression must not be excluded from our inquiries into social affairs, that this experience too is a source of knowledge, insight and understanding.

Summary

Feminist theories of the 'silences', omissions and distortions in conventional research procedures have deep analogies with many of the central arguments in favour of action research. The cultural 'silencing' of women by the processes of conventional social science (opposed by feminist theory) has parallels with the silencing of care workers and service-users in the formulation of professional knowledge and practice, which is opposed by action research. And both are aspects of the institutionalised politics of knowledge, in which the citizen's 'voice' is silenced by the power of managerial and academic definitions of acceptable research agendas and procedures. It is also important to remember that the potential problems of 'cultural silencing' do not immediately disappear just because one is doing action research. Although in theory the action research ideal is of collaboration between 'equal' participants, in practice the status hierarchies of the wider society (based on gender, ethnicity, class, age, etc.) always threaten to distort this ideal. Unless we bear this in mind, therefore, and remain continually alert to the danger that certain individuals or groups will not be fully 'heard' within the process of the inquiry, the relationships of an action research project, like that of conventional social science, could echo and reinforce societal patterns of dominance and oppression.

8 Action research and anti-racist research

The impossibility of a 'value-neutral' social science

One of the most significant dimensions of critical thinking about health and social care policy, research and practice in recent years focuses on the oppressions and injustices created by racism. Like action research, the anti-racist perspective emphasises the need for practical change and a generally *critical* stance towards current practices and the forms and relationships of knowledge and research which reinforce them. Like feminist research, anti-racist research involves a particular emphasis on the politically structured power relationships underpinning our knowledge and our modes of inquiry, and this is an important message for action research, as indicated in this final section.

Let us begin by noting some anti-racist criticisms of the methods of conventional social inquiry and comparing them with the arguments we have presented in favour of action research. An early example is Joyce Ladner's book *The Death of White Sociology* (1973). Ladner describes the way in which conventional social science researchers determine the topics and methods of inquiry and impose them on the 'subjects' of their inquiry as a relationship of 'oppression', analogous to the oppression by colonialists of a 'subject' people (ibid.: 419). And Gorman (1999: 178) corroborates the point: 'researching others' is 'a form of oppression among stigmatised groups'. For example: white sociologists present negative interpretations and explanations of black family life in terms of their assumptions and political fears that such 'inadequate' families constitute a potential threat to social order (Billingsley, 1973). More recently, Hugman also notes the use of white norms and black deviations as a framework for interpreting differences in styles of parenting (1991: 167), and Billingsley's general argument is corroborated by Troyna (1998). Troyna confesses that that the conceptual scheme he had used (in an earlier piece of work) to classify the 'lifestyles' of Afro-Caribbean teenage boys unwittingly interpreted their lives in terms of his own (white) assumption of a *unified* underlying 'mainstream' culture and how far the boys' lifestyles did or did not pose a 'threat' to this unity (ibid.: 104).

The anti-racist research tradition thus builds on Gouldner's argument that the notion of a politically neutral, 'value-free' social science is a 'myth' (1962, quoted by Ladner, 1973: 421): there are always political interests and values behind the selection of topics, methods and conceptual schemes (Ladner, 1973: 419–22). Blair (1998), writing on racism and research methods in the context of education, also rejects the claims of social science to political neutrality. Ladner herself concludes that, since her *interest* is researching people with whose problems she identifies, her research must include advocacy and commitment to practical change on their behalf: mere observation from a position of detachment would mean implicitly accepting existing patterns of disadvantage (1973: 422). Ladner's 'colonial' analogy thus provides a precise historical and political perspective on what we have written so far on action research's desire to involve participants in practical change, on their own behalf, through 'participatory', co-operative, 'emancipatory' forms of inquiry. Dalal (1997) gives an interesting psychoanalytic explanation of why researchers might seek to claim 'neutrality': when we make formal interpretations of social events (e.g. when we speak as 'researchers' or 'analysts') we adopt an identity in which we feel we can speak with 'authority'. And in order to do so, we unconsciously split off and project onto others all those aspects of our own selves that we wish to deny.

Social research and oppressed identities

The question of identity is clearly central in all research: conventional, 'positivist' researchers wish to establish a *different* identity from their 'subjects' (an identity of detached authority), whereas in feminist and anti-racist research and also in action research, the emphasis is on acknowledging or creating a *shared* identity (based on common experience). Identity, of course, is a complex issue. Ethnic categories in themselves are often too broad to be helpful and indeed often reproduce the cultural stereotyping at the heart of racism (Ahmad and Sheldon, 1993). Other dimensions of identity such as gender, age, class and even cultural 'style' can in particular circumstances be equally significant (Mirza, 1998; Troyna, 1998).

However, within a research process the identities of those involved are important because they affect relationships, communication and interpretations, and the anti-racist research perspective serves as a particularly dramatic reminder that for many people in many social contexts their identity leads to a real experience of oppression. Black patients are regularly subjected to racial harassment in healthcare organisations (National Health Executive [UK], 1998: 3), their 'problems' are exacerbated or even actually created by the racist context of service delivery (Hugman, 1991: 165), and black staff regularly experience discrimination and abuse on the part of (white) managers, colleagues and patients (Healy, 1995). Attempts to set up collaborative relationships between white and black workers are often fraught with resentment and disrespect (Jackson *et al.*, 1999) and attempts to address such matters are often publicly ridiculed as a naïve and unrealistic search for 'political correctness' (Singh, 1994).

The main lesson from anti-racist research is not, however, simply its emphasis on how we perceive and manage identity (sameness and difference) during the process of inquiry, but its recognition that there are powerful *conflicts* at work within a culturally diverse and politically unequal society, and that not all participants may wish to acknowledge this. The anti-racist perspective emphasises not simply that differences in culture must be valued and appreciated ('multi-culturalism' – Gerrish *et al.*, 1996: 15) but that the relationships between different cultures are rooted in, and still influenced by, longstanding historical patterns of oppression. The anti-racist emphasis on the long history of colonial exploitation (Stevenson, 1992; Chomsky, 1993) serves as reminder (in the context of action research) of other deep-rooted and ancient patterns of oppression – of women, of the poor, of people who are homeless and people who have mental illness, physical disability, or learning difficulties, etc. The anti-racist perspective reminds action researchers that the attempt to establish patterns of equality and collaboration in order to resolve conflicts of interest and perspective will not be easy, will probably encounter resistance, and requires a broad awareness of deep-seated political divisions. In this context, Neil Thompson's (1993) 'PCS' (Personal/Cultural/Structural) model of 'anti-discriminatory' practice is helpful. Working within an action research project will require us to understand the links between our Personal Practices and Prejudices, the Cultural Consensus within which we locate ourselves and to which we tend to Conform, and the Structure of Sociopolitical divisions and the Social forces of power in which we are embedded (Thompson, 1993: 19–20).

Empowerment: processes, relationships and communication

So how does the anti-racist perspective relate to action research principles concerning the *relationships* of research and practice development? First of all, the important emphasis is not on simply 'acquiring knowledge about' different cultures but about careful and empathetic *listening*. Hugman (1991) observes that *power* is a dimension of both care and control, so that the caring professions always have a complex task in seeking to be 'democratic'. More precisely, he argues, the experience of 'autonomy', implicit in a democratic model of professionalism, must not be just an experience for professionals themselves but for professionals and service-users working in partnership together (ibid.: 216–17). Ahmad (1990: 39–42) gives an example of such a partnership relationship, emphasising that it must lead to 'empowerment' on the part of both the (black) client and the (white) professional worker involved. Ahmad presents the interaction as a process in which each learns from the other, with the social worker recognising the limitations of her knowledge, the client recognising the pain and disappointment of the social worker faced with criticism, and both parties accepting responsibility for developing good practice. Similarly, Turney argues that non-oppressive interpretations of situations can only emerge through dialogue between those involved ('dialogic understanding'), in which both recognise that they do not know about important aspects of the situation and therefore need to 'allow for the possible truth of other views' (1997: 118). This model of understanding based in open and critical dialogue is, of course, implicit in much writing on action research, as we have seen (e.g. Carr and Kemmis, 1986: 31). But the anti-racist perspective warns action researchers against excessive optimism: cultural and political divisions in the situations with which we are concerned mean that 'dialogue' risks being undermined by deep-seated defences (Cooper, 1997).

Gerrish *et al.* (1996: 24–32) present the problem in terms of 'inter-cultural communication' and the skills and qualities it requires. The starting point must be 'reflexive honesty', self-understanding concerning one's own sense of ethnic identity (ibid.: 20) and a general recognition that our communications are indeed attempts to *cross* cultural boundaries (rather than familiar moves within a single culture). We all therefore need to adopt the cautious, tentative, analytical stance of 'the stranger' (ibid.: 24) – i.e. treating our current knowledge concerning the situation as *probably* inadequate and therefore in need of continuous checking and revision (Schutz, 1964). This suggestion echoes the argument that for action research 'reflexivity' is a key principle: we need to be ready to see our own current interpretations of events (and our role in them) as data-to-be-analysed (Winter, 1989: 38–46; 1996: 18–20; Section 6 above). It is also a reminder that 'empower-ment' within the research process is not always or simply a matter of being able to give direct voice to previously 'silenced' spontaneous thoughts and feelings (see Section 7): our spontaneous interpretations are influenced by historical and political pressures and therefore need to be subjected to *critical* analysis (see Section 6).

Summary

The anti-racist perspective can thus be seen as reinforcing the central action research themes of empowerment and collaboration, and as contributing to a model of action research an emphasis on relationships based on self-questioning as well as questioning others. But it also suggests the scope of the difficulties we are likely to encounter, both at a personal and a wider political level, through its emphasis that particular interactions within an inquiry are always structured by historical, political and cultural forces.

Conclusion

Although each of the sections above describes either a different research context or a different aspect of action research, it is clear that, together, they present a number of common themes, values and principles. In each case there is an emphasis on the value of the experiential knowledge of practitioners and service-users and, in particular, of the knowledge created through the experience of being 'marginalised' in some way, either within the social and political structures of society or within an organisation. Equally, there is an emphasis on developing this knowledge in collaboration with others. Consequently, there is as much emphasis on the process of the research as on its final outcomes, because it is within the process of the research that both the learning and the practical change occur. Action research is just as much about social relations as about the formulation of 'new knowledge'.

Some of the sections explicitly highlight and address the power relations within which research is conceived and conducted, and others do so more implicitly. But in all cases they bring our attention to the wider structural relations that impact at a local level within a particular study. Thus, there is also a general emphasis on the importance of critical personal reflection, on clarifying one's own position in relation to the study – in terms both of one's position in the social hierarchies of status, gender and race and of one's personal value commitments. *All* the social contexts of action research are structured by hierarchies of some sort, and the attempt to create new forms of understanding and practice within such contexts therefore involves action researchers in a project of both personal and political development.

Part II

Examples
The variety of action research

Introduction: some themes and contrasts

What do the general principles presented in Part I look like in practice? The chapters in Part II provide a variety of answers to this question. They do include general reflections on aspects of action research (in some cases elaborately and in others only very briefly). But this is incidental to their main purpose, which is to describe the processes and outcomes of a particular project – what was done and what was learned through the doing. The examples have been carefully selected to include as much variety of approach as possible (to avoid any sense that there is only one way to do action research, or only one way of writing up a report) since 'action research' includes different 'traditions' (see Chapter 3), each with a slightly different emphasis. Consequently, if you study the examples in conjunction with the 'Practical guide' (Part III) you will notice that each of the examples illustrates some, but by no means all, the points contained in it. So (a further important point) the examples are not presented as models to be followed but as a variety of starting points for your own consideration when you proceed in your particular project.

Individual readers will therefore find their own points of interest in the examples, and it would be impertinent for us as editors to try to pre-empt what will be helpful in each one. So the following brief notes are simply intended to draw attention to some general themes, common to work in very different contexts, as well as some interesting contrasts.

An important feature common to most of the examples is their *narrative* form: they present a *sequence* of events, each stage developing from the one before (see in particular Chapters 10 and 11). Sometimes the narrative describes a very *personal learning process*, either concerning unexpected difficulties (Chapter 7) or unexpected success (Chapter 8). The important role of *service-users in defining service provision* is a theme of many of the chapters (especially Chapters 8, 11, 12 and 13), and most of the examples also emphasise the *empowering effect* of the project on those involved – Chapters 9, 12 and 13 are particularly explicit on this point. A number of the examples emphasise the contribution of a whole *team* of participants (e.g. Chapters 4 and 8), so – consequently – the process of *facilitation* is another important theme (especially in Chapters 4, 5 and 10) and also, inevitably, the *problematic* nature of 'collaboration' (Chapters 5 and 7).

'Theory' plays a varying role and takes different forms: sometimes it provides an overall conceptual framework (e.g. Chapters 9 and 10), sometimes it arises 'spontaneously' from the practical work (e.g. Chapter 7), and sometimes it takes the form of a 'background' body of prior research findings (e.g. Chapter 4). In some cases the *precise focus* of the work only *emerges* in the course of the project (e.g. Chapter 6), and indeed, most of Chapter 9 describes the *initial process of defining the themes for the inquiry*, since it draws mainly on the 'co-operative inquiry' aspect of action research methodology, where this is of central importance. In some of the chapters the theme of the work is explicitly *political* (Chapters 9, 10 and 11), whereas in other cases the focus is on a *practical/technical problem* (Chapter 4). One of the chapters makes extensive use of *numerical data* (Chapter 5), whereas others consist largely of *analytical reflection* on participants' comments (e.g. Chapter 6).

Finally, in their different ways, each of the chapters 'tells a story'. Chapter 9 explicitly emphasises 'telling stories' as a general purpose of 'research', and the different chapters illustrate how stories may be told at different 'levels': the national-political (Chapter 11), the personal (Chapters 7 and 14) and the local (Chapters 10 and 12). Chapter 10 also shows how community development work in itself exemplifies many aspects of the action research process (illustrating the argument made in Chapter 3, Section 2). Chapter 14, written from a carer's perspective, is particularly interesting in that it uses the format of a story to evoke the complex, subtle human reality so easily and frequently hidden behind abstract professional vocabularies. It reminds us with particular clarity that action research is essentially about developing understanding through *personal encounters*.

But perhaps we have already gone too far. The real importance of these examples is that they will (and are intended to) stimulate different interpretations and responses, depending on the reader's individual concerns and purposes at the time of reading. One person may respond to an example by thinking, 'Yes, I'd like our project to be rather like that', whereas other readers might feel that the same example illustrates exactly what they hope to avoid. And many readers will probably conclude that they would like their own work to combine, if possible, the features of several of the examples presented: this is inevitable, since every project has its own uniqueness.

Chapter 4

Developing nursing practice

Introducing knee-length anti-embolic stockings

Noreen Kennedy

Introduction

The purpose of practice development (PD) is the development of nurses and nursing to ensure both the quality of patient services and the nurturing of innovation in practice (Manley, 1997). The practice setting of the work described here is a thirteen-bedroom mixed acute surgical ward in a large London teaching hospital, where I am ward sister. In this report I describe the use of an action research strategy (which, I feel, has many parallels with the aims behind PD) to investigate whether or not patients should wear knee-length anti-embolic stocking as part of the preventive measures taken to reduce the incidence of deep venous thrombosis (DVT) in surgical patients within our ward. Within nursing, action research has often been seen as an appropriate way to try to bring about changes in clinical practice. Towell and Harries (1979) suggest that action research builds on people's own motivations to change, gives authority to a programme of change, and offers support and resources to those trying to develop new ways of working. Canavan (1996: 9) argues that there is a great need for nurses capable of managing change. Liddy (1996: 3) and Rispel (1995) argue that nurses must sit at the table where policy is made. In my current position, as ward sister, I find that management do involve key leaders when making changes and developing policies, and that I am in a key position to motivate my nursing team, to identify areas of practice and care that need development and improvement, and to increase collaboration and unity among members of the multi-disciplinary team.

Justification for using action research

Greenwood (1994) argues that 'traditional' positivistic nursing research is failing to realise its aim of improving practice, and that clinical nurses do not perceive research findings as important because they cannot see their relevance to their own practice. From my nursing experience I have found that management and researchers have consistently remained aloof from the practitioners intimately involved in the daily routines of patient care, although this trend has been changing slightly since 1995. Previous dissatisfaction with the knowledge generated by research has persuaded practitioners to turn to strategies that aim to produce knowledge that is seen to be valid in helping people to improve a practical situation. As Nolan (1993) argues, if there is to be any substantive change in the current climate, the 'top-down' generation of knowledge so characteristic of traditional research will need to be substituted with a more open and participative 'bottom-up' approach such as action research. Action research provides a sense of ownership, while also focusing on values, beliefs and team-building among those involved. Carr and Kemmis (1986: 162) define action research as: 'A form of self-reflective enquiry undertaken by participants in social situations in order to improve the rationality and justice of their own practices, their understanding of those practices, and the situations in which those practices are carried out.'

Although action research may not necessarily be the optimum choice in all settings, it is particularly appropriate where problem solving and improvement are on the agenda. Lewin (1946) identified a framework for action research, including a four-stage spiral of steps: planning, acting, observing and reflecting. Nurses are thereby able to analyse problems, devise programmes of action designed to solve problems or improve standards, carry out and evaluate these plans, and learn more about research in the process. Elizabeth Hart (1995: 4) suggests that action research offers a means of narrowing the gap between theory and practice, promoting the development of the nurse as 'practitioner researcher', and empowering nurses and users to bring about change in their lives and work. Hart and Bond (1995: 3) also suggest that many practitioners will already be familiar with an action research approach, even though they might not explicitly label what they do as such. This corresponds with my own experience: following a seminar on action research, I concluded that I was familiar with the empowerment strategy of action research and had used it as a problem-solving approach but without identifying it as the method I had been using.

In contemporary action research the emphasis is on researchers and practitioners working collaboratively, with a special focus on awareness-raising and empowerment. It would appear that nursing is very slowly beginning to turn away from the top-down approaches to implementing change in nursing practices. Macke (1995) describes collaboration as one of the key skills that nurses need as we enter the twenty-first century. He suggests that transformational nursing processes will push collaboration to the forefront, as nurses participate in the transformation of the health service. Thus when a planned change theory is being chosen, provision for collaboration between researchers and practitioners needs to be one of the key characteristics.

Preventing deep venous thrombosis: identifying the problem

Sandler and Martin (1989) found that deep vein thrombosis (DVT) and subsequent pulmonary embolism (PE) (i.e. clotting of the blood obstructing the flow of blood to the lungs) remain a significant hazard to hospital patients. This pathological process was responsible for 10% of deaths of patients in hospital, and post-operative surgical patients accounted for 24% of this series. Not only do DVTs predispose to PEs, they are also painful, they delay discharge, they are linked to the formation of leg ulcers (Lowe, 1992) and they are estimated to cost the NHS £600 million per year (Thomas, 1999). A number of studies have shown that anti-embolic (graduated compression) stockings are effective in increasing blood velocity and reducing the incidence of deep vein thrombosis (Allan *et al.*, 1983; Caprini *et al.*, 1988; Porteous *et al.*, 1989). Jeffrey and Nicolaides (1990) suggest that the use of these stockings on their own reduces the incidence of deep vein thrombosis by approximately 60%, and that when used in combination with other methods of prophylaxis (such as low-dose heparin or intermittent calf compression) there may be a reduction of up to 85%.

The nursing practice issue in the work reported here relates to the use of knee-length anti-embolic stockings rather than thigh-length stockings. All patients on my ward, irrespective of age, illness, surgery, gender or medication, wear thigh-length anti-embolic stockings, are encouraged to mobilise daily and receive low-dose heparin. This 'triple therapy' is insisted upon by both medical consultants. However, manufacturers also provide knee-length anti-embolic stockings, and studies by Porteous *et al.* (1989) found no significant difference between thigh- and knee-length stockings in their ability to prevent DVT.

The initial idea for this project was suggested by a second-year student, Mark Webb, who came from an area where patients only wore knee-length anti-embolic stockings. His questions to us (the nursing team) highlighted the fact that in using thigh-length stockings we were simply following medical instructions without questioning the practice. We continued to discuss this at intervals throughout the day with all the staff on duty, and decided to put it on the agenda for the next ward meeting. In our ward the nurses display the agenda two weeks in advance of the ward meeting, so that people have time to think, speak to others, and gather articles, information and other experiences, and thus make the meetings more productive. Persons who add to the agenda discuss the issues themselves at the meetings. I have found that this strategy has increased confidence among the nursing team, so that they are unafraid to express ideas and concerns. Thus, all projects undertaken on our ward are led by their innovators with the support of the rest of the nursing team.

Prior to the ward meeting, Mark contacted the two companies which supply our stockings, to ask them to give a teaching session on their products. He also did an Internet search on the ward to seek information from other companies we were not familiar with. As he was not very experienced with the Internet, he involved other members of the nursing staff to help him do the search. Another of the nursing staff, Corinne Martorell, was undertaking a research module as part of her degree pathway, and suggested that that she would undertake a literature review on knee-length versus thigh-length anti-embolic stockings and also use this topic for one of her assignments.

A well-recognised dilemma in action research is how to 'empower' others to take the initiative in bringing forth and identifying the 'problem'. (The word 'problem' implies there is something wrong, whereas in action research a 'problem' is merely a recognition of the need for a specific change.) In this case my 'empowerment' work began by supporting the student nurse in identifying the problem, encouraging discussions, literature searches and the idea of asking the rep from the supplying company to educate the team. These approaches commenced prior to our first formal discussion at the ward meeting, so that the nursing team were already interested and geared up to tackle the issue.

The first action research cycle

The first ward meeting

At the ward meeting many nurses fed back ideas, experiences and literature related to anti-embolic stockings. At this stage I introduced them to the idea of action research, 'selling' it as a 'collaborative strategy to change practice'. Some felt that we used this approach anyway, while the others were willing to 'give it a go'. At the meeting we also examined the possible 'forces' for and against using knee-length stockings (Tiffany and Lutjens, 1998). Initially numerous 'forces against' were identified, e.g. lack of time, difficulty of finding information. But after further consideration and discussion of the literature and research findings we minimised the 'forces against' to comprise only the influential opinions of our medical consultants. However, nurses are very quick to spot and discuss the disadvantages of a situation, and at this early stage the project might not have continued had we not critiqued the literature prior to the meeting and felt comfortable and confident that the change in practice was possible.

Data collection

Gathering the data was easier than anticipated. One nurse had contacts in other hospitals, another volunteered to speak to patients, and others spoke to staff on other wards. I volunteered to speak to the consultants. The following is a list of the different data collection processes at this stage.

- A questionnaire was completed by nursing staff on other wards about their use of anti-embolic stockings.
- I interviewed the nursing staff on our own ward about their knowledge and methods of application of anti-embolic stockings.
- Questionnaires were completed by patients, relating to how comfortable and 'user friendly' they found the thigh-length anti-embolic stockings.
- Another member of the nursing team, Briony Grant-Parke, had discussions with staff in another hospital on their practices related to use of the stockings.
- Finally, I agreed to have discussions with our own medical consultants, to gain their views on the possibility of a change to knee-length stockings.

Results presented to the second ward meeting

At the next ward meeting one month later, I presented the findings to the staff. Action research does involve a collaborative approach; however, due mainly to time constraints, I offered to take a lead in compiling and presenting to the group the various data that had been collected by the team. I also wanted them to see me presenting it using the 'power point' computer-based technology, so that in future they could use it themselves for other presentations. The following summary of the results of our inquiries was presented.

I   Interviews with fifteen nursing staff on our own ward (use of thigh-length stockings)

The majority of nurses usually used guesswork to estimate correct size, and on the occasions when patients' legs were measured, the results varied enormously. Some staff were unaware of how often the stockings should be changed and in some cases exact pressure points were unknown. Only one nurse knew how to apply the stockings according to manufacturer guidelines. When patients complained of stockings being uncomfortable or too tight, staff did not always re-measure or change them.

2   Questionnaires from ten patients (experience of thigh-length stockings)

The majority of patients emphasised that the stockings never fitted properly and made them very hot and uncomfortable. The stockings were either too constricting at the thigh level or fell down to their knees. When they complained about their discomfort they were told that the stockings usually were uncomfortable. Stockings that are too loose are left hanging from patients' thighs. Only one patient had been measured for a stocking.

3   Other findings

- A neighbouring ward had commenced using knee-length stockings, but without research evidence to support the change.
- Some wards do not use any anti-embolic stockings if a patient is only in for minor surgery and a speedy recovery is expected, but no guidelines were available on how this decision was made.
- Neither nursing staff nor patients were aware of how frequently the stockings should be changed.
- Some wards used both lengths of stockings: the nursing staff decided without guidelines or policies.
- Staff in another hospital also seemed to be unaware of proper practice: for example, they washed and reused the stockings.

4 My discussion with the medical consultants

I had spoken to both Medical Consultants and asked for their support. In approaching them I made sure I was well informed on all aspects of the problem, identifying the huge variance in practice, the probability that knee-length stockings are just as effective as thigh-length, the patients' discomfort with thigh-length stockings, the cost implications and the reasons behind this project. They were most supportive and one of them gave me the name of a professor who had done research in this area and also gave me other suggestions. I informed him I would keep him up to date with my progress, provide him with my conclusions and implement any change with the consultants' support.

The support and collaboration of the medical consultants had a powerful effect on our research group and gave a great sense of empowerment to all involved. Overall, the questionnaires had highlighted patient discomfort and poor patient compliance. The interviews with nurses had highlighted huge variations in practice and a lack of knowledge.

Changes in practice

Following further discussions with our consultants we developed and implemented a change in practice on our ward. The new practices we implemented involved:

- ensuring that patients' legs were measured according to the guidelines of the stocking manufacturers;
- increasing our knowledge in relation to all aspects of anti-embolic stockings, through reviewing research articles and teaching sessions by company reps;
- allowing patients to wear either knee- or thigh-length anti-embolic stockings.

Prior to implementing these changes we added information about anti-embolic stockings onto our patient information leaflet. We also invited nurses from other wards to a teaching session given by a company rep on the correct use of the stockings, since many of the team felt strongly that there should not be such variances in practice in the hospital and that inviting other nurses might encourage them to question their practice.

Evaluation of the changes

Eight months later, in order to evaluate the changes we had introduced on our ward, further data were collected. A summary of these findings is presented below.

I Questionnaire returns from ten staff

Nursing staff and healthcare assistants were using the tape-measures supplied by the company to measure patients' legs. When patients wore knee-length stockings staff did not need to spend as much time 'fixing' them or pulling them up. Staff felt that they were able to give more positive explanations for patients regarding their practice, and that, in general, they were using anti-embolic stockings more appropriately: they had clear guidelines and felt their knowledge had increased.

2 Interviews with ten patients who had worn knee-length stockings

Patients reported that:

- the knee-length stockings did not fall down;
- they were not as hot and itchy as thigh-length stockings;
- they did not form little gathers or creases;
- they were much easier to put on and take off.

3 Comparison with findings from other research

This information, especially the data from the patient interviews, equates with recent published research findings. Agu *et al.* (1999) found that knee-length stockings are as effective as thigh-length stockings, and that they are cheaper and better tolerated by patients. The above-knee segment of a thigh-length stocking often rolls down, either hanging loosely around the knee or exerting a garter-like tourniquet effect (Whitley, 1988). Williams *et al.* (1996) found that patients who had worn both lengths of stocking revealed that they found knee-length stockings more comfortable and that they often rolled the thigh-length ones down. There is both theoretical and clinical evidence that compression of the thigh as well as the calf does not give extra benefit (Lawrence and Kakkar, 1980; Porteous *et al.*, 1989).

Conclusion

The main conclusion of our research is that knee-length anti-embolic stockings are preferable to thigh-length stockings, although we would accept that further studies are required to provide more scientific evidence. Our next step will be the development of new policy and guidelines within the surgical directorate in relation to the use of the knee-length stockings.

Overall, action research has the potential of closing the research–practice gap, although, as Meyer (1993) points out, action research has limitations, including the difficulty, in reality, of addressing the power relationship between 'experts' and practitioners. Its success, therefore, depends on the degree and type of collaboration between researchers and practitioners and the amount of key stakeholders' support. As the ward sister initiating this project, I feel I was able to be both an 'insider', holding the same values and beliefs as the practitioners, and also an 'expert', able to educate the nursing team about action research as a strategy and to facilitate its implementation. However, as a result of this experience I would certainly advocate the use of external emotional support for those initiating practice development at ward level. This is an issue I overlooked, and when I needed further advice about the strategy I realised I had left it too late to involve someone to support me, as the project had already started. In general, I have found that much of the literature on action research omits to identify the necessary skills and maturity the researcher requires in order to co-ordinate the approach. Without well-established management and leadership skills it is questionable whether it would be possible to obtain support from all the healthcare professionals and to deal with the inevitable conflicts and issues of non-compliance within the project.

As mentioned in the introduction, PD critically explores what nurses do in order to enhance patient care. I see action research as a means for critically exploring patient care in order to formulate new strategies to improve its quality, and for narrowing the theory–practice gap. Manley (1997: 5) suggests that PD is eclectic and complex, and provides the mechanism for integrating all other professional functions for the benefit of patients. Thus, it is a prerequisite for clinical effectiveness, quality improvement and the development of a culture which facilitates radical action. The project reported here has attempted to implement a process of practice development by systematically using the combination of problem identification, data collection and analysis, reflection, collaboration and staff empowerment which make up 'action research' as a strategy for change.

Acknowledgement

I would like to thank all members of the ward nursing team for their support, ideas and enthusiasm during this collaborative project.

References

Agu, O., Hamilton, G. and Baker, D. (1999) 'Graduated compression stockings in the prevention of venous thrombo-embolism', *British Journal of Surgery*, 86: 992–1004.

Allan, A., Williams, J., Bolton, J. and Le Quesne, L. (1983) 'The use of graduated compression stockings in the prevention of post-operative deep vein thrombosis', *British Journal of Surgery*, 70: 172–4.

Carr, W. and Kemmis, S. (1986) *Becoming Critical: Education, Knowledge and Action Research*, Lewes: Falmer Press.

Canavan, K. (1996) 'ANA asserts attack on practice threatens safety', *American Nurse*, 28, 2: 1, 9.

Caprini, J., Scurr, J. and Hasty, J. (1988) 'The role of compression modalities in a prophylactic program for deep vein thrombosis', *Seminars in Thrombosis and Homeostasis*, 14, supplement: 77–97.

Greenwood, J. (1994) 'Action research: a few details, a caution and something new', *Journal of Advanced Nursing*, 20: 13–18.

Hart, E. (1995) 'Developing action research in nursing', *Nurse Researcher*, 2 3: 4–23.

Hart, E. and Bond, M. (1995) *Action Research for Health and Social Care*, Milton Keynes: Open University Press.

Jeffrey, P. and Nicolaides, A. (1990) 'Graduated compression stockings in the prevention of postoperative deep vein thrombosis', *British Journal of Surgery*, 77: 280–3.

Lawrence, D. and Kakkar, V. (1980) 'Graduated static external compression of the lower limb: a physiological assessment', *British Journal of Surgery*, 67: 119–21.

Lewin, K. (1946) 'Action research and minority problems, *Social Issues*, 2: 34–46.

Liddy, K (1996) 'Urgent visit nurse practitioners', *Indiana State Nurses Association Bulletin*, 22, 1: 3.

Lowe, G. (1992) 'Risk of prophylaxis for venous thrombo-embolism in hospital patients', *British Medical Journal*, 305: 367–74.

Macke, E. (1995) 'Professional collaboration imperative' (President's message), *Start Taking Action Today* (newsletter), Indiana: Indiana State Nurses Association.

Manley, K. (1997) 'Practice development: a growing and significant movement' (editorial), *Nursing in Critical Care*, 2, 1: 5.

Meyer, J. (1993) 'New paradigm research in practice; trials and tribulations of action research', *Journal of Advanced Nursing*, 18, 4: 1066–72.

Nolan, M. (1993) 'Action research and quality of care: a mechanism for agreeing basic values as a precursor to change', *Journal of Advanced Nursing*, 18, 2: 305–11.

Porteous, M., Nicholson, E. and Morris, L. (1989) 'Thigh length versus knee length stockings in the prevention of deep vein thrombosis', *British Journal of Surgery*, 76: 296–7.

Rispel, L. (1995) 'Challenges face nurses in Republic of South Africa', *Image: Journal of Nursing Scholarship*, 27: 231–4.

Sandler, D. and Martin, J. (1989) 'Autopsy proven pulmonary emobolism in hospital patients: are we detecting enough deep vein thrombosis?', *Journal of the Royal Society of Medicine*, 82: 203–5.

Silva, M. (1977) 'Philosophy, science, theory: interrelationships and implications for nursing research', *Image: Journal of Nursing Scholarship*, 9: 59–63.

Thomas, S. (1999) 'Graduated external compression and the prevention of deep vein thrombosis', *Journal of Wound Care*, 8, 1: 41–3; 8, 2: 93–5; 8, 3: 133–9.

Tiffany, C. and Lutjens, L. (1998) *Planned Change Theories for Nursing: Review, Analysis and Implications*, London: Sage Publications.

Towell, D. and Harries, C. (1979) *Innovation in Patient Care: an Action Research Study of Change in a Psychiatric Hospital*, London: Croom Helm.

Whitley, A. (1988) 'Elastic stockings', *British Medical Journal*, 296: 413–14.

Williams, A., Davies, P., Sweetnam, D., Harper, G., Pusey, R. and Lightowler, C. (1996) 'Knee-length versus thigh-length graduated stockings in the prevention of deep vein thrombosis', *British Journal of Surgery*, 83: 1553.

Chapter 5

Introducing bedside handovers
Changing practice on a coronary care unit

Fergal Searson

Introduction

This research originated from the desire on the part of a sister in a hospital coronary care unit (CCU) – Sister Rachel Sagar – to change the handover system when nurses change shifts. She had been dissatisfied with the current, traditional system for a while and wanted to introduce bedside handovers. While this is not a particularly new idea in nursing practice, the format that she was proposing, involving the patients in the process rather than just leaving them as passive onlookers, was new in her 'high-tech', short-stay hospital environment. This approach has been more frequently found in longer-stay, rehabilitation-type wards where the emphasis is on nursing care more than medical intervention.

The unit in question is a five-bedded CCU in a district general hospital serving a population of approximately 250,000 people, with a workforce of thirteen staff, all qualified nurses. It takes all potential heart attack patients as well as patients with severe heart failure and abnormal heart rhythms requiring specialist invasive interventions. Patients remain on the CCU for anything from twelve to forty-eight hours, depending on illness severity and pressure on beds. I used to work there as a charge nurse and continue to work on the 'bank', coming in when there is a staff shortage. My 'main' job is that of course leader for coronary care courses in the nursing department at a local university which takes some of its students from this unit. As I was looking to do some research for my dissertation, Rachel had asked if I could help with the introduction of a new system.

Prior to the work reported here, the handover took place at the nurses' station with each nurse handing over her patients to the next shift staff. Rachel Sagar felt that this system was old-fashioned and inefficient, tending to be medically oriented and retrospective in nature, and liable to reinforce patient stereotyping. Strange (1996), when considering the ritual of the handover, says that nurses 'justify its presence by claiming it facilitates continuity of care and allows information regarding that care to be easily transferred'. However, there are problems concerning the nature of such information and the 'transfer' process. Much of the information passed on is judgemental in nature, providing the incoming nurses with preconceived ideas about the patients. The communication process is one-sided, with the report-giving nurse in control, little participation from the incoming nurses and little if any discussion of future care plans (Sherlock, 1995). Moreover, the patient is viewed as a 'condition', not a person. The only patient involvement, on a unit that espouses a patient-centred, holistic approach to nursing care, is their unavoidable eavesdropping on the report as a distraction from boredom or reflection on their illness. This report describes the introduction of bedside handovers, focusing also, in a final commentary, on issues of facilitation and collaboration.

Change

One of the main problems related to the proposed change in practice was the very fact that it was a change. People are often resistant to change and in this case Rachel Sagar was convinced that her staff would be very resistant. The handover in its traditional format is at the very heart of nursing. In many cases it has survived the onslaught of such innovations as 'the nursing process', the 'named nurse' initiative and 'patient-centred care'. To be told that it is to be revised and changed to include active patient involvement and possibly control can be very disconcerting. While most nurses are all in favour of patient involvement in care the processes usually advocated are under the control of the nurse; the proposal described in this project, in contrast, offered the patient the chance to wrest back some of that control.

Responses to the idea of change can vary from outright enthusiasm on the one hand to outright rejection on the other hand. Between these two groups are those who don't openly accept or reject the idea but have valid concerns about the change. They are what Weil (1992) refers to as the 'yes buts'. She goes on to assert that these are the people who should be targeted in an attempt to change scepticism into support. They must be satisfied that the change procedure is going to take on board their perceptions and worries. If this can be accomplished, then potential poachers can be converted into gamekeepers.

Aims

The aim of the research then was to introduce a change in the nursing report style from a traditional, minimally interactive process, taking place at the nurses' station, to an interactive bedside handover which would actively encourage patient involvement. Some of the key questions that needed to be answered were:

1   Does the bedside handover improve the quality of nursing care delivery to patients?
2   Does it lead to patients becoming more involved in their care management?
3   Is it more informative for the new shift nurse?
4   Are nurses comfortable with it?
5   Do nurses feel that it enhances their care giving?
6   Do patients feel that it enhances care delivery?

A couple of secondary aims emerged during the course of the research. The first of these was to see whether active involvement in the process would encourage the nurses to think about initiating research into their practice on their own account. The second was to analyse how I manage my role as nurse tutor and research facilitator.

Theoretical considerations

What was needed was an approach which encouraged and supported the involvement of those participating in the project while at the same time providing evidence about the effectiveness or otherwise of the change in practice. Action research would appear to offer this opportunity. It can provide a framework to analyse the problem in the first place, help to design programmes of action and review, carry out the programmes and at the same time enhance understanding of the research process (Webb, 1989). One of the consequences is the active involvement of those affected (Fawcett, 1998). The emphasis is on the current situation, with immediate implementation and evaluation, rather than the delay between evidence collection and reporting in more conventional research approaches. As there is close co-operation between the researcher and the practioners it will hopefully contribute to the narrowing of the theory–practice gap. Potential difficulties associated with action research include problems around possible power relationships between researcher and practitioners, with the practitioners feeling that they are being coerced into co-operation. This could be overcome by the development of a 'relationship that is equal and based on openness and honesty' (Webb, 1989: 408). The use of two-way communication with continual feedback to and from participants should help to overcome questions of lack of informed consent in relation to unknown outcomes (Meyer, 1993). Hunt (1987) also points out the dangers of ignoring the interests of the 'supplicants' (in this case, patients) at the expense of the drive by 'experts' (in this case, nurses) for increased professional standing.

The model chosen for this project (Figure 5.1) was that utilised by Fawcett (1998) which was developed from the stages of action research identified by Laurie (1982). By representing the process as a cycle as opposed to a list, she emphasises that there should be continuity in the process, not just a quick review and implementation which doesn't allow for review and adaptation.

The preliminary diagnosis had already been made by the sister in her identification of the shortcomings of the present system. Nevertheless there was a need to identify the attitudes and beliefs of the rest of the staff in relation to the traditional, office-based handover; this would be accomplished by asking them to complete a questionnaire (stage 1). The results of this questionnaire were then to be fed back to the staff at a focus group session held during unit meetings. This would help to initiate discussion about the current system, introduce the concept of bedside handovers, and involve the staff in formulating an initial approach to its implementation (stage 2). This initial focus group meeting would also be used to design a comment sheet to be completed after handovers. This would allow for

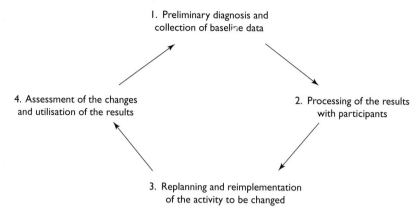

Figure 5.1 Stages of action research
Source: Fawcett (1998: 91).

the immediate recording of opinions and concerns about the bedside handover which could then be addressed in further focus groups sessions; on-going analysis of comments would also provide early indications of any perceived improvements and acceptance (stage 3). Because of the difficulties that surround trying to get staff together it was decided to utilise unit meetings for the focus groups. Final evaluation of the bedside handover would occur at a final focus group session when the results of a further questionnaire, to garner individual views on the new system, would inform a discussion on the effects of the change on staff and patients (stage 4). The patients' perspective would be obtained by interviews on the medical ward after their transfer from CCU.

The initial questionnaire

This was used to obtain information about the staff nurses' attitudes and views in relation to the traditional handover. It mostly utilised Likert scale questions with statements for them to choose a response to: strongly agree/agree/disagree/strongly disagree. It was initially piloted on nurses from other CCUs prior to its administration with all thirteen staff on the unit completing a questionnaire. With such a small number of respondents, the aim of the exercise was merely to get a 'feel' for the opinions to feed into the first discussion. The analysis presented is therefore descriptive rather than statistical. The main findings are shown in Table 5.1.

The first focus group

This was used to give the staff feedback on the questionnaire and to introduce the concept of bedside handovers to the unit. The nurses were asked if they were prepared to 'give it a go' but before they made their decision they were given some ground rules about the research:

- I wasn't telling them how to do it;
- they had to design it;
- they had to implement it;
- they could adapt it as they went along;
- the trial period would be three months;
- they had ultimate sanction on whether to adopt it permanently.

Table 5.1 Findings of questionnaire on attitudes to the traditional handover

1. It involves subjective comments about the patient.

Strongly agree	Agree	Disagree	Strongly disagree
1	12		

2. It encourages you to involve patients in the evaluation of care.

Strongly agree	Agree	Disagree	Strongly disagree
2		11	

3. The patient should be involved in the handover.

Strongly agree	Agree	Disagree	Strongly disagree
2	7	4	

4. Could the current system be improved upon? (Yes = 12; no = 1)

5. If yes, how and why?
   - Bedside handover would be preferable. (7 responses)
   - More time needed. (1 response)
   - More privacy needed. (1 response)

6. If no, why?
   - You need to observe patients during handover. (1 response)
   - Providing more privacy could endanger patients. (1 response)

The purpose of these rules was to demonstrate to the nurses that they had control of the process, from the initial decision on whether to start it right through to the final choice on whether to accept or reject bedside handovers. This led to a discussion on the pros and cons of bedside handovers based on journal articles on their use and other areas of concern. The main one of these centred on confidentiality. On the one hand, there were the United Kingdom Central Council (UKCC) *Code of Conduct* (UKCC, 1992) and *Guidelines for Professional Practice* (UKCC, 1996), but, on the other hand, nurses and doctors already conduct twice daily 'ward rounds', and also collect detailed personal data from patients at the bedside during the 'admission' process. There was concern about the presence of relatives during the handover when sensitive issues such as HIV status might be discussed; and the question was raised whether patients would feel comfortable with a system in which the discussion of their case might be overheard by other patients. Practical issues were also discussed, such as which nurses should be at the bedside for the report, should they stand or sit, and whether every handover should take place at the bedside. Following a decision by the nurses to proceed with the trial, its initial format was agreed upon, a feedback sheet was designed and a date fixed for the start.

Examples of the types of comments made during the focus group are: 'If you're on the phone talking to a relative then Joe Bloggs will say "Was that my wife?"' 'So how are we going to tackle the complicated patients with a lot going on that needs explaining?' 'What about a situation like where the family are sat around or whatever?' 'I think we could always ask the family to leave . . . I think we should ask the patient.' 'Sometimes when you're at the station you tend to gossip, don't you?' 'I think we're a lot more tactful than the medics anyway.'

Development

The progress of the new system was monitored by the use of the feedback sheets which were to be filled in after each handover by both the nurse giving the report and the nurse receiving it. The results of these were then fed back into the discussions on progress at the following two focus group sessions. The following are examples of comments that were written down: 'They [patients] are better informed now.' 'It helps address sensitive issues.' 'It makes a good introduction between new staff and patients.' 'It works for some patients but not for others.' 'Some patients aren't interested.' 'It shouldn't be done just for the sake of it.'

Some of the issues that arose and the ways they were dealt with are listed below:

1   It's too technical – some of the medical terminology was bypassing the patients and discouraging involvement. So it was decided to reduce the use of jargon and try to use words the patients could understand.
2   It's too simplistic – nurses were finding that they were unable to pass on all the technical information they needed. So it was decided to use a 'mini' (technical) handover at the nurses' station prior to the bedside handover. However, this resulted in two of the nurses slipping back into the traditional format, so the mini-handover was abandoned and the meaning of technical information was explained to the patient at the bedside.
3   Some patients who were on the ward for longer periods seemed to experience the process as tedious, saying, 'Not again!' At the same time, some of the nurses highlighted the value of the traditional handover for the passing on of general and management information, the chance of a gossip ('team-building'!) and a 'brew'. So it was decided that the morning handover would be at the nurses' station – many patients were still asleep at this time anyway.

The patient's perspective

Following ethical committee approval, I interviewed the patients to ascertain their views. This took place on the medical ward to which patients were transferred as their condition improved. Verbal consent was obtained for both the interview and the use of a tape recorder. Patients were merely asked if they could remember the bedside handovers, and if they could they were asked what they thought of it. As the ward operated an open visiting policy this meant that sometimes relatives were present during the interview; any decision about their presence was made by the patient. Some patients couldn't remember the handover or had problems resulting from language barriers or deafness which had excluded them from the report. In all, ten patients were successfully interviewed with nobody refusing either the initial request or the use of the tape recorder. Of those who could remember the handover, all thought it was a good idea. Their comments included: 'The patient is more involved.' 'It's a good thing, I knew they were caring for me . . . they told me what was happening.' 'It's better than going in the office like they used to do . . . you always wondered what they were saying about you.' 'It's nice to talk to people . . . it's helpful. You know what's happening, you are more informed.' 'I think it gives the patient more confidence in the end.'

The final questionnaire

The final questionnaire, canvassing the opinions of the nurses about the bedside handover, was distributed with ten of the possible thirteen responding. The section of the questionnaire dealing with the bedside handover, including the responses, is shown in Table 5.2. Another part of the questionnaire, concerned with the nurses' general feelings about their involvement in the project, is discussed later.

The final focus group

These findings, along with a review of the patients' comments, were fed back into the meeting. The nurses were asked to discuss their current feelings about the bedside handover and to come to a decision about whether to keep it or revert to the traditional format. This discussion revealed that while some of them thought that initially it had been forced upon them (see later discussion), in general they now liked it: 'you get a more informed handover at the bedside'. One example of the advantages was given. A patient was complaining of high levels of chest pain, but although the nurses were treating him for this they were not convinced about his claims of its severity. This 'labelling' of the patient at a traditional handover could well have coloured the new nurses' judgements, but because the report took place at the bedside it was easier to raise the subject with the patient, and this led to the discovery of underlying personal issues which were affecting the patient.

At the end of the discussion a decision was taken by the nurses to adopt the new system and to review it on a regular basis via their unit meetings.

Discussion of results

The main aim of the research was to support the introduction to the coronary care unit of a bedside handover which included patient participation. This was

Table 5.2 Results of the bedside shift handover questionnaire

Questions 1–11: Please place a tick in the box which most corresponds to your experience. There is provision at the end of the questionnaire to add further comments.

1. How long does each shift handover take on average?

	5–10 minutes	11–15 minutes	16–20 minutes	21–25 minutes	26+ minutes
Morning (traditional)	1	4	4	1	
Afternoon	2	3	5		
Evening		4	6		

Questions 2–9: In comparison to the traditional shift handover:

2. Are you more or less informed about the patient's condition?

Much more informed	More informed	No change	Less informed	Much less informed
	1	8	1	

3. Is the patient more or less informed about their condition?

Much more informed	More informed	No change	Less informed	Much less informed
	6	4		

4. Do you have a better or worse idea of the patient as a person?

Much better	Better	No change	Worse	Much worse
	5	5		

5. Is care delivery enhanced or hindered?

Much enhanced	Enhanced	No change	Hindered	Much hindered
	2	8		

Table 5.2 continued

6. Are patients more or less involved in their care?

Much more involved	More involved	No change	Less involved	Much less involved
	8	2		

7. Are nurse/patient relationships better or worse?

Much better	Better	No change	Worse	Much worse
	3	7		

8. Is nurse/patient communication better or worse?

Much better	Better	No change	Worse	Much worse
	5	5		

9. Is nurse/patient rapport better or worse?

Much better	Better	No change	Worse	Much worse
	5	5		

10. 'Patients are generally comfortable with the system.'

Strongly agree	Agree	Disagree	Strongly disagree
	10		

11. 'I am comfortable with bedside handovers.'

Strongly agree	Agree	Disagree	Strongly disagree
1	9		

Table 5.2 continued

12. Do you think that there are any other advantages or disadvantages not identified here? Please write on the reverse of the questionnaire if there is insufficient space.

- The decision to conduct handover at the bedside should be at the nurse's discretion.
- Sometimes staff or patients feel uncomfortable.
- Sometimes patients like the attention.
- Patients know there are no hidden agendas.
- Bedside handover can take longer if the patient is chatty or if there's delicate information.
- Confidentiality.
- It could enhance anxiety, e.g. if there are multiple handovers. The patient might get fed up.

successfully done, with the nurses in the final focus group meeting taking the decision to adopt this form of shift handover whenever appropriate. Answers to some of the key questions were supplied in the focus groups, the feedback sheets, the final questionnaire results and patient comments:

- *Does the bedside handover improve the quality of nursing care delivery to patients?*
  Answers to Questions 3 and 4 (in Table 5.2) show that at least half the respondents felt that patients were more informed and that nurses had a better idea of the patient as a person. Nobody thought the situation was worse with the new handover format. Concerning Question 5, although only two out of ten thought that care delivery was enhanced, once again, nobody thought that it was hindered.

- *Are patients more involved in their care management?*
  Question 6 indicates that eight out of ten felt this to be the case with the other two respondents finding no change. Patient comments certainly indicate that they felt more involved.

- *Is the new format more informative for the new shift nurse?*
  Question 2 shows that eight out of ten thought that there was no difference while one thought that it was better.

- *Are nurses comfortable with it?*
  Discussion in the focus groups and analysis of the feedback sheets shows that, while at the beginning of the trial they were uncomfortable, by the end they were comfortable with the system. This is supported by answers to Question 11 with nine out of ten nurses agreeing and one nurse strongly agreeing.

- *Do nurses feel that it enhances their care giving?*
  Certainly some of the nurses feel that this is the case, as shown in Question 5. This is also touched on in the focus groups where nurses talk about its use in clarifying or resolving communication problems, e.g. the patient with severe pain.

- *Is there a problem of maintaining patient confidentiality?*
  The answer to this has got to be 'yes', as evidenced by the mention made in Question 12 of the final questionnaire by two of the nurses. However, this is a problem in all aspects of both nursing and other professionals' interactions with patients – it is not peculiar to bedside handovers. It is up to nurses to be aware of it as an issue in all aspects of their work with patients and relatives, and to use their professional training and discretion to make decisions on an individual patient basis.

- *Do patients feel that it enhances care delivery?*
  The answer to this can be found in the patient interviews, which were all positive in their discussion of the bedside handover. It could be argued that the patients, even though they are no longer on the CCU, are still recipients of nursing care, and are therefore perhaps unlikely to be critical for fear of 'reprisals'!

To sum up, then, two of the ward sister's reasons for wanting to do away with the traditional handover were the issues of stereotyping and the 'medical' approach to the patients' condition. Both of these concerns have been addressed, the former apparently more than the latter: (1) by holding the handover at the bedside the incoming nurse is not receiving any preconceived ideas from the report-giving nurse; any stereotyping or labelling is purely of the nurse's own making; (2) Involvement of the patient in the process often leads to discussion of his/her needs and worries rather than just a review of the medical management.

Overall commentary: 'facilitation' and 'collaboration'

One of the problems that I had with this research was that it took a top-down approach to the implementation of a change in practice, even though it was initially presented as a 'collaborative' process. This issue was highlighted by a few of the nurses in the final focus group session. Because I used to work on the unit and still help out as a bank nurse, I thought that I would be seen as an 'insider', i.e. one of the nurses, and that this would help them to see me as merely a 'facilitator' rather than an authority. However, because I now teach coronary care nursing at the local university and am an ex-charge nurse on the unit, I was probably seen more as an outsider and as one of the management. Williams, talking about the researcher as facilitator, suggests that in the process of trying to help and 'emancipate' one runs the risk of being seen as patronising:

> Even an insider nurse who is facilitating other nurses may be an outsider in the sense that he or she has a closer affiliation with, say, a management or educational setting than the setting in which the change is being facilitated, such as a clinical setting.
>
> (Williams, 1995: 52)

From this it could be argued that the work described here is not a fully collaborative utilisation of group decision-making, as it is was used as a technique to lead or direct the nurses in a particular direction. It assumed that the management stance is the desired goal to be attained. This is more akin to what Lewin called 'rational social management' in which 'action research' is utilised to smooth the introduction of management initiatives. Other writers on action research do not believe in setting such a specific agenda, maintaining that participants should be more fully involved from the outset. For instance, Soltis-Jarrett (1997: 45) distinguishes between 'social action research', which is researcher designed and is trying to solve a particular problem, and 'participatory action research' which is designed by *all* participants (including the researcher-facilitator) and which focuses on concerns which have been highlighted by their own reflection. In this project, for example, the nurses were not originally told that the focus of the work was to be on introducing the bedside handover, although several had guessed as much from the slant of the questions being asked in the initial questionnaire.

With hindsight, although this probably did provide for more accurate recording of opinions unbiased by thoughts of future change, it may well have engendered feelings of being manipulated, something which some of the nurses highlighted at the end of the research. However while it is certainly true to say that this piece of research was utilised to point the nurses in a certain direction, this 'engineering' was done merely to 'kickstart' a process which later became 'owned' by the nurses and self-perpetuating. According to Elliott (1991: 53), a felt need to initiate change is a 'necessary precondition of action research', and in this case it was initially the sister, not the nurses, who felt the 'need' for the change in the handover process. Nevertheless, most of the nurses involved in the project did feel that they had had some control over the process, saying (in their responses to the section of the final questionnaire not presented earlier) that they had had 'a chance to air their views' and to 'change things if they were not working'.

There were also some moral and ethical considerations. In relation to the issue of informed consent in this study, there are problems around when consent was obtained and to what the participants were consenting. The staff were originally asked to fill in a questionnaire about traditional handovers, and it was only when feedback to this had been given at the first focus group meeting that any kind of request for consent to be involved in an action research programme was raised. In a sense they had been led blindly down the garden path and were now having their blindfolds removed and being asked to continue on their way. Second, to whom were they giving consent – to me as a colleague, to me as an independent researcher, or to me as a university coronary care course teacher? Was consent to be involved given out of a fear of management repercussions (it was known that sister had initially raised the issue of problems with the traditional handover) or fear of possible 'reprisals' for current and future course students? Ultimately, nurses' final decision to continue with bedside handovers may possibly have been taken out of a feeling of personal loyalty to me as an ex-colleague, because 'my' research would fail if they refused.

Certainly, in my conversations with Sister Rachel Sagar since the research was completed, she has expressed the opinion that it was seen by some of the staff as a management initiative rather than any truly collaborative research process, another view supported by some of the comments in the final questionnaire. However, Hart (1996: 12), in an exploration of these issues of power and control in relation to collaborative research, points out that 'the alternative is to research at a distance, which does nothing to build bridges between researchers and practitioners, professionals and users'. And Sister Sagar also feels that, in retrospect, in spite of its difficulties and limitations, the work has been worthwhile. In her words: 'By this process [the bedside handover] the patient is drawn into the care team as an active member in their care, rather than the previous role of passive recipient.'

Conclusion

The use of action research helped to introduce the change to the use of bedside handovers within the coronary care unit. The system adopted was designed by the nurses and they dealt with any on-going problems as a group. In other words, it successfully involved the nurses in the change process and in the research process. Feedback from both the nurses and the patients suggests that bedside handovers involving the patients provide an improvement in nursing care. The Royal College of Nursing (1987: 2) states that 'each patient has a right to be a partner in his /her own care planning and to . . . become involved in his/her own care', while Nolan (1998: 57) highlights the government's 'emphasis on capturing the patient's experience of health care and reflecting such experience in future quality measures'. Bedside handovers which involve the patient have possibly been viewed in the past as something more typical of non-acute rehabilitation settings, where the emphasis is on nursing interventions rather than on high-tech care. This research has reaffirmed that it can also work in critical care areas. The bottom line is that the project improved the nursing care and patient satisfaction, an achievement made by these nurses.

The nurses also indicated that as a result of their involvement in this project they would consider carrying out research into their practice, while indicating that they would want help in the process, something they didn't think was available at the moment. Healthcare organisations need to look at ways to make their research and development support more visible and accessible to staff on the wards. If research is a pudding, then the proof of this pudding will not be in its eating but in whether the staff in the coronary care unit go on to start baking puddings of their own in the future.

References

Elliott, J. (1991) *Action Research for Educational Change*, Milton Keynes: Open University Press.

Fawcett, J. (1998) 'Care planning: best tool for the job?', *Nursing in Critical Care*, 3, 2: 89–97.

Hart, E. (1996) 'Action research as a professionalizing strategy: issues and dilemmas', *Journal of Advanced Nursing*, 23: 454–61.

Hart, E. and Bond, M. (1995) *Action Research for Health and Social Care: a Guide to Practice*, Buckingham: Open University Press.

Hunt, S. (1987) 'Evaluating a community health project', *British Journal of Social Work*, 17: 661–7.

Laurie, S. (1982) 'Development of the nursing process through action research', *Journal of Advanced Nursing*, 7: 301–7.

Meyer, J. (1993) 'New paradigm research in practice: the trials and tribulations of action research', *Journal of Advanced Nursing*, 18: 1066–72.

Nolan, M. (1998) 'Outcomes and effectiveness: beyond a professional perspective', *Clinical Effectiveness in Nursing*, 2: 57–68.

Royal College of Nursing (1987) *In Pursuit of Excellence: a Position Statement on Nursing*, London: Royal College of Nursing.

Sherlock, C. (1995) 'The patient handover: a study of its form, function and efficiency', *Nursing Standard*, September 20, pp. 33–6.

Soltis-Jarrett, V. (1997) 'The facilitator in participatory action research: les raisons d'être', *Advances in Nursing Science*, 20, 2: 45–54.

Strange, F. (1996) 'Handover: an ethnographic study of ritual nursing practice', *Intensive and Critical Care Nursing*, 12: 106–12.

United Kingdom Central Council (1992) *Code of Professional Conduct*, 3rd edn, London: UKCC.

United Kingdom Central Council (1996) *Guidelines for Professional Practice*, London: UKCC.

Webb, C. (1989) 'Action research: philosophy, methods and personal experience', *Journal of Advanced Nursing*, 14: 403–10.

Weil, S. (1992) 'Learning to change', in Office for Public Management, *Managing Fundamental Change*, London: Office for Public Management, pp. 9–17.

Williams, A. (1995) 'Ethics and action research', *Nurse Researcher*, 2, 3: 49–59.

Chapter 6

Empowering the supporters

Enhancing the role of unqualified support workers in a housing scheme for people with mental health problems

Philip Kemp

Introduction

One of the consequences of community care policies has been the growth of unqualified support workers in a range of care contexts (Johnson *et al.*, 1997). Support workers now make a substantial contribution to the care of people who have experienced mental health difficulties as well as other vulnerable groups. There is some evidence to suggest that this contribution is valued, at least by users of mental health services, although professional staff have mixed feelings about their role (Murray *et al.*, 1996). One issue of concern is the level of training support workers receive and how well they are supervised, particularly when they have been left responsible for people experiencing serious difficulties (Davies *et al.*, 1995).

One area of service delivery which support workers have expanded into is supported housing. The UK government 'community care' initiative has seen the development of a range of small-scale supported housing as a means of meeting the care and accommodation needs of people with mental health problems. While examples of small-scale supported housing date back many years (Abrahamson, 1993), given the extent of its recent expansion it can be considered a relatively new but significant form of service delivery and location of care.

The research reported in this study is a practitioner action research project, primarily concerned with the activities of unqualified support workers in a supported housing scheme for people who have experienced serious mental health problems. It is a continuation of an earlier action research study (described in Kemp, 1997) which suggested some ways of meeting the learning and support needs of staff working in this care setting. One key proposal was the implementation of a learning programme for support workers. It is this that forms the starting point of the investigation recounted here.

Central to this research is a fundamental area of tension within community mental health services. On the one hand, a group of people with serious mental health problems have become an increasing focus for public concern (Muijen, 1995). On the other hand, a group of unqualified staff are taking on a larger role in the burden of care and are sometimes placed in demanding situations. The significance of this contradiction and how it manifests itself in the particular care setting that is the subject of this research is an important theme in this study. This contradiction influenced a series of practice developments that contributed towards a mediation of this tension. It also resulted in a reorientation of my own role as manager.

The starting point of this study was the implementation and evaluation of a learning programme for support workers coupled with a system of practice advice-giving which was the outcome of the earlier study. However, the evaluation of this action phase led to a reanalysis in the course of the study as to how staff could best be supported. This acted as a trigger resulting in a broader understanding of the support workers' role and how they can be supported. The focus of the research shifted to how they related to professional staff in the mental health system. There was thus a realisation of the more complex context within which support workers operate and an understanding that the initial action steps had been too narrowly set.

The research setting

The setting for this study was a social service department-managed supported housing scheme for people who have experienced serious mental health problems. In recent years the scheme had undergone expansion and development. There are currently sixteen establishments providing a range of supported housing options for up to forty individuals. The properties included single-person-occupied flats, shared accommodation for two or three people, and two larger establishments, 'Dickson Road' and 'Harrison Road', accommodating five and eight people respectively.

The residents of the accommodation were all people who had had much contact with mental health services over the years. A small number of residents were former long-stay patients who no longer required twenty-four-hour staffed residential care and took up the opportunity to move to accommodation where they could live more independently. A similar rationale applied to residents who had previously been living with carers, usually ageing parents. Others, for a variety of reasons, had experienced significant problems in sustaining themselves in their previous accommodation on their own.

One of the major developments intrinsic to the expansion of the accommodation scheme, and the main focus of this study, was the establishment of a team of support workers to support the residents. The supported accommodation team consisted of nine unqualified support workers with me as manager of the scheme. Most of the support workers had no or minimal experience of people with mental health problems on taking up their appointment. One of the fortunate aspects for the purposes of this study, and more importantly for the users of the service itself, is that the staff group proved stable with minimal turnover. Thus by the time of the commencement of the study a number of the support workers could claim up to three years' experience in this work setting.

My role was manager of the supported housing scheme as a whole, including line management of the support workers. My own professional background was in mental health nursing before I moved to work in the social service department managing the scheme.

Gathering evidence

A wide range of sources of evidence were used in this study. The central sources, however, emanated from the primary participants in the research setting. It is the personal encounter with experience and participants that is a central source of validity in action research. It allows for the generation of other views to stand alongside my views and the 'official' or 'institutional' views expressed, for example, in policy documents. These 'multiple perspectives' of how reality is experienced can then be analysed in a systematic way in order to make sense of them.

Evidence was gathered from contexts that arose in normal daily practice, for example team meetings, supervision sessions, care review meetings, house meetings and a multiplicity of informal interactions. Additional methods of exploring particular emergent themes were used, such as tape-recorded discussions of team meetings.

A key tool was maintaining a 'reflective diary', recording personal accounts of observations, feelings, reflections and interpretations. The diary provided the necessary pause from the day-to-day routine for this reflective process to take place. Included in the diary were what Elliott (1991) referred to as 'analytic memos', used after a period of 'reconnaissance', containing new ways of conceptualising a situation, emergent ideas and hypotheses, and suggestions for further evidence-gathering. Kept in a loose-leaf binder, entries could be rearranged into particular themes that emerged.

Practice development 1: a learning programme for support workers

The earlier study (Kemp, 1997) had revealed an important area of contradiction. The rationale for the accommodation was primarily conceived as a means of providing *practical* support to enable residents with various levels of dependency to sustain themselves in a community-based setting. However, the principal benefit of the accommodation experienced by the residents was very much to do with *social* aspects of support. This contradiction was reflected in the advice and guidance that support workers sought from me as manager. On the one hand, they were seen as providing mainly practical assistance to residents, but on the other hand, their predominant requests for guidance in their work concerned issues of social support.

This relationship between how residents experience 'being supported' and the learning and support needs of support workers was explored with a view to implementing practice developments that would respond to the tension between practical support and social support. A learning programme was devised as a major step towards achieving this. Thus, as a direct outcome of the earlier exploratory study a regular weekly training session for support workers was initiated. This was intended to be tailored to the day-to-day practical work experiences of support workers covering topic areas generated by continuing reflection on practice. This was supplemented by frequent practice guidance (based on similar principles) provided by me, often on an *ad hoc* basis, as the support workers carried out their day-to-day work.

Initially, in implementing the training initiative some important principles were adopted. First, the provision of a rationale (theory, related research, etc.) accompanied the practice guidance that was given. Second, the practice guidance provided consisted of a small number of key suggestions that could be readily applied by support workers back in the work setting. They would be 'bite-sized' pieces of guidance. Third, the training was intended to be on-going, with new topics included as they are identified. It was not intended to be a set programme with a set number of sessions, as in in-service training programmes. Fourth, and most importantly, it was very specific to the actual work the support workers were engaged in and to the people they were caring for. This was an attempt at ensuring that the training had a direct and immediate relevance to the work situation.

The training was implemented in the following way. Each Monday a weekly team meeting was held. This was the only occasion when all team members were able to meet as a whole group. We agreed to spend forty-five minutes on team business, with the remaining forty-five minutes available as a 'training slot'.

The format for each session was as follows. I began by covering some theoretical background material or research on a given topic, generating discussion as support workers related the material to their own observations of the residents and their work with them. An example of this was the concept of 'expressed emotion'. The concept of 'expressed emotion' emerged as a result of research with the families of people with schizophrenia, suggesting that the emotional atmosphere at home can exert an influence over the course of the illness (see, for example, Vaughn and Leff, 1976; Kuipers *et al.*, 1992). Families characterised by high levels of expressed emotion (EE) feature a relatively high frequency of critical comments, a higher degree of hostility expressed verbally and non-verbally, and higher levels of face-to-face contact. Such families have been found to be associated with increased rates of relapse compared to more tolerant 'low EE' households. This research suggests some useful guidance on the style of interaction with people with schizophrenia. Through one of our sessions support workers came to see the relevance of applying the concept within group home accommodation.

The next step in the session was to discuss some practical guides that support workers could apply in their work. Often this might take the form of suggesting both general and specific strategies, i.e. ways of interacting that can reduce levels of expressed emotion. For example, 'If Steve is not helping with the cleaning, try saying something like, "While you vacuum your room, I'll get the kettle on for us to have a cup of tea."'

With each topic covered, I supplied support workers with two handouts. One, coloured blue, covered the theory/rationale element in bullet-point form. The second, coloured yellow, detailed the practice guidance. They were provided in clear plastic covers which were retained in a ring binder. The intention was that over time each support worker would acquire a portfolio of guidance material over a range of practice-related topics that could be easily referred to.

Critique of the learning programme

As the learning programme was implemented questions arose stemming largely from trying to consider how to evaluate its effectiveness. Reflecting on the overall objective of the study (developing ways of supporting support workers in order to improve the quality of support they provide) suggested some limitations of the learning programme and a concern that its implementation had become an end in itself; some limitations were also exposed in respect of my guidance-giving to support workers. The team and the range of the accommodation had expanded significantly. I was no longer in a position to provide such a close level of supervision. Moreover, I felt that I had fostered an over-dependency on myself in terms of providing guidance and support. This was essentially 'internal' to the team and my role within it. Concerns about insularity caused me to reflect on how support workers related to other staff within the mental health service. I had conceived my role as mediating this relationship and being the main point of contact, and this appeared to me to impose limitations on the role of support workers.

The following points summarise some of these reflections (diary entry, 24 August 1997):

1   While the learning programme is of value as contributing to the support of support workers and in *promoting* good practice, it is probably insufficient in *sustaining* good practice.
2   Similarly, the practice guidance and supervision that I am directly providing is making an essential contribution to the support of support workers in their work, but it is also limited. It is a narrow interpretation of their support needs. Insufficient advantage is being taken of potential 'external' sources of support available.
3   A possible side-effect of the above is that it is having a limiting effect on the role of support workers. If support workers were more robustly engaged with mental health professionals in the local mental health service, it could be both a means of helping them feel more supported in their work and improving the quality of care they provide by enhancing their role.

So far I have described an evaluation of the implementation of the learning programme which identified some limitations in terms of the overall objectives of the study. It also gave rise to a new focus: an exploration of relationships between support workers and professional staff. I envisaged that it would be in this area that further practice developments would arise, but for this further evidence-gathering and analysis would be needed. In the next section I describe a method I adopted for analysing such evidence, before proceeding to describe the additional practice developments that were implemented as a result of this analysis.

Analysing evidence: focusing on critical scenarios

One of the challenges in carrying out action research is to be able to analyse the evidence in a systematic manner so that some sense can be made of it. The result of such an analysis should be the development of new ideas that were not previously evident. This is important because, first, it is such a process that contributes rigour to a study. Second, unless new ideas or ways of thinking are developed, no power is generated to stimulate considered practice developments. At best, all that is achieved is evidence which confirms existing practices. A means is required to force the practitioner to examine their practice for new insights and interpretations within a context that is otherwise familiar and within which the practitioner is at ease.

One method that can be adopted in trying to make explicit and analyse assumptions is the use of 'critical incidents'. These refer to events or occasions that give sufficient cause to stop and reflect. They act as punctuation marks in the narrative of the day-to-day work routine. Critical incidents act as catalysts for learning, as incidents are recounted about actions within an individual's own professional work. As such, responses to critical incidents 'stand alone as primary data sources giving insights into learners' assumptive worlds in expressions that are indisputably the learners' own' (Brookfield, 1990: 180).

I selected a series of such critical incidents (I preferred the term 'scenario' to suggest a longer time frame and the clustering of incidents around a common theme) partly by re-examining my reflective diary entries under the more concentrated focus of the professional/non-professional relationship, and, in particular, at points of intersection between support workers and professional staff. The following critical scenario is discussed in some detail, and illustrates both the method and the developing focus of the study.

Mary's scenario: relationships between support workers and 'professional' staff

Mary, one of the support workers, contacted me from her home expressing anxiety about a meeting I had asked her to attend about a resident who was causing concern. The source of Mary's anxiety was her perceived status of the other staff who were also to attend: 'They are a much higher level than me.' The others attending were a community mental health team manager, a community psychiatric nurse (CPN) and me as the supported accommodation manager. The fact that Mary had met the others before did not reassure her. The degree of anxiety she expressed was somewhat surprising as she is ordinarily a confident, outgoing person. I explained to Mary that the reason for asking her to attend was that she was the person who had most contact with the resident and her observations and opinion would be valuable.

Most of the discussion focused on Mary's input concerning the care of the resident. She made the central contribution to the meeting and her views as to what action to take were keenly elicited. This seemed to be a recognition that Mary was an important repository of detailed information about the resident. Her distinctive expertise (relative to the professional staff involved in the meeting) was the knowledge that stemmed from the nature and frequency of her interaction with the resident, as illustrated in the following example. The resident concerned was known to have volatile mood swings. At times he was sociable and responsive to conversation. At other times he would be unaccountably irritable, angry and abusive, and prolonged conversation would often make matters worse. Professional staff (CPNs, psychiatrists, etc.) who called in, whether by appointment or otherwise, could experience either mood and the outcome of such 'one-off' contacts would thus be influenced by the mood that the resident displayed at the time. Mary too had experienced the resident's volatility, but over time was able to determine whether conversation was possible and how far it could be prolonged. She was able to fine-tune her interaction with this resident because of her knowledge of his behaviour, acquired through the frequency of her contact. One consequence of this was that Mary had developed a rapport that no one else appeared to have established. It also meant that if there was useful information to pass on to the resident, suggestions to make, or information to elicit, Mary was best placed to undertake it and determine the appropriate timing.

Following the meeting I was able to discuss the experience with Mary. I underlined the value of her input. As anticipated, she did not find the meeting such an ordeal. However, she did repeat the reason for her discomfort, namely the disparity she perceived in professional status. I drew the following conclusions from this scenario (diary entry, 8 September 1997):

1   On the one hand, Mary's perception of her inferior status relative to professional staff implied a devaluation of her role. On the other hand, her central contribution to the meeting underlined the *value* of her role. Moreover, it was a value the professional staff involved recognised and acknowledged.
2   If experienced support workers find such events anxiety-provoking, what do users of mental health services feel?
3   This is an area for training. Given the value of support workers' contributions to such meetings and other contacts with professional staff, how can their input be made most effective?
4   The support workers seem to operate in a 'gap' between the user of the service and professional staff involved in their care. Their practice can be seen to be able to bridge this gap.
5   This suggested some ideas as to how the position of support workers could be enhanced to increase their effectiveness.

This scenario raised a number of issues around support workers' contact with professional staff which I thought warranted further exploration. I therefore facilitated an audiotaped discussion with the whole team of support workers with an agenda including the points listed above. The following quotations are extracts from this taped discussion (19 September 1997).

- Support workers appeared to recognise a value in their role relative to professional staff: 'Even though they are doctors and CPNs, they do not see as much of the client as we do.'
- But they were nevertheless conscious of what they perceived as a disparity in status that could affect their interaction with professionals: 'It is a confidence thing really – it's a problem on my part.' 'You feel intimidated I suppose.' 'Yeah, you feel they're a professional and I'm not.'
- Support workers, however, felt that other professional staff valued their input, although they appeared to discriminate between specialist mental health professionals and non-specialists such as GPs. For example, discussing residents' appointments with one GP, they commented: 'He doesn't talk to them, he talks to you.' 'He treats them like idiots.' 'Dr —— won't see any of the Dickson Road residents unless we are present.'
- In contrast, the support workers had more confidence in CPNs and social workers: 'They know more about mental illness.' 'You can talk to them easier.'
- As for psychiatrists: 'I've always been welcome when I've [accompanied a client to see the psychiatrist]. They think they can get bits of information from you. That's the reason. That's the difference from GPs: they're frightened they're going to freak on them.'

Thus, support workers perceived a professional/non-professional disparity that was to some extent intimidating, but they also recognised that many professionals appeared to acknowledge their value in the care of clients, and in particular their input in 'formal' professional–client contacts. In addition, the perceptions of the support workers, as will be shown later, were echoed by users of mental health services.

In this same discussion (19 September 1997) we went on to try and specify in more detail the value of the support workers' role in 'formal' contacts with professional staff.

An important aspect of the role which support workers felt they played in respect of 'formal' contacts with professionals was *mediating* the experience for users. They recognised that if they could find dealing with professional staff intimidating, it might be much more of an ordeal for users. In addition, they felt that there was a potential for shortcomings in communication that could have a bearing on a user's care, as indicated more precisely in the points below.

First, while support workers appeared to harbour doubts about GPs, there was an acknowledgement that they are sometimes very busy and might be overwhelmed by the numbers of patients they have to see. This was seen as a good reason for support workers being present at an appointment: 'They might not have the patience to spend time talking to someone like Malcolm.' Residents would also have difficulty 'taking in' what a doctor might have to say. Thus the support workers saw themselves as facilitating more effective communication between GP and resident.

Second, in general, support workers also saw their presence as important in supporting communication *from* staff *to* residents. As already indicated, psychiatrists can elicit helpful information from support workers, which was one of the reasons why they liked them to be present at out-patient appointments. Also, the support workers were frequently responsible for ensuring that advice was acted upon, for example for obtaining a new prescription for medication.

Third, support workers often found they had to compensate for residents' difficulties in articulating what they wanted to say. These difficulties can be so great that the whole reason for the appointment could be lost: 'Take Martin. He needs someone like us to go there and calm him down. . . . Martin can go in with his foot and end up talking about his throat. Just to make sure what is wrong is said.' 'Edna wouldn't say anything. She just used to say "I'm fine".'

Fourth, support workers did not always find this role easy to perform. This seemed to be partly because of the professional–non-professional disparity which has been discussed. It was also because of a sensitivity to the residents: 'Sometimes you don't know whether to butt in or not.' Moreover, at doctors' appointments (whether with a GP or with a psychiatrist at an out-patient appointment) 'going in' with the resident was not taken for granted. Support workers usually asked residents if they wanted them to go in, and normally residents did prefer support workers to be present.

Fifth, one support worker pointed to another area of difficulty that sometimes arose. She gave the example of a 'conflict of interest' during a resident's out-patient appointment. There were concerns about this resident's safety, given the medication he was taking, because he was driving a car and had already been involved in a traffic accident. (There was also a legal issue.) When the resident did not seek advice from the doctor about the matter as previously agreed, the support worker felt compelled to raise the issue herself. She nevertheless felt she had been 'disloyal' to the resident, even though he was quite amenable to the doctor's advice to discontinue driving. This can be viewed as an exquisite example of the tensions of working within the space between the professional and the service-user (i.e., in this case, the resident).

The professional–non-professional relationship

The observations generated by the critical scenarios contributed to a reformulation of the role of the support worker. This revolved around the identification of an area of 'expertise' arising from their *location* in the delivery of care rather than a technical expertise.

Support workers, though valued, are not accorded the status of professional staff. They do not have the emotional attachment of caring relatives but because of their proximity to the residents they can potentially exercise a considerable influence over the quality of care. They can therefore acquire a detailed knowledge of the residents not always readily accessible to professional staff.

Thus the support worker is able to operate within a 'conceptual gap' between the residents and the professional staff. Harnessing this source of expertise by bridging this gap provided an impetus for the practice developments that were subsequently put in place. The crucial issue was to achieve a balance within the role of the support worker that ensured good-quality care and that they performed safely within their capabilities.

Practice development 2: promoting 'informal' support worker–professional staff contacts

On the face of it, this was a simple initiative. Rather than always deferring to me, support workers were encouraged to make direct contacts with professional staff, in particular with care programme approach (CPA) keyworkers, when they felt their involvement was warranted.

In the course of their work, support workers had chance informal contact with professional staff involved with a particular resident. Perhaps a community psychiatric nurse would visit at a time when a support worker was also present. Otherwise, intentional contact with professional staff tended to take place at 'formal' occasions such as CPA review meetings or out-patient appointments.

However, many professionals recognise that often the most useful contacts with other professionals occur 'informally' on an unscheduled basis. Support workers did not appear to view such contacts as within their realm, still less did they initiate such contacts themselves. They also had fewer opportunities, given the relatively small amount of time spent in the office. Such contacts, though informal and often *ad hoc*, are nevertheless intended and thus not merely chance happenings. Quite often they take place over the telephone.

The effect of promoting such contacts was to foster a closer working relationship between the support worker and professional staff. It also had the effect of encouraging direct contact in the opposite direction, from professional staff to the support worker. Judging from the feedback from professional staff, this appears to have enhanced the value of support workers in the eyes of the professional staff. One reason for this appeared to be that the role and activities of support workers became perhaps more evident to professional staff through face-to-face discussion.

Informal contacts between support workers and professional staff also brought a change in approach on my part. My usual response to a support worker was now 'Can you meet up with resident X's CPN to discuss our concern?' rather than 'I'll discuss that with resident X's CPN.' This might seem a rather simple and obvious practice development. However, underlying it were a number of significant issues.

First, informal contacts of the sort described above were infrequent until they were actively promoted and support workers recognised them as a legitimate aspect of their role. Then informal contacts became a frequent occurrence. This increased frequency was reinforced by professional staff initiating direct contacts with support workers.

Second, this development was a manifestation of a significant change in approach on my part. I had perceived myself in a mediating role between the support worker and professional staff. As described above, this placed limitations on the role and effectiveness of support workers.

Third, the inhibitions that support workers experienced in respect of contact with professional staff were being reinforced by our previous practice.

Fourth, the change in practice had the effect of contributing to the integration of support workers into the care delivery system. They were increasingly seen as integral members of the multi-disciplinary team. For example, individual support workers began receiving invitations to CPA review meetings in their own right. In the past it would have been me who was invited and I would then ask the appropriate support worker to come along too.

Finally, we were also faced with a changing situation. Many of the support workers were becoming increasingly experienced and continually gaining in expertise. If there had been some merit in my position as the over-riding point of contact with professional staff in the early days of the team, it was now less appropriate.

Practice development 3: preparing for formal support worker–professional staff contacts

The team agreed that the preparation of support workers prior to *formal* contacts with professional staff (out-patient appointments, CPA review meetings, appointments with local doctors, etc.) would put in place another 'connection' in terms of plugging support workers into the system.

The first step was to include 'Contacts with professional staff' as a subject in a team training slot. The taped discussion was used as a basis for the formulation of a set of guidelines for planning contacts, paying particular attention to the perspective residents had articulated about their experiences. Second, a briefing session was built into our regular practice prior to the contact. Third, we agreed that when a discussion about a particular resident was to take place, for example at an appointment to see the psychiatrist, a list of questions and issues to be raised would be agreed in advance with the resident concerned.

Overall, support workers said that they felt more confident about their contacts with professional staff, and these became a more clearly defined part of their role. For some residents it proved a means of facilitating the articulation of their views.

Practice development 4: resident summary sheets

A further practice development which I suggested was the introduction of 'summary sheets'. When a client's situation continues unchanged for long periods, as is often the case in long-term care environments, contact with professional staff can become infrequent or indeed cease as cases are 'closed' (from the point of view of the community mental health team (CMHT)). We were looking at finding additional ways of increasing support for worker–professional contacts so as to take the greatest advantage of support worker expertise. One way of doing this proactively, without the inhibitions imposed by disparities in professional status, was to institute regular written feedback from support workers to professional staff.

The method used was as follows. Support workers would write summary sheets (on blue paper so as to be easily identifiable in community mental health team cases files) at regular intervals, typically three monthly. These would be circulated to the relevant CPA keyworker or to the CMHT manager if the case was 'closed'.

Initially the summary sheets were free text accounts of perhaps half a page. However, after a time support workers said that they were often unsure what to include and some had difficulties in structuring them. We agreed to a suggestion from one of the support workers that we should change the original format by including a series of relevant headings with a 'comments' section at the end. An added benefit was that this facilitated a consistency of reporting. A further refinement, which I suggested, was that we decided to time the completion of the summary sheets to coincide with CPA review meetings, so that they would form a useful preparation for support worker input into the meetings.

Concluding thoughts: my role as manager

My role as manager (and the only 'professional') of the team underwent a significant reconceptualisation as the various practice developments were formulated and implemented.

An important consideration here was the small-scale, geographically dispersed nature of the service and the organisational and professional 'distancing' tendencies that have been indicated. The implications of this were: (1) the high burden of responsibility experienced by support workers, as evidenced by the frequency of their guidance seeking (Kemp, 1997); and (2) the difficulty of finding the most effective means of supporting them, given the configuration of the service.

Examination of further critical scenarios arising from the intersection of support workers with professional staff helped to specify these issues more precisely. One issue, for example, was how support workers dealt with 'urgent situations', especially outside 'office hours', where there was a potential conflict between the support workers' intimate knowledge of a resident and the type of response a professional duty worker (who was likely to have no previous knowledge of the resident) might suggest in trying to exercise their overall responsibilities. As support workers gained experience they began to exercise increasingly refined judgement as to the appropriateness of whether to call a duty worker in situations that arose.

A second frequent scenario was described by a support worker as 'dumping'. This would invariably take place near the end of a span of duty when a support worker would unburden concerns about a resident to me just before going home.

Very often relatively innocuous observations would be made, yet there was always a small chance that they might be precursors to something more significant. More often than not a process of seeking affirmation was at stake, whereby the support worker would seek confirmation that the steps he or she had taken were appropriate.

Thus, just as there is a 'practice gap' between professional and residents within which support workers operate, there is also a 'supervision gap' in terms of my relationship with support workers as their professional manager. In a hospital ward or a residential care home setting, this gap can be viewed as relatively narrow, since there is usually a hierarchy of personnel working in close proximity over a twenty-four-hour period. In the setting of the supported housing scheme that is the subject of this study, this 'supervision gap' can be considered as relatively wide, because of the dispersed and fragmentary characteristics of the service. The practice developments introduced in the course of this research were intended to help bridge this gap, to overcome the resulting tensions, and to supplement the previous arrangements for formal and informal supervision and for team meetings.

Thus, to sum up, an important outcome of the work I have described here was to put in place a number of supporting linkages between support workers and professional staff, and thus to reduce the dependence on me as the sole source of support. These linkages also had the effect of enhancing the role of support workers, as evidenced in their increased involvement in the overall delivery of care in the ways described, and their higher levels of confidence in areas of work they previously found daunting.

References

Abrahamson, D. (1993) 'Housing and de-institutionalisation: theory and practice in the development of a resettlement service', in M. Weller and M. Muijen (eds) *Dimensions of Community Mental Health Care*, London: Saunders, pp. 208–32.

Brookfield, S. (1990) 'Using critical incidents to explore learners' assumptions', in J. Mezirow (ed.) *Fostering Critical Reflection in Adulthood*, San Francisco: Jossey Bass, pp. 177–93.

Davies, N., Lingham, R., Prior, C. and Sims, A. (1995) *Report of the Inquiry into the Circumstances Leading to the Death of Jonathon Newby (a Volunteer Worker) on 9 October 1993 in Oxford*, Oxford: Oxfordshire Health Authority.

Elliott, J. (1991) *Action Research for Educational Change*, Buckingham: Open University Press.

Johnson, S., Brooks, L., Sutherby, K., Thornicroft, G., Johnson, C. and Loftus, L. (1997) 'Sending in the paras', *Health Service Journal*, 11 September, pp. 30–1.

Kemp, P. (1997) 'Supporting the supporters: the learning and supervision needs of unqualified support staff in a supported housing scheme for people with mental health problems', *Educational Action Research*, 5, 2: 193–210.

Kuipers, L., Leff, J. and Lam, D. (1992) *Family Work for Schizophrenia: a Family Guide*, London: Gaskell/Royal College of Psychiatrists.

Muijen, M. (1995) 'Britain in moral panic – Part five: Care of the mentally ill', *Community Care*, 7–13 September, pp. i–viii.

Murray, A. and Shepherd, G. (1996) 'Suspicious minds (support workers in the community)', *Health Service Journal*, 106: 27.

Vaughn, C. and Leff, J. (1976) 'The influence of family and social factors on the course of psychiatric illness', *British Journal of Psychiatry*, 129: 125–37.

Chapter 7

What does an elephant look like?

Problems encountered on a journey to innovation in child protection

Valerie Childs

Introduction

Have you ever got on a bus believing you knew where you were going and the route you'd take, and then suddenly found you were going to places you'd never been before? What happened to me felt like that. This is how it all began.

I have been in social work for twenty years, working mainly with adolescents in residential units. This involved significant amounts of groupwork, with a variety of focuses.

I am a social worker, for social services, in a Family Centre, whose remit under the UK Children Act, 1989, falls within Section 17 – Children in Need. The service is for children aged 5–12 years and their families. We offer a wide range of packages including groupwork for adults and children.

During initial interviews for a behaviour management programme for parents and carers, we noticed that 100% of the 'problem' children had witnessed domestic violence. The centre's student at the time had run a women's group and found domestic violence was a significant factor for most of the participants in her group. This raised the question: 'Who was offering a service to the children who had lived with family violence?' Our centre surveyed the local area social work teams about the kinds of interventions for which their current caseloads indicated a need, and we found there was a demand for such a group for children. This was interesting, as we had not received any referrals for this service prior to our inquiries.

This all coincided with an opportunity, as part of a post-qualifying study, for me to work for five weeks in Newfoundland, Canada. Part of my undertaking to the centre team was to look out for information on groupwork for children who had witnessed family violence. At the time of writing (1996), the impact of domestic violence on children has received little acknowledgement or support from statutory agencies (*Childright*, 1995). Higgins (1995) found that children often felt caught between their parents and had difficulty in talking to either of them. However, she also found that, given the opportunity to talk to someone who would listen and support them, the children made progress.

During 1994 (the International Year of the Family) the National Children's Homes' (NCH) 'Action for Children' initiative commissioned research into the impact of domestic violence on children. The research noted the lack of written material on this aspect compared to a substantial amount written about women and domestic violence. It was noted that most of the published research came from North America (NCH, 1994).

On the whole, statutory social work intervention in cases of domestic violence tends to take place when social services departments are concerned that a child living in a violent situation is at risk of 'significant harm'. In this instance there is a statutory duty under the Children Act, 1989, Section 47, to initiate child protection procedures. 'Children seeing domestic violence are not, by law, classed as child protection cases' (Mapp, 1995: 24). Also, children living in refuges are not usually deemed by the local authority to be 'children in need' (Children Act, 1989, Section 17), which effectively prevents them from being provided with the range of support services available under Part Three of the Act. The 1989 Act refers explicitly to three abuses (physical, emotional and sexual abuse), and child protection conferences consider adding children's names to the Child Protection Register under these categories. But there is no 'psychological' abuse category, which would acknowledge domestic violence as the 'fourth abuse'. However:

> Children who live in a battering relationship, experience the most insidious form of child abuse. Whether or not they are physically abused by either parent is less important than the psychological scars they bear from watching their fathers beat their mothers. They learn to become part of a dishonest conspiracy of silence. They learn to lie to prevent inappropriate behaviours and they learn to suspend fulfilment of their needs rather than risk another confrontation. They expend a lot of energy avoiding problems. They live in a world of make-believe.
>
> (Walker, 1979: 46)

So much for the background. From my placement in Newfoundland I brought back a copy of Yawney and Hill's (1993) model of groupwork intervention for child witnesses of family violence. A very organised and detailed binder containing philosophy, research, sessions plans, exercises and notes for group leaders. At the back of the folder were comprehensive lists of written and video materials, with distributors' addresses and formatted questionnaires for carers and children for use at pre- and post-group interviews.

I felt I had found not only ideas for my team, but something much more than I expected. With the benefit of hindsight the phrase 'heading for a fall' has a certain resonance. I didn't see that I was already questioning aspects of the Canadian model, or consider how this would impact on my co-workers when they appeared to believe I was presenting them with answers. My plan was to be part of a collaborative project, involving all of us and using the Canadian model as a guide, which would develop and implement a groupwork programme for families who have lived with domestic violence.

Periodically, over many weeks, I raised the matter of the group process, and eventually acknowledged that I was struggling to avoid getting too involved in thinking and planning before co-workers were identified. I worried that I would begin at a different place in the process and this would be unhelpful – it didn't occur to me at the time that I was already in a different starting place. Obvious, you may say, and I would agree. The question 'Why didn't I think of that?' has become very familiar to me, and I will always associate it with my action research project.

I had enrolled in a university action research course with a view to using the groupwork project as my focus. I felt it would maximise my learning and assist in the evaluation of working with child witnesses of family violence. However, as I progressed, the question of 'innovation' became a central issue, in particular the aspect of communication. It is therefore these matters which are given specific consideration in this chapter, within the context of the groupwork programme.

Innovation: a gift or a burden?

Although the innovation had been requested, there were still the complex processes of collaboration and implementation to contend with, such as the impact on the 'natural order of things' in a team. 'Attitudes, values and practices, organisation and structures have their own in-built inertia which may be very change resistant even when an innovation is potentially acceptable to those concerned' (Sweetingham, 1981: 95).

The team of which I am part is small, and there is a core group who have been together for around seven years. Who was bringing this initiative? The newest team member. People in general are creatures of habit, and there would be an impact on each and every one of us if a new initiative was instigated. The 'resistance to change' element was not something I considered in depth at the outset, although this seems a very obvious omission now. I think my own enthusiasm for the 'project gift' on the one hand gave the innovation process an impetus, and on the other hand 'blinkered' me to some of the 'project burdens'.

In retrospect, I feel it would have been interesting to have had team discussions (encompassing the handy person – responsible for minor repairs, maintenance and the garden – the administrative clerk and the domestic) at the starting point and at various other junctures along the way. I think the wheels of the process might have been oiled if everyone had felt they had an explicit invitation to communicate their thoughts and ideas, and to express any anxieties about the impact of the innovation from their particular perspective.

I had conversations/meetings with individuals and received valuable contributions. For example, when the social work staff were struggling to find a name for the project, I mentioned my frustration to the handy person. He asked what the difficulty was. I explained that our thoughts about a name for the project had been around 'peace' and 'doves', and it felt as if we were stuck, trying to 'sanitise' the notion of violence. Later the same day, he came up with the suggestion of 'The Minorsaur Project'. Brilliant! He had made a different connection – a play on the word *minorsaur* (pronounced 'minor saw'), that is *children* who have *seen* a large creature who had the capacity to physically dominate a smaller creature, and also a current topic within films, books and videos for children. Thus, the project logo became a dinosaur. The domestic was present when I was discussing group snacks with the assistant social worker, and offered to make individual cakes for each session and a special 'dinosaur cake' for the last meeting.

My experience in residential work had taught me the value of the contributions and perceptions of non-social work staff, but I lost sight of the importance of communication, explicitly of the balance between the 'gift' and 'burden' aspects of an innovation. Looking back over my diary notes, I can see how later comments, such as 'That paint was all up the walls and over the carpet. What will people think when they come in here for their meetings?' and 'These kiddies can't just run around the building: the noise was terrible' and 'Oh no, it's Thursday!' were perhaps attempts to highlight the fact that the 'burdensome' aspect of a new group had not been explicitly recognised.

The comments did, however, impact in other ways. For example, the children running around the building at the end of the group had been of concern to us, and we addressed it through my suggestion of a 'merit point' system. The children were asked, after the session and before they left the room, if they wanted to try and achieve a merit point by leaving the building in an orderly manner – a behaviour modification approach which we had not previously considered. It worked well and leaving the building became less stressful for everyone. This change also led to the development of an idea for a 'prize-giving' at the end of the project.

The project

Although we sent information packs to the area teams who had participated in our original survey of interventions required, we received only nine referrals and in some ways this felt disappointing: the Canadian programme suggested a group membership of twelve. We set up the four family interviews. The children were to be interviewed on a one-to-one basis by the group workers, using the questionnaire which we had adapted slightly from the Yawney and Hill model. During the child(ren)'s interview, the parent(s) were seen, in another room, by one of the carers' group workers, also using an adapted version of the Yawney and Hill questionnaire.

In the annual groupwork programme for the centre the best fit for a twelve-week schedule would be to start in November, with a break during the school Christmas holidays and therefore ending in March. Time was becoming a real issue – little did I realise the significance of that thought! There were familiar difficulties – one letter didn't arrive, we had been given the wrong address for the family, another family had an emergency and wanted to rearrange their time, and so on. Looking back, I have come to see that we did not all have the same belief or perception about the time needed for a given task or activity or an individual's learning process.

The interviews were completed. One family with two children and another family with one child did not attend the interviews. They were offered alternative appointments and although they accepted, they did not attend or contact us, as we had requested if there was an unforeseen difficulty. The third family had three children referred to the project, but on the day of the interviews the eldest boy refused to leave his mother and so was not interviewed with his siblings. He agreed to come the following day and be seen separately. At the end of the appointment, he was clearly saying he did not want to be part of a group, but might want to work individually. This was discussed between workers and with his mother, and it was agreed he would be offered individual sessions.

Thus, there were five children and two mothers for the project. I didn't realise it, but I was about to make one of the biggest 'simple omissions' of the entire process. Even as I look at this now, I can't believe I didn't think about the impact of the children's 'group' actually being composed of only two families: these children were coming from shared histories and were anticipating shared futures.

This realisation is resonant with the development of theories of family therapy. There are obvious parallels between small groups and families, and this led family therapists, in the early years, to treat families as though they were just another form of group. They were assisted by a vast body of knowledge and literature on group dynamics and group therapy. However, as they gained more experience with family work, they discovered the group therapy model was not entirely appropriate for families. Therapy groups are made up of separate individuals, strangers with no past or future outside the group. Families, on the other hand, consist of intimates who share the same myths and beliefs, and are already involved in a shared life script. In addition, families are not peers who can relate democratically as equals: generational differences create hierarchies which cannot be ignored. Thus family therapists eventually abandoned the group therapy model and replaced it with a variety of 'systems' models (Nichols and Schwartz, 1991). Ludwig Von Bertalanffy, a prominent biologist, developed a model which was mistranslated from the German as general systems theory (GST) in 1950. He had intended the last word to be 'teaching', as his ideas were not so much a theory as an approach, a way of thinking which could be applied to all kinds of systems (Davidson, 1983). When applied to families, his approach suggests that a family system should be seen as more than just a collection of people, and that therapists should focus on the interactions among family members.

The idea of a parent/carer group to run alongside the children's group was born out of the centre's previous experience of the usefulness of this notion in other children's groups, not from the Yawney and Hill model. (This became significant in my thinking later on in the programme.) A male and a female worker were interested in facilitating the adult group. The five of us were joined by a male facilitator as a consultant.

There was an assumption that, as the person who found the model, I wanted to be part of the children's group. This was true. However, the lack of explicit discussion about the various roles of personnel contributed to all kinds of other assumptions not being voiced. The team leader, a keen supporter of the initiative, felt she had time to be a co-worker, and her student had already expressed a specific interest in experiencing groupwork and working in issues around domestic violence. These were the children's workers.

Time was very tight and I persuaded myself to take the initiative in drawing up some ideas. I passed these to my fellow passengers and was surprised to find few suggestions for change. I had snatched conversations with various combinations of the other project workers, and so we progressed. At this time I still believed I was part of a collaborative process: naïve, you may feel, but the benefit of hindsight is a marvellous learning opportunity. I didn't see that I was holding the responsibility and rapidly becoming 'the perceived expert'. What followed, I can now see, was inevitable, but at the time it felt painful and (it was suggested) 'bewildering'. I felt this was a useful term because I had been naming my feeling 'confusion', meaning chaotic and orderless; the notion of bewilderment, meaning puzzling, gave me a different insight into my feelings. Later on in the process I made a connection with the notion of 'curiosity', from the model of systemic family work by the Milan Associates. A branch of this team developed the idea that therapy needed to become more of a research *expedition* which the therapist joined. This meant that the therapist was released from responsibility for any certain outcome and could take on an attitude of 'curiosity' (Cecchin, 1987).

I had been feeling a particular responsibility, because I had found the model and brought it into the team. I thought my role had been 'searcher and finder', but then perceived an expectation that I should also be 'implementer'. This was not an explicit communication from the other workers and I did not attempt to check out the accuracy of my perception at this point because, I think, I was unsure of how much responsibility was involved. On some level I feel I may have been unaware of the difference between the two tasks – (first) implementing an innovation and (second) organising and running the group. In the event, by not communicating my thoughts I feel the two became mixed up together until about half way through the sessions. Not explicitly communicating with one another led to a series of assumptions being made and perpetuated. Our unspoken thoughts about who was responsible for which part led to feelings of frustration and at one point anger and hurt on my part.

Changing perceptions

My journey had become bewildering in the extreme. I wondered what I was trying to do in the group. In the first session the children were invited to tell us about their day during the snack. Notable comments were: 'My teacher's a lesbie', 'My teacher used to be gay and a pervert, but he's all right now he's married', 'I know about shagging', 'What about your knickers?' There was also much bottom pinching and going to the toilet. What did this mean? The 'sex' theme continued through five sessions. What did this have to do with family violence? Why was I doing this group? Why was I doing it with these people? Perhaps the problem was me? Then came what I retrospectively consider my 'going through the pain barrier'.

It started when I got up one Monday morning. I sat in the kitchen drinking my tea and pondering my floor. The carpet fitters were coming, but before they could lay the new flooring they had to board one end of the room and screed the other. This set me thinking. Why was I paying all this money to have board put upon floorboards? I knew the answer: the surfaces were uneven and needed levelling, a shame because the floorboards were actually very sound. I sorted through my papers, getting ready to go to my action research learning set, when all of a sudden I started linking my 'floor' thoughts to my project.

I do have skills in social work, working with children and working in groups – the floorboards. Why, then, was this group so different? What was I trying to achieve? The problems of the uneven surfaces? So what needed to happen? What were the boards and screed? It was so beautifully simple – I just needed to find where the gaps were! I wrote a list:

> *What are the issues for a social worker trying to set up/implement an innovation?*
> Common understanding of the aims
> Individual roles/relationships
> Knowledge and gaps
> Strategies for struggling
> How different people learn – starting from different places
> Responses to conflict
> Use of a model – structure from different places, structure as disabling/ disempowering
> Importance of coherence – not assimilation
> Being scared of what I don't know
> Success/failure
> Resistance in the team
> Perceptions/realities – communicating to learn (Elephant story) (see below)
> Experiences and contributions
> Reinforcing vulnerabilities/expectations
> How does what I know impact on my ability to deal with the unknown?
> (The new flooring – how does what's underneath need to change to accommodate the new finish?)

For weeks I had been agonising, in the throes of confusion and chaos which turned into bewilderment, but on that day, during the action research course meeting, I got out my list and talked with what I felt was clarity about the reflective process of my learning to date. This was when the question 'Why didn't I think of that?' became an important part of my new perspective.

A part of the whole

There is a Buddhist story about three blind men. These men, each touching a part of an elephant, were asked what an elephant looks like. The man touching the trunk thought it resembled a snake, the man touching the leg was sure it was most like a tree and the man touching the tail said it was like a brush. That's how I was feeling. The team leader, the student and I were all touching a part of the whole, but the difficulties arose out of the tension between believing you are touching all of it and understanding you are only touching some of it and therefore knowing there is more. Collaboration is about explicitly recognising what we each know and don't know. It's about valuing one another's perceptions and ideas without feeling a need to own the only reality and attempting to persuade others to that particular view. Like the men in the story, once we had recognised and talked together about the pieces we had and the gaps between them, we could see that although jointly we had more of the picture than we did individually, we could also see that the elephant we were touching was neither a snake, nor a tree nor a brush, but a combination of all three and more. This was a very exciting breakthrough for me.

We hadn't previously had conversations about which knowledge we each held and which gaps in our learning we thought might be filled by the project. I felt a pressure from my co-workers to have and hold the knowledge of this groupwork model, which meant I felt I couldn't consider what my gaps were. Their feeling that they had only or mostly gaps may have meant that they didn't recognise the knowledge they each had to contribute. All this made it feel very hard to share the responsibility for the group, to work collaboratively, as I had envisaged.

These thoughts also freed me to consider who else had knowledge which would be useful: the mothers. As a result of this thinking I was able to suggest that we give some written feedback to the carers' group, and this precipitated some unforeseen outcomes. First was the impact on the children: this was very positive because it showed the children we were all communicating. Second, acknowledging to the women that they were the experts on their own children had an empowering and enabling effect upon their group. Third (in one case), the feedback gave one of the mothers time to reflect on matters at home which had been worrying her, which in turn enabled her to talk to her daughter, and this facilitated a disclosure allegation of sexual abuse from the child.

It seems obvious now that we had each made (but not communicated) assumptions about what strategy we would adopt if we felt we were struggling in the children's group. My assumptions had been that the three of us would meet with the carers' group workers, to see if they could assist. And only if that failed would we approach the consultant for an extra appointment. But after the chaotic sixth session the team leader initiated an extra meeting with the project consultant without prior discussion. I felt very angry, initially, that someone else's 'struggling strategy' had been implemented, partly because we had not discussed it together. But beyond that was a worry that there was something seriously wrong, which I hadn't seen and no one had pointed out to me. If I was being seen as responsible for the project, why was the team leader taking responsibility for this part? Was she 'pulling rank' because of a dreadful error on my part? That thought hurt. During the extra consultation, I voiced my assumption about the 'struggling strategy' and found that others had also made the same assumption, but we hadn't talked to one another. The feelings of individual isolation dispersed and became an opportunity to explore some other unspoken assumptions.

It was interesting to reflect how this behaviour veered around the stages of 'Forming', 'Norming', 'Storming', 'Performing' and 'Adjourning' (Tuckman and Jensen, 1977). Somehow, I had never thought about the process of the workers *becoming* a 'group'. I had probably assumed we *were* a group, because we worked together in the same team and various combinations of us had already co-worked with groups of children. It seems obvious now, but we all had multi-roles with the project, the team and the organisation, but didn't talk about how/if these multi-roles might conflict and how we could support one another at times of tension.

Salvador Minuchin is recognised as the pioneer of structural family therapy, and has written extensively on its theory and practice (Minuchin *et al.*, 1967; Minuchin, 1974; Minuchin and Fishman, 1981; Elizur and Minuchin, 1989). Retrospectively, it would have been interesting to consider how a structural model of systemic family work, applied to teams and organisations, might have impacted on understanding the innovation process. Structural theory has three essential components: structure, subsystems and boundaries. Structure is seen as the organised pattern in which the system interacts. These repeated interactions determine who, how and when the members relate. The structure also involves a set of rules which govern the transactions; changing or challenging the rules may or may not change the structure, but changing the structure will affect all transactions.

Figure 7.1, below, uses Minuchin's ideas to present an organisational hierarchical depiction of the personnel involved in this project. Figure 7.2 is my perception of the system's structure, up to the point when the team leader called for the extra consultation, as described above. At that point I felt the system shift from Figure 7.2 to Figure 7.1 – although that is not an explanation I would have given at the

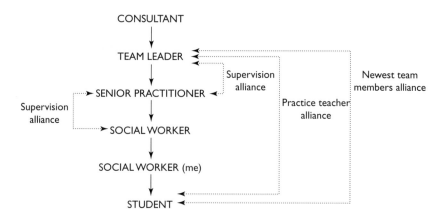

Figure 7.1

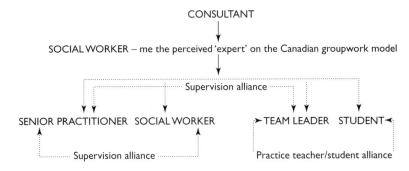

Figure 7.2

time. I think it would have been very helpful to make some simple drawings like these. Then we could have contributed our perceptions of our own and others' positions, in the context of Minuchin's structural model, at the beginning of the project and updated it throughout the process.

The vulnerability of learning

Someone once said, 'While carrying out my own creative effort, I depend on that which I don't know and that which I haven't yet done.'

Another problem for the team, I think, was that we did not share our beliefs about the way we each learn, the time we need to learn, and things which help and hinder our learning. The impact of this, for me, was feelings of isolation, frustration, insecurity and loss of confidence in my own skills and abilities. At times I also felt lost and hurt and afraid. There had been no explicit recognition that we had all joined the journey at different times, in different places.

This led to a thought about difference and conflict. The tension which arises out of difference can be very creative, freeing and enabling, but if the likelihood of it arising is not acknowledged, the tension can become fraught, unhelpful and disabling. A kind of tug-of-war develops, a competitive edge, leading to unhelpful coalitions and feelings of unconnectedness with co-workers. To say, 'I don't know', does mean becoming vulnerable. I wanted to say, 'I don't know.' I wanted to give away part of the responsibility, but I don't think I was communicating this well. I wonder why I felt responsible for this communication gap? I made a decision not to attend a planning session. Then, I reasoned to myself, the others would have to take responsibility. A part of me felt like a recalcitrant adolescent, perhaps because adolescence is to some extent about becoming appropriately responsible and learning to be independently dependent. This notion has a connection with the family life cycle (Carter and McGoldrick, 1989).

Retrospectively, there was also my position in relation to being alongside the children, feeling their chaos, perhaps because it didn't make sense to them any more? The children were wanting to make their own unique and personal connections with the theme and I wanted to be alongside them. However, although we had had conversations about the two families, I don't feel I gave enough consideration to the wider issues of having all female leaders for the children's group, or working with black children in groups.

In one way the fact that the children's group leaders were all women reflected the children's situation in single-mother households. What I didn't connect until later was how this fed into the 'families' issue. Family B and I made a connection from the beginning, which Family A and I didn't. Why? I'm not sure. There were external factors: for example, the B family interview did not start with a protracted debate, as all the children wanted to come to the group. However, the children in Family B were more challenging during the interview. Did I feel I could learn more from those who made me think and challenge some of my own thoughts?

During the group exercises, the 8-year-old boy from Family B and I often worked together on the periphery of the group. He wanted to do many of the individual tasks in a different way. For example, when the others were drawing their body shapes, he joined in initially and then tore up his work, saying he wanted to play football. I got alongside him and we went to the back of the room. He asked for a piece of paper and drew a figure, then filled it with a variety of colours. He looked to me (quite literally) during group time to be 'with' him, whether it was to reaffirm boundaries, which he continually tested, or during group exercises. He and his sister balanced each other like a see-saw. When he was quiet, she was loud and vice versa. If he was doing some work, she wasn't, and so on. I found myself 'running' between the two. In a later conversation with their mother, she described herself as doing the same. I had unknowingly played out the family patterns.

The children from Family B had a dual heritage (a black mother and white fathers); the children from Family A were white, but did have three dual-heritage half-siblings. This factor reflects society's exposure to colour – where black people have more exposure to whites than the other way round. The fact that all the leaders were white is also reflective of the lack of black people in positions of power. Was the connection a matter of colour? Personality? Expression of self? Did the children perceive my struggle to work anti-oppressively as an adult in relation to children? Or as a white person in relation to black people? Did I communicate my aware- ness of difference positively? What did I do and how did I do it? Was working with the 8-year-old child individually within the group sensitive practice or oppressive behaviour?

This part of the process, I think, links with the notion of 'risk' (Winter, 1989: 60–2). I wanted to take the risk of going alongside the children on their journeys, instead of Yawney and Hill's journey. Were the children there to serve the model or was the model there to serve the children? In other words, had the tension between the model we were using and the children not conforming made us too preoccupied with trying to make the children fit? Put another way, I felt the map had become the territory (Korzybski, 1942), and this seemed to me to be oppressive, unhelpful and not something I wanted to perpetuate.

More changing perceptions

I shared (with my co-workers) the story of the blind men and the elephant, and the connections I thought it had to us and what we were doing. I was delighted with the outcome of the ensuing conversation. We talked together about some of the issues I've already highlighted. We all agreed we wanted to 'throw the book out of the window'; it had just taken us different amounts of time to come to the realisation that it was more of a hindrance than a help. One of my co-workers talked about her need for structure and therefore the appeal this very prescriptive model had for her. I was able to discuss my frustration with session plans which did not allow for 'going with the flow' with the children. With this new level of communication we were able to negotiate some structure for the session, but not too much. I was told by one of my co-workers that she didn't feel she had the same confidence as I appeared to have to invent things 'on the spot'. I found that surprising; I must have made an assumption that it was possible to improvise, without consulting my co-workers. It was agreed that each session would have a theme and that we would have some pre-session discussion about the way we would present the idea. It was further agreed that I would be responsible for the 'on the spot' alternatives, but that I needed to communicate more openly with my co-workers about what I was proposing.

The recording after that session had a very different 'tone'. The team leader commented, 'That's the best I've felt . . . I felt more in control . . . this was one big learning, something I've not experienced before . . . I don't think I handled [child's name] very well, I couldn't find the words.' I thought these comments posed an interesting contradiction: in giving away control, more control had been gained. This theme seems to continue into the idea of 'big learning'. By acknowledging our gaps, we create a space for learning. This recalls of the adage, 'You have to speculate to accumulate', and that there is an inherent risk-taking in the process.

Endings

The idea of the prize-giving was something I held on to from the first phase. It seemed important to mark in a tangible way the families' attendance and achievement. It's interesting how once we freed ourselves from the confines of a previously trodden path, we became open to different creative ideas.

The children had been asked to choose what they would like their merit points converted to. They each chose something different, i.e. money, a toy, make-up, something to wear, and drawing materials. I found their choices fascinating. They reflected individuality and uniqueness. Sibling rivalries and emulating others did not seem evident, as it had been in the group exercises. I began to consider the post-group interviews with a degree of excitement. Had we made connections? How would the feedback challenge/confirm our perceptions? I had no doubt it would be interesting and it no longer mattered what the feedback was: I knew I could learn from it.

In addition to the merit awards, I suggested, we could create certificates for each child and parent. I had not anticipated how much these would mean, particularly to the adults. Comments made included: 'I'm framing this and putting it on the wall', and 'No one tells you when you do something right as a parent, but they're quick to jump on you when you get it wrong', and 'This is the first certificate I've ever got.'

The final meeting had a party atmosphere, and I wondered what we were each privately celebrating. Was it a measure of 'success'? Or the joy of starting a journey together and still being together at the end? Was it the end or the beginning?

Summary comments

Do I know what an elephant looks like? Well, I had more idea at the end of what this elephant looked like, but not all elephants look alike. In considering an innovation, I've learnt the value of taking nothing for granted, the importance of clear communication and the excitement of doing something new and different. Looking at the 'culture' of the team, I have realised that individuals are associated with the groups they most frequently run. Would this innovation have met with less resistance, then, if an established team member had taken the lead role? Once people become intrinsically linked with a particular practice focus, they become the 'perceived expert'. How much, then, of my experience was influenced by my becoming assimilated into the team culture? Does this culture have a protective element for the team? Would we be overwhelmed if we each went through the pain of becoming involved in every group innovation? By keeping somewhat removed from it, are the team helping to keep a healthy balance within which to work?

This 'new' experience has connected with me on another level. The word 'new' still evokes some scary feelings within me, which perhaps connect with my lack of confidence at the beginning of this innovation. Having considerable experience in residential work, mostly as a team leader, I then became a student for two years and from there joined a fieldwork team specialising in adoption, immediately before my current post. The impact of those three and a half years had a large deskilling component. The lack of support and supervision in a new setting with a new role compounded the disabling scary feelings associated with the 'new' but did not provide the balance of the excitement of learning in a safe environment. So perhaps this was my own subconscious contribution to the 'resistance to change'. There are also the status labels which are so prevalent in our society and laden with oppressive undertones: 'student'; 'new'; 'junior'; 'senior'; 'worker'; 'client'. How much had I internalised over recent time the belief of being 'less than'? What effect does this kind of experience and internalisation have on children? And on black children?

After the last project session, other team members commented, 'I bet you're glad that's over', and 'Would you do that again?' But I was sad it had ended. I can remember commenting earlier in the process, 'At the end of this, I'd like to run a group for child witnesses of family violence.' Perhaps I knew on some level that I was just starting to concentrate on the group rather than the innovation. Perhaps an interesting question to consider during the next group programme might be: 'What can systemic family therapy ideas teach us about group work?' Hmm, I wonder what kind of animal that would turn out to be . . .

References

Carter, E. and McGoldrick, M. (1989) *The Changing Family Life Cycle: a Framework for Family Therapy* (2nd edn), Needham Heights, Mass.: Allyn & Bacon.

Cecchin, G. (1987) 'Hypothesizing, circularity and neutrality revisited: an invitation to curiosity', *Family Process*, 26: 405–13.

Childright (1995) 114 (March).

Davidson, M. (1983) *Uncommon Sense*, Los Angeles: JP Tarcher.

Elizur, J. and Minuchin, S. (1989) *Institutionalising Madness: Families, Therapy and Society*, New York: Basic Books.

Higgins, G. (1995) *Children Living with Domestic Violence*, London: Women's Aid Federation England (WAFE).

Korzybski, A. (1942) *Science and Sanity: an Introduction to Non-Aristotelian Systems and General Semantics* (2nd edn), Lancaster, Pa.: Science Books.

Lewin, K. (1946) 'Action research and minority problems', *Journal of Social Issues*, 2: 34–46.

Mapp, S. (1995) 'Violence and innocence', *Community Care*, 7–13 December, pp. 24–5.

Minuchin, S. (1974) *Families and Family Therapy*, Cambridge, Mass.: Harvard University Press.

Minuchin, S. and Fishman, H. (1981) *Family Therapy Techniques*, Cambridge, Mass.: Harvard University Press.

Minuchin, S., Montaliro, B., Guernery, B., Rosman, B. and Schumer, F. (1967) *Families of the Slums*, New York: Basic Books.

NCH (1994) *The Hidden Victims – Children of Domestic Violence*, London: National Children's Homes.

Nichols, M. and Schwartz, R. (1991) *Family Therapy: Concepts and Models* (2nd edn), Needham Heights, Mass.: Allyn & Bacon.

Robinson, L. (1995) *Psychology for Social Workers: Black Perspectives*, London: Routledge.

Sweetingham, P. (1981) 'Special needs: support for change', *Classroom Action Research Network*, Bulletin 10, Cambridge: Institute of Education.

Tuckman, B. and Jensen, M. (1977) 'Stages of small group development revisited', *Group and Organisation Studies*, 2, 4: 419–27.

Walker, L. (1979) *Battered Women*, New York: Harper & Row.

Winter, R. (1989) *Learning from Experience: Principles and Practice in Action Research*, Lewes: Falmer Press.

Yawney, D. and Hill, B. (1993) *Project Child Recovery*, Alberta: Society for the Prevention of Child Abuse and Neglect.

Chapter 8

Developing client-focused work with people with profound learning disabilities

Brenda Dennett

Introduction

I am the manager of a day centre for people with profound learning disabilities, which for this report I will call the 'Grasmere Road Centre'. The aim of the project reported here was to ascertain whether the services we provide are properly client-oriented and focused, with a view to implementing a fully needs-led service for our clients.

The current day-care programmes for service-users have developed in myriad ways. At one time, clients with profound learning and physical disabilities were not expected to do much more than sit or lie, preferably quietly, and to accept the care ministrations of the staff. In the early 1980s many were just beginning to come out of long-stay hospitals, and any community presence was felt to be an improvement upon institutionalised living. In contrast, many younger users had not been subjected to such hospitalisation, and increased awareness, improved educational facilities and pressure from service-user movements began to raise the expectations of users, parents and staff. Suddenly, it was not enough for a child with profound learning disabilities to leave school and stay at home. Thus, day-care facilities were established (called 'special care units' because of the perceived needs of users), but often without overall plans about how such services should or could develop.

Teaching sessions in the Grasmere Road Centre have evolved with time, and are dependent to a large degree upon the skills and interests of the current staff group. Care workers are rarely recruited in the way that teachers are recruited, where training in particular skills and knowledge would be a requirement. The main specification for care workers tends to be experience and willingness to work with the client group. Any additional talent, such as the ability to do craft work or play an instrument, is considered to be a bonus. As a result, programmes are often adapted to the abilities of the staff rather than the needs of the users. More recently, however, close co-operation with the community adult education department has changed this to some degree, as has the use of community facilities such as leisure centres, leading to a broadening of interest and adding professional teaching input.

In July 1993, the King's Fund began a national consultation exercise on the trends in service provision for people with learning disabilities. As a result of this exercise, day care was identified as a priority area for change and development (Wertheimer, 1996: Preface). The King's Fund team were joined by the national Development Team and funding was obtained from the Gatesby and the Joseph Rowntree Foundations in order to define what people with learning disabilities wanted from their 'day-care' facilities. This, in itself, was an amazing breakthrough, with the emphasis on user-perceived needs as opposed to service-providers' concepts of need. It rapidly emerged that 'day care' was not really what users wanted; rather, they felt the need for community presence, meaningful work, and sufficient support to use community-based facilities, and to be treated with respect and dignity (ibid.: 2–3); in short: social inclusion.

A similar county-wide inquiry revealed that service-users with learning disabilities have the same aspirations. In her book, *Changing Days*, Wertheimer says that people with behaviour perceived as challenging or with serious physical needs tend to spend their days in special-care units. She urges staff not to feel so defeated by the sheer weight of the health and care needs of such people that they fail to begin to make the changes to services suggested by the needs articulated by those with less profound disabilities (ibid.: 71–4).

The catalyst for my dissatisfaction with the daily sessions offered to service-users at Grasmere Road was the growing frequency of disruptive behaviour. Centre-users are non-verbal, and if you believe that behaviour is communication, people hitting out or falling asleep during sessions must be interpreted as the powerless 'voting with their feet'. I was not able to define what my uneasiness related to, but simply that it was present. This feeling was accentuated by changes in legislation to protect staff. Such changes as Manual Handling Regulations and the protection of new and expectant mothers effectively lowered our staffing ratios. I applaud this legislation, since it protects staff from injury and harm. But the fact that it is frequently introduced without making financial means available to enable managers to provide the necessary services and to support other staff seemed to symbolise, for me, that the needs of our clients/service-users do not always come first, and helped to focus this topic as the basis for the action research project described here.

The action research process

The basic shape of the action research process, as I initially understood it (based on my reading of Kemmis and McTaggart, 1982) is shown in Figure 8.1. I entered this process at the OBSERVE stage. My vague uneasiness with services that I had felt satisfied with previously made me spend more time in the working areas of the centre. I observed some work that was of good quality and I observed much that related very little to clients' needs. With growing awareness of changing trends both nationally and locally and my own unease, I was forced to REFLECT upon

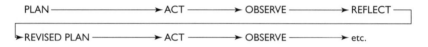

Figure 8.1

what I had seen. I felt that in service settings like the Grasmere Road Centre, too little time was being spent on reflection and, following this tradition faithfully, I had spent insufficient time reflecting.

So I decided to PLAN. We had a meeting where I introduced my interest in action research and asked staff if they felt that the clients in sessions they were working in were all correctly placed. The resounding answer to this question was 'No'. We pondered how to find out which sessions best suited which clients. This is not easy to do when people have no verbal communication. At this point we were not considering radical changes to the sessions or their subjects; we merely wanted to make minor changes to the people attending them.

The staff thought about the dilemma, and the following morning an assessment sheet arrived on my desk. This had been developed by staff to try to gauge service-users' reactions and involvement in sessions (see Figure 8.2, Observation chart). We decided to use this sheet because it was a simple tick chart and had some graphic details that we hoped would help users to participate. This seemed a very minimal way of empowering centre users but we were baffled as to how to do better when working with clients with very profound disability. (It is also debatable whether this really was 'empowerment' at all. Dowson (1997) would argue that if people are not able to take power, it might be considered mere tokenism to 'give' it, leaving all the power with us, the service providers.)

Data collection

It was now time to put the *action* into the process. (Fuller and Petch (1995: 5–6) in defining action research, emphasise the importance of the research informing the development of *practice*.) It was important to us all to begin the practical tasks and to work towards the practice changes that we thought we would see as a result of the process.

The first thing to evolve spontaneously from the first meeting was a group of interested people. Similarly, there was also a group of nervous people who doubted the process, or their own ability, and who were not seeking involvement. Staff not wishing to be involved were asked if they would like to give some comment on what they felt about the current services. I hoped that this would give them a voice, engage their interest and possibly give me something to consider when making changes and when assessing whether the changes reflected the perceived weak service areas. Their comments and suggestions are included below.

SESSION:

DATE & TIME:

STAFF:

CLIENT NAME:	🙂	😐	🙁	😠	😴	COMMENTS:

<u>**SESSION COMMENTS:**</u>

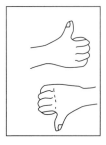

Figure 8.2 Observation chart (developed by George Brown, Senior Day Centre Officer)

Grasmere Road Centre – positive aspects
The building is on one level.
There is a high level of qualified staff with a variety of skills to meet the needs of all clients.
Staff care about clients and are enthusiastic about changes (even though they often receive negative feedback).
We are good at liaising with parents/carers about problems.
We are good at dealing with fits and seizures.
There is a good standard of care for clients' hygiene and clothes.
There is good communication with clients.

Grasmere Road Centre – negative aspects
Lack of staff training.
Time restraints make everything a rush.
Inadequate staffing levels make time restraints worse.
Staff are not able to use their own initiative, and when you do you feel that you are undermined.
Interaction between clients isn't encouraged. For example, we don't encourage them to sit next to others whom they get on with.
Staff 'pull rank' among each other.
We feel that we always have to go to a senior even when minor problems arise.
We could use more facilities in the community, e.g. education and other facilities.
We could encourage more independent skills.
We should employ a qualified teacher to structure the day for clients and staff and to oversee the work done.
We should engaged in more advocacy on behalf of clients.

With these comments as a starting point, we agreed, rather casually, to 'collect data'. Although this section is written as though it only happened once, it was a continuous 'feedback loop', rather like a painting that the artist thinks is finished until, from a distance, another view is revealed and the painting is changed, sometimes so as to alter the whole vista. Growing awareness in one area tended to have 'knock-on' effects in other areas as the whole project continued to grow.

Much of the data were collected by using the specially designed observation/ assessment sheets (see Figure 8.2). The purpose of the sheets is to assess individual service-users' responses to the sessions, and they were filled in immediately after the session concerned. It was intended that users should be as involved as possible in this process. From my own observations, this happened rarely. Not all staff were committed to doing this, and pressure, I felt, would damage the collaborative approach essential to action research (Winter, 1989; McNiff, 1994). This method of data collection still leaves us with the dilemma of our own subjective view of what people's reactions and facial expressions mean. There is also the subjectiveness of collecting 'credit ratings' for your own work: it is a confident and secure soul who can say 'I did that wrong; nobody benefited'.

A key incident

One session analysed in this way led to some particularly interesting developments. The analysis recorded by the staff member running this session was that most clients enjoyed it ('a music session planned to be without words'), and that users found the session soothing and relaxing. He named users individually and recorded their response mostly with 'smiling faces'. I had begun by merely observing, 'sitting and watching' (Delamont, quoted in Simpson and Tuson, 1995: 16). This wondrous detachment lasted a very short time, as the group erupted into a variety of dramatically challenging behaviours, including one client who pillaged the box of musical instruments. We also had a sleeper. On the recording sheet, this session was recorded as a success and the one person deemed 'not to have enjoyed it' was the pillager, who, by *my* reckoning, was the one who had shown most interest and desire to join in.

In supervision later, the staff member admitted that he had not prepared for the session. What I found disconcerting was the wide disparity between my observed view of the session and the staff member's recorded view. However, if I view my observation reflexively I would have to say that I (generally) did not hold the work of this staff member in the highest esteem and that my general 'vibes' towards him are less than positive. So how much did my own subjectivity colour the information? Of course, I am not simply 'the researcher' – I am also a part of the group (Winter, 1989: 56–7). My view is only one aspect. The senior staff member concerned felt that the staff member leading the session was unsure *how* to plan, and needed support to do so. The session leader accepted this view and the help that was offered. Thus, by considering a variety of views, in a rather casual form of 'triangulation', we were forced to look more carefully at what had happened.

Dialectically, I also had to look more widely at the *context* of the incident. Why could this staff member not manage this group? Some discussion and thought revealed that he had no control over *which* service-users were in the group. A hierarchical series of managers decided this, though they did not take part in the session. There is a centre 'ethos' of not moaning about that 'icon' known as 'the rota', the planned daily programme that allocates staff and clients to particular sessions. (Is this because the managerial planners feel protective about their brainchild?) It would therefore be very difficult for the 'mere' leader of a particular session to say, 'Look, this is a very motley group of people whose behavioural difficulties trigger each other, *and* the staffing is inadequate to ensure full participation.' This, of course, throws a different light on perceived staff failure and service-users' challenging behaviour. So, with this tiny piece of data, it seems we learned quite a bit about clients and their needs in a direct sense. We also learned that people do not know instinctively how to teach or how to lead, and might need development input rather than criticism; also that there was far too little consultation with the people destined to implement the grandiose plans of remote 'others'.

Developments

Partly as a result of this incident, I initiated a staff consultation process about the programme, in which all members of staff were invited to put forward their ideas about their own and others' sessions and their views regarding their understanding of users' needs. At first this was done in a series of meetings, but we found that this led the more vocal people to 'hold sway', so I also began to include the discussions as part of the supervision process, and to give staff private planning time to develop their ideas on paper. In many other instances, the data collection sheet proved useful, highlighting people who gained/did not gain by particular activities. Certainly for the cookery leader, it showed clearly that service-users could not manage the fine motor skills needed for the 'rubbing in' method whereas melting and stirring could be achieved by most. This resulted in a change of planning. We also realised that the cookery session 'ended' before the participants had had a chance to eat the goodies, and a change in timing resulted in some wonderful 'Mad Hatter'-type tea-parties, with others (including managers) invited to join in.

While much of the 'observation' type of data collecting was of a sit-and-watch nature, the behavioural therapy student (Gail Fisher) undertook far more structured observations. Her methods were far more formal and she used schedules developed as part of her course at the Tizzard Centre, Kent University. She observed one client, Robin, in order to learn more about the behaviours that we had considered 'challenging'. She was seeking information regarding his behaviours of incessant clapping, usually a prelude to great agitation, blowing his nose in his hand and smearing the mucus, overturning furniture and attacking other people. She began by using a method of observing for one minute in five. This revealed almost none of the behaviours. After further discussion with the staff team, we decided to keep 'ABC' charts. This involved recording the *Antecedents* (prior to the targeted behaviour – e.g. 'the room was noisy'), a factually based recording of the *Behaviour* (not 'he was angry' but 'he tipped over the table'), and the *Consequences* (e.g. 'I asked him to stop', 'I took him from the room'). A fortnight of this sort of data collection revealed that Robin's most vulnerable times were transition times, i.e. moving from one session to another, coming into the centre, and going home. Gail then changed her method to continual observation for set periods at the identified crucial times.

All this revealed a great deal about Robin's behaviours. It also revealed a great deal about centre dynamics, session planning and suitability, e.g. the fact that people deemed to have 'challenging' behaviours are left alone if quiet, on the understanding that one doesn't 'poke tigers'. It also showed that service-users often did not understand the communications staff used with them. Gail also asked me and Robin's 'key worker' (Joanne Morris) to observe alongside her, and we compared notes afterwards in order to check accuracy and validity. There weren't too many discrepancies, but there certainly were some, and this indicated the human frailties in all such undertakings. One example of a discrepancy was the fact that one of us defined the noted behaviour as 'attention seeking', another as 'task avoidance', and the third person missed the whole event. This form of observation also revealed that for 74% of the time there is *no* interaction between staff and clients, for 9% of the time there is negative interaction and for 19% of the time the interaction is positive. Gail also assured me that the figures for the Grasmere Road Centre are somewhat better than average.

We also used recorded staff meetings and individual discussions as a way of getting information and seeking people's views. This was also interesting. I usually minute staff meetings and tend to write what I think of as brief, succinct minutes reflecting our decisions. Reading them with a more 'analytic' eye, I realised that they also tend to reflect the issues that I regard as important. When Joanne Morris took notes alongside me, her notes revealed a more 'chatty' style' and her emphasis was different. Thus, I noted the need to have more activities in the base groups (an issue dear to my heart), and while Joanne gave this a mention too, she also listed many small details suggested by the staff group to enhance their sessions and to reduce challenging behaviour. I therefore decided that minute-taking should also be a turn-taking activity for those keen to do it.

It is important to note that much of the data that became available through our work were not 'new' data, collected for this research, but data that were already there but not used or acknowledged. The data collected by the language and speech therapist during her assessments of clients' language and comprehension ability are one example.

Data analysis

Fuller and Petch (1995: 81–6) present some very sophisticated tables and charts and a system called 'coding', into which our shambolic data refused to fit. Nevertheless, although our approach to research was rather 'unstructured', our staff meetings and the topics *were* planned and staff members knew the issues to be discussed. We also tried to keep minutes of the meetings to give to people who were not present. Eventually these were given out to all those involved, present or not, and we also occasionally tried to have two note-takers in order to record varied views (see above). Many other discussions were informal in the extreme, and often involved staff stopping in the office or a corridor to say, 'By the way, I was thinking last night about . . .', and much of the information gained like this was extremely valuable. However, it had the disadvantage of making it difficult to keep all group members informed about all the ideas and information being generated.

One example of such information shattered the view previously held by me and most of the staff group, that there is not enough planning time for 'good-quality work'. Staff arrive for work at 9 a.m., and the service-users begin to arrive at about 9.10. Staff work until 4.30 p.m., and service-users tend to leave the centre at 3.45.

This leaves a little time at the end of each day for tidying, staff supervisions and staff meetings. One staff member suggested collecting some of these small, not very useful periods of time, adding them to Tuesday's working hours to make a finishing time of 5 p.m., and going home a little earlier on Thursdays and Fridays. This had the effect of helping us to celebrate 'le weekend' while giving us a more useful period of time for work planning on Tuesday afternoons. Mondays and Wednesdays remained the same to allow for staff meetings and supervision time.

I have a lingering regret that our research 'data' are so informal and lack the perceived authority of the 'white-coated research expert'. However, I am aware that such research would have been received with scepticism, and that ours has been accepted by staff precisely because it is just that, *ours*, and has come about by a process of evolutionary development. It would also have been extremely difficult for data like ours to have been collected from non-verbal clients by a researcher unfamiliar with the group. The problem may be stated using Goffman's theory of communication (Puddicombe, 1995: 29–30). Goffman distinguishes between two forms of communication – 'giving' and 'giving off'. 'Giving' communication is the straightforward use of words to be understood by the other person in the way in which they are spoken. 'Giving off' is less deliberate, less clear and more to do with the perceptions of the listener. As people with no language have no practice or tools for using 'giving' styles of communication, our service-users are left with the more ambiguous style of 'giving off', which requires the communication partner (e.g. staff) to be able to suspend their own complex techniques for long enough to find ways to understand. This is a daunting task for any researcher, but infinitely more so for one with no knowledge of the often very idiosyncratic communication systems of people with severe learning disabilities.

The research group

In my project proposal, I anticipated that the action research would be carried out by a fairly small group of staff and associated members. This group was to include several members of staff from the various base groups, the speech and language therapist, a manager from another centre who is also a behavioural therapy student currently studying at Kent University, two parents and me. There was a significant lack of service-users' input in this group, and this was a situation that I did not resolve, although much of the data collected does (I hope) reflect service-users' views.

I was also aware of the conflicts of my own role as both manager and research group member. There was a strong possibility that I would only see and hear what I wanted to or would only be told what people wanted me to know. There was also the staff perception that to make criticisms of an area of service provision could feel like 'grassing' on one's colleagues. I also had the action research input at college and began my project with a vague feeling of intellectual superiority of which

I was soon disabused. Several staff were attending courses on teaching adults and bandied about such phrases as 'lesson plans' and 'teaching outcomes', where I was considered to be a babe in arms. My confidence regarding the eventual success of the action research process was also, at this stage, not very high. Most important of all, the project ceased to be 'mine' almost immediately, and was claimed by a lot of other people, in some very diverse ways.

For example, Gail Fisher, the behaviour therapy student, based several of her university assignments upon the work she did in Grasmere Road, and in return gave us invaluable information about our clients, our services, and the dynamics of our group. She also devised a process for changing the service for one client (Robin, see above) that helped us in our thinking about many others. She also gave several teaching sessions for the whole staff group about autism, challenging behaviour and its management, and set up systems for evaluating the whole process. This evaluation involves keeping records of user behaviour, participation and awareness, both before intervention and after intervention. She also helped us to analyse what we collected by way of evaluation material.

The parents in the group, who had been involved with Grasmere Road staff in a 'partnership' initiative to evaluate our services, also showed a deeper understanding of our difficulties than I had expected – including the staffing difficulties, the larger political arena and the issues relating to such a large centre, with such diversity of needs. They participated less than I would have liked in our action research project, but as one mother explained: 'We have been involved in the teaching and education of our children much longer than "normal" parents. Now that he is 30, I rely on you to care, and I try to get on with my life.' I have to accept that as an important statement.

The language and speech therapist was invaluable. She had completed some in-depth assessments as part of her working role with users, and made these readily available to us. She also highlighted some staff development issues, and this resulted in some training in total communication methods, with more in-depth training planned. She also worked with the staff to develop some visual timetables for users, but more of that later.

I had envisaged that some staff would be very interested and involved, and that some would not participate at all. This was not an accurate view. Certainly a small group of staff have been intensely interested and have done a great deal of work, well beyond anything their employment role would require. However, most staff have had some degree of involvement, certainly in discussions regarding changes to the daily rota programmes, and much of what they had to say has been very valuable. One of the group met with others in the county to develop craft sessions with viable products that users could take to a selling outlet. She also worked with the language and speech therapist to develop communication books and visual timetables. Another group member investigated the MOVE process (motivation via education), which enables severely physically disabled people to achieve maximum movement and thus to enhance their areas of control, choice and autonomy. One senior member of staff returning from a long maternity leave said,

'The place feels different, staff seem much more involved, more positive. I don't know why.' This member of staff also had some useful suggestions for involving the more reticent people in the planning.

The results of the action research process

The above heading should be firmly qualified by the words 'so far', as the process has, like Topsy, 'just growed'.

The data gathered by Gail Fisher, the behavioural therapy student, made me feel suddenly overcome by a 'light on the road to Damascus', but this light, far from being blinding, was illuminating. We had actually got it wrong. We were still working to our traditional programme, and we were 'tweaking' it to make it 'fit'. Our precious rota was actually standing in the way of the changes that Gail was suggesting, based on her work with Robin.

I had considered Robin in my original assignment proposal. He seemed ill-served by the sessions and the teaching that he was receiving, and he was repeatedly disrupting sessions, appearing aggressive, smearing mucus and often seemingly agitated and distressed. Her investigations had shown that his condition ('Fragile X Syndrome') is frequently accompanied by autism. Recent research at the Center for the Study of Autism in Salem, Oregon, USA (http://www.autism.com/), suggests that people with this condition are affected in three areas of function: they have serious communication difficulties, difficulties in social functioning, and impairment of imaginative function. Why, then, were we offering him art and craft sessions, music sessions in large and complex groups, and sessions with no clear beginnings, middles and endings that must torture his mind in its desire for concrete activities? Why, too, was such a young man with this particular condition leading such a sedentary life? Further investigation revealed that many syndromes have autism as an additional effect, suggesting that at least ten of our twenty-five clients might have autistic tendencies.

The language and speech therapist assessed many of our client group as having a language understanding based on single words. This means that sentences were confusing to them, and that the key word in every sentence needed to be clearly stated, or they would be both confused and implacable when asked to do things. It also meant that they have little concept of what is going to happen to them, of when they are to start an activity or when they are to finish. This meant that though staff practice was good and clients are *told* what is going to happen, they may actually have very little comprehension of what they are told. Therefore their day is a muddle over which they have little control or knowledge. The speech therapist and key workers therefore developed an 'object-of-reference' timetable. This is a set of hooks, on which small objects are hung with string. For example, Robin is currently working with a small plastic cup (to indicate having a drink), a trainer shoe (to indicate going out for a walk), a sponge bag (to indicate washing his hands), and a spoon to indicate food/lunch time. Robin puts items onto his board at the beginning of the day with the help of staff, and as each session is due to take place the object is removed (by Robin himself, if possible), spoken about and returned to the storage box after the activity has happened.

We also decided that many of our sessions were too similar to those offered to children in nursery schools. This is a familiar feature of activities for those with profound learning disabilities and ignores the adult status of the recipient of such services. It also does not teach skills to enable social inclusion. We therefore agreed that programmes and activities should reflect real tasks, rather than invented ones. These included teaching people to wash their cup after a drink, to collect their own knife and fork for lunch (a very appropriate 'object of reference' for lunch) and to clear the table when the meal is over. Because Robin blows his nose into his hand, a hand-washing programme also seemed appropriate for him. These tasks are immensely complicated for our service-users and require many teaching sessions.

We also rerouted the centre bus, enabling those who were capable to walk some of the way into the centre. This has had the effect of calming much of the agitated behaviour, since it uses surplus energy and improves fitness, including that of the staff member who walks with the clients.

For staff at the centre there have also been changes.

1   Staff identified a need for training in 'total communication' systems and more use of communication aids. Training in both areas has taken place.
2   Staff have been consulted about the people in their sessions, and have been invited to make proposals for changes to the sessions. Key workers have also put forward specific ideas for their own clients.
3   Staff identified difficulties in carrying out physiotherapy input for clients, especially as the health authority had withdrawn professional support due to financial restraints. In this area too, staff have received support and training. One senior member of staff, identified as being particularly skilled in this area, was scheduled to undertake staff training and oversee the clients' physical programmes.
4   Changes were proposed to the 'sacred' rota, so as to allow more time in 'base groups' to develop services and sessions more in keeping with clients' identified needs. (When this has been introduced we will then begin again the process of data collecting, to see if we have got it 'right'.)
5   One of the day centre officers, Maureen McCarthy, is seeking to involve occupational therapy and physiotherapy professionals in her work on the MOVE process mentioned above. This would enable many of our physically disabled users to achieve a standing position for periods of time each day, thus giving them a 'normal' view of the world while building stores of calcium into unused bones and relieving stress upon internal organs.
6   Groups of staff will receive help to enable them to undertake specific tasks such as leading communication and choice sessions, and (physiotherapy-based) stretch and exercise programmes preceded by massage and relaxation sessions.

However, we are only just beginning and have a long way to go yet. These changes are just a pilot scheme for a few people who are not physically disabled. Another group, with very limited mobility, wait in the wings for changes specific to their needs.

Evaluation: dilemmas and issues

1   I have not found it possible to involve profoundly disabled service-users in a way that is based on *their* declared needs for service. We have tried, by collecting data, reading body language, developing 'objects of reference', photograph books and symbol timetables, to involve users in their service provision, but it all remains very subjective: users can only choose from the symbols *we* provide.
2   The national government and European agencies are moving towards making monetary grants for work with people with learning difficulties dependent upon success in areas of supported employment. Managers are being asked to consider using artwork etc. as a saleable commodity. In contrast, I am moving away from this towards basic self-care skills. Am I moving users away from sources of money that will develop services? Grants and finance depend upon 'output', but how does one measure a decrease in severely challenging behaviour and an increase in positive communication, in order to seek a grant? I also have a duty towards a department that is 'strapped for cash'.
3   I cut my social work teeth on theories of 'normalisation', but 'the normal' (for clients with profound learning disabilities) now looks very simple and basic: people in their thirties and older learning how to ask for a drink. I seem to have narrowed client choices, as research suggests that people with autism and profound learning disabilities have great difficulty coping with wide areas of choice. We have tried to make their world feel safer by making it more concrete. However, most of us live happily in worlds that are shades of grey. Suppose we are wrong?
4   Parents and carers often want very sheltered services for people with such profound disabilities. We have followed a policy of parental involvement and information. Sometimes this means spending a great deal of time with parents, reassuring them and persuading them to let their sons or daughters spread their wings a little. But who am I to add complications to already complicated lives?
5   There is the dilemma of working within a large bureaucracy. Recruitment is slow and bound by a policy of nil external advertising. This leads to limited applicants for posts. But this project has made me feel that there needs to be a change in some of our recruitment procedures, in order to obtain a more proactive staff group.
6   Staff were recruited for very different requirements and their job is changing. Many are eager to push the changes forward but some are having difficulty, feeling merely tolerated rather than valued, and I feel a duty of care towards

them. But I also have a duty of care towards clients, whom staff are there to serve. This presents a difficult dilemma for those who find change hard. This is especially fraught at present, with a day care review in full swing and people already concerned about job changes and possible losses. There are staff training and development issues that need addressing and my own feelings towards changes in my own job make me wary of beginning.

Conclusions from the project so far

In a personal sense, I am amazed at the awareness engendered by the project. For my own part, I had not realised how controlling I like to be. I had fully absorbed statements like 'person-centred life planning' and 'client-centred services', and yet still managed to maintain a traditional, hierarchical approach to decision-making, which actually made it difficult to provide 'client-centred' services. Fuller and Petch (1995: 9) would call this 'habit blindness'.

The project has also made definite differences to the way we provide services. It has made it possible to explore the ideas of many of the staff group, as opposed to just a few. It has also been possible to delegate some of the responsibility for the way services are given. I feel that I can ask others to investigate issues, and they usually do this very well. Looking back at the initial staff critique of the Grasmere Road Centre (see p. 120 above), we have picked up on the time restraints, and staff have participated in the data collection and have contributed to the development of new services. Hopefully, we are also beginning to encourage a genuinely client-centred emphasis on independence and ordinary life skills. For better or worse, it would not be easy, now, to take the initiative away from staff who have picked it up so willingly, even though I found it so hard, at first, to 'let go'.

It is also an amazingly inexpensive way to develop services, involving mind shifts as opposed to new buildings or equipment purchase. Despite the inadequacies of buildings and budgets, there is little we have been unable to do because of those constraints. Even the need for additional staffing will probably be achieved, to some degree, by different deployment of staff.

On the deficit side, it has also been a time of anxiety, as change is not easy to cope with and routines give a feeling of safety. But this is just the beginning of the project. Who knows where it will end?

References

Dowson, S. (1997) 'Empowerment within services: a comfortable delusion?', in P. Ramcharan, G. Grant, J. Berland and G. Roberts (eds) (1997) *Empowerment in Everyday Life*, London: Jessica Kingsley, pp. 101–19.

Elliot, J. (1993) *Action Research for Educational Change*, Milton Keynes: Open University Press.

Fuller, R. and Petch, A. (eds) (1995) *Practitioner Research*, Milton Keynes: Open University Press.

Kemmis, S. and McTaggart, R. (1982) *The Action Research Planner*, Geelong, Victoria: Deakin University Press.

McNiff, J. (1994) *Action Research Practice and Principles*, London: Routledge.

Puddicombe, B. (1995) *Face to Face*, London: Values into Action Publishers.

Simpson, M. and Tuson, J. (1995) *Using Observation in Small Scale Research*, Edinburgh: Scottish Council for Research in Education.

Wertheimer, A. (1996) *Changing Days*, London: King's Fund.

Winter, R. (1989) *Learning from Experience*, Lewes: Falmer Press.

Chapter 9

Researching the experiences of black professionals in white organisations
An example from social work

Cathy Aymer

This chapter looks at how a group of black professional workers used the 'co-operative inquiry' methodology to research their experiences in the social work profession and in higher education. It outlines the development of the inquiry process from the initial ideas through to the practical strategies and how these led to new understandings and new questions about how black professionals can survive within white organisations and find a place that honours their contributions. Thus, it describes the beginning of a research process which was part of a larger research programme. Although many people were involved in this inquiry this is my account of the process and my attempts to make sense of what happened (see Acknowledgement, p. 144).

Thinking and formulating questions

The research grew out of a conversation in the corridor, at work, between a colleague and me, two black women, both of whom are teachers of social work in a university. It began in the form of an exasperated question. 'Why is it that when we read about the experiences of black students on social work courses they are always negative?' We were able to ask such a question because we knew from our experiences as lecturers working with black students that while there were some who viewed their experience as negative, there were many for whom the experience had been extremely positive and yet others for whom the experience had been mixed. We also recognised that while, in public, students would sometimes be critical of their experiences, these same students would seek us out in private to let us know about the positive effects that the course had had on their lives, as well as on the lives of their children. So we had knowledge that black students had positive or mixed stories to tell as well as the negative ones that were so often and so well documented. The silence surrounding black people's achievements and successes on social work courses and in the profession was deafening.

We were very concerned that if these stories were not being told, how would the black community know of its successes? How would other black people be encouraged to follow the path into higher education and into the professional world if the experience was relentlessly portrayed as negative? We wanted to be able to tell stories that did not leave out the positives and would challenge the dominant story about how black people should experience the world. We wanted to gain authorship of a different set of stories that we felt had come out of our experiences, and that, we were certain, other black people were experiencing. Schon's (1983) view of reflective practitioners, people who formulate and explore their tacit knowledge and understanding of their practice, is of utmost importance here. Coupled with this is the ability to hold a self-critical stance towards one's professional practice.

The first task that we engaged in was to write down our thoughts separately and then come together to talk and share our ideas, so that we could lay the foundation stones on which we could build our work. The nature of these early conversations created a great deal of energy and excitement for us. We were in fact beginning to share our stories together for the first time, preparing the groundwork for collaboration and co-operation with each other. What was remarkable was that although we had been working together for about four years and were friendly in our interactions, it was only in the process of these discussions and early writings that we began to know something of the other and learn more about our individual identities. As we approached the questions we were asking we had to go through a process of formulating, clarifying and re-clarifying our ideas and in so doing I became more confident about my personal and professional identity.

We asked ourselves questions about what it means to be black as professionals and as lecturers working in higher education. For example: 'What are the assumptions we hold about other black people as we encounter them in the world?' 'How do we know what other black people think when they encounter us in the world?' Needless to say, we also asked similar questions about our encounters with white people. We tested our ideas tentatively at first, but as we became more confident in our intentions, purposes and motives we were able at times to 'say the unsayable'. What I mean by this is the recognition that in the discourse of race there is a private world and a public world, that some things may not be said in public for fear of accusations of disloyalty and fear of being ridiculed by other black people, and in the belief that some things must be kept private within the black community. Not only did such discussions focus our thinking, but we came to ask ourselves fundamental questions about the nature of black people's psychological development. We were able to think about how that psychology, mediated through the damaging effects of racism, might limit our development and cause black people to be unable to fully encounter each other in either the private or the public arenas we inhabit.

Much later, my analysis of this phenomenon of conflict between the public and private domains was helped by reading Fukuyama's book *Trust: the Social Virtues and the Creation of Prosperity* (1996). Although I do not share Fukuyama's orientation to think of progress in terms of economic growth, his analysis of high trust and low trust societies assisted my thinking by focusing my attention on the general notion of trust. Inequalities, social division and the pervasive influence of racism at all levels within British society all help to create a low trust society.

How can black people 'trust' their experiences in British society, when so much of what happens to us is diminishing and spiritually disruptive to the self? The obvious effect of this low trust society is that relationships between black people and white people are entered into with a legacy of suspicion, anger and mistrust. At the same time there are no mechanisms by which black people can encounter each other in a truly authentic manner, free from the damaging effects of racism, so black–black encounters often have some of the same characteristics as black–white encounters.

While people work in organisations to satisfy their individual needs, the organisation also draws people out of their private lives and into the wider social world, so that it becomes a place where they seek to have their dignity recognised (i.e. evaluated at its proper worth) by others. Living in a low trust society means that people who are not related to each other will only co-operate under a system of formal rules and regulations. Race relations and equal opportunities legislation testify to this, but this legal apparatus serves as a *substitute for trust* and creates what Fukuyama terms 'transaction costs', so that low trust societies levy a type of 'tax', which represents an emotional and spiritual burden on all its members, and one which particularly affects the lives of black people in organisations. I suppose I am suggesting that this tax is too much to pay and I really have no wish to continue to pay it.

To sum up, it is only by the creation of some sense of moral responsibility, either in a society or in an organisation, that there will be any degree of trust between people of different races. Underlying this research, therefore, is a search for a cultural renewal, which is about developing a type of morality that will allow 'trust' to re-enter the system.

This emphasis on the theme of trust places our work within the debate about insider versus outsider research. There are some black researchers who believe that only researchers from the same social group as the 'subjects' of the research can be adequate interpreters of their experience. There are others who, not unlike some white researchers, challenge the claim that insiders have a monopoly on understanding the social groups from which they originate. This is not a new debate; it mirrors earlier debates about women researching the lives of women. For myself, I am absolutely convinced that my autobiography, my identity and the historical context in which I live not only matter, but will influence what I observe or do not observe, how I think and how I make sense of material and what type of knowledge I am able to make.

At the start of this inquiry, therefore, I had implicitly accepted the insider position and continue to do so. But I also continue to hold with the idea that identity, historical context and biography are contingent, and therefore I may not hold this position for all time. It was with the acknowledgement of this insider stance that we set out to bring a group of black people together in order to set up the research. The fact that we were black people researching with other black people did not mean that we did not run the risk of just confirming the status quo about black lives, nor does it mean that our scholarship will be given a positive reception.

Hindsight

Some time after the project was well under way, my colleague and I were giving a paper about our research at a seminar where there was one other black person, a woman in the social work education field. The paper had been distributed beforehand and as she sat next to me I could see that she had underlined the term 'black on black' in the text. She was the first person to comment, questioning directly why we had described this as a black on black study. I was rather taken aback by this as it had seemed such a natural thing to do. Now, I had to question the taken for granted: research is never described as a 'white on white' study because 'white' is seen to represent the norm and is thus, in some sense, 'not an ethnicity'.

Preparing the ground

The next phase was to consider how we could gather together those stories that we knew existed out there in the world. While continuing our general thinking, we started to devise a methodology for our work. At first we devised a three-part strategy:

1   to write to black students who had qualified from our course asking whether they would be willing to take part in a research project in which we would interview them about their experiences on the course, and to ascertain their career trajectories and experiences within their organisations;
2   to study the personal files of the students in these cohorts;
3   to contact prominent black practitioners and managers, and conduct interviews about their experiences.

During the early discussions I had had a vague idea about 'doing something with groups' but this could not be articulated properly until we discovered the work of Heron (1996) and Reason (1988) and the ideas surrounding co-operative inquiry in particular and action research in general. The ideas appealed to us strongly, and we immediately picked up the ball and began to run with it. We maintained our three-part strategy but we subsumed it within the larger project that would be built on these ideas of co-operative inquiry and the building of a community of inquiry. This methodology seemed ready-made for us: what better way to understand this than to start a co-operative inquiry group of our own?

The invitation

Another colleague joined us and we sent out invitations to two cohorts of our ex-students to tell them about the ideas we had for research and to ask if they would be interested in being contacted again to work with us on the project. Even though it is notoriously difficult to get answers to unsolicited questionnaires, the response from this group was over 50%. There may be at least two reasons for the high response. First, each person knew one or other of us and felt some personal commitment to respond to a known individual, and second, as we believed, this was an idea whose time had come.

During our earlier discussions we had postulated a typology of adaptations that black students went through when on the social work course, and we had posed the question as to whether these adaptations are seen in practice settings (Aymer and Bryan, 1996). So we invited two other groups of black professionals at different stages in their career development to inquire with us into our experiences. So, implicitly, we were investigating the possibility that different levels of professional maturity may create different experiences and different ways of being within an organisation as well as in personal life. The professional groups were middle managers, and social work lecturers and trainers.

In the end we invited a group of fifty people to spend a day with us, exploring ideas about black people's experiences in organisations, both as students and lecturers in institutions of higher education and as practitioners and managers in social work agencies. We used the term 'seminar' at that time, but in reality we were inviting people to join a co-operative inquiry group, in which the inquiry process would have parallels with the storytelling tradition in our own backgrounds. We were hoping to set up the possibility that these black professionals would feel a resonance with this, and want to engage with us in the telling of their (and also our) stories. Choosing those to invite is the start of the process and is itself a political and ethical choice.

The first 'seminar' meeting

Preparations

If we were really to manage the process of what we believed co-operative inquiry to be and in particular the first stages, the type of experience that we would have on the day would be a complex one. We devised a programme that looked like this:

- We would give input that outlined our starting point, our interests and our motivations. This would also introduce the participants to the methodology of co-operative inquiry.
- Participants would then divide into groups which would focus on an area of interest. Each group would be led by one of the facilitators (see below).
- The whole group would come together to share experiences and devise further questions for the inquiry.
- Out of this we would establish the possibility for 'inquiry groups', made up of practitioners, managers and educationalists (lecturers and trainers).
- This would be followed by final feedback from the discussion groups, to draw out the themes that would later be developed and explored in the three inquiry groups.

- Participants would then be invited to join one or other of the inquiry groups. We were aware of the need to include definite information about what they would be contracting into.
- This would be followed by the setting of a new date, when those who wished to proceed could come and make an actual commitment to start an inquiry group that would be in existence for approximately six months.

We also discussed how to raise awareness with colleagues of what we were trying to accomplish with this research, i.e. the need to make interventions in the work environment. So I posed the question, 'How would the inquiry affect my professional practice in the day-to-day work in my department?' This was an important aspect for me to bear in mind and review as the inquiry developed.

The other questions that arose concerned the process of the inquiry and the organisation of the day. How should we handle negotiating the contract with the group? Should we just let it emerge? What exactly were the purposes of the group? As the discussions went on, it became clear to me that our preparations should concentrate on mapping the issues and the path, instead of posing and answering the final questions. It was apparent that we needed to think about different strategies for creating the maximum amount of data, as well as the practical functions that my colleagues and I would have to carry out over the life of the groups. These practical considerations included: (1) getting the group to sanction the use of tape recordings of the discussions; (2) the type of group facilitation that we would adopt that would demonstrate our collaborative intent while leaving space for our individuality; (3) thinking through and handling the issues of authority and trust that might be uncovered.

The outcome of this type of thinking and planning was to help us to name the process (for the participants and for ourselves), and to pose questions about the nature and quality of the reflection that would be necessary to make sense of the work we were embarking on. This was one aspect of the process of legitimation for this type of research and for data gathered in this manner.

Inviting facilitators

We decided that we could not manage the seminar process on our own, and agreed to invite a group of people we knew to be experienced facilitators to assist us with co-ordinating the day's activities. We envisaged them acting as enablers, drawing out stories from the participants in a sensitive manner. However, the facilitators became a vital part of the design of the broad strategy, although we had not anticipated how absorbed they would become in the whole process. The setting up of the facilitators' group was another aspect of the process of legitimation. We chose five people to assist us as facilitators, all of them black. They were: a management consultant known to my colleague and not a member of the social work profession; a lecturer on another social work course known to both of us; a senior manager in a voluntary organisation; a senior manager in a statutory organisation; and a course director of a youth and community course.

The meetings of the facilitators' group

The intention was that this group of experienced facilitators would only meet for a short time to discuss the mechanics of the day. Instead, we met for half a day on four occasions to discuss our stories and experiences, and the meetings of the facilitators' group created further material for the main inquiry. The people working in higher education told similar stories to my colleague and me about their work with students, and these were also echoed in other people's experiences. Some of the stories generated a general mood of fun and excitement as we recounted tales of survival, transcendence and, above all, the desire to move beyond our present situations and develop something new and exciting. There was real energy in the facilitators' group: enthusiasm for the project was overwhelming and the discovery of connectedness was refreshing and sustaining.

These meetings highlighted one of the main functions of the facilitators' group, namely to listen for emerging questions and record their essence. In this project much emphasis is placed on the notion of storytelling. But storytelling can lead to the notion of victim. Why should black people meet to reinforce stories of being victims? It is necessary to remember that any one story is only part of the picture, so the notion of storytelling as a research approach was one that needed to be explored. What type of narratives would be told and how would we begin to analyse them? This deserves greater exploration and is taken up again later. The facilitators' group became a process of *owning a responsibility* to black professionals and *recognising* that by wishing to tell a different story we were engaging in a subversive act. How we would define and measure success was an important question left unanswered. Finding the question was more important at that point than finding the answer.

At the final meeting of the group before the day of the seminar, we devised a set of 'prompts' for the facilitators to assist them and us in managing the group process.

- Why do we talk ourselves out of success?
- Why are we fixated in a victim role (do we believe different things in public and in private)?
- What areas of life do we have control over and how do we know that we have?
- What are the criteria for trusting, and how long does it take you to trust your fellow black student/colleague?
- What stops anyone from taking the risk of forming an alliance with another black person?
- If we are not in total agreement with each other, how can we find ways to disagree?
- How can we reduce the suspicion that creates barriers between us?

Part of the purpose of these questions was to help us to focus on the idea of returning to an intuitive /authentic self which could interact with another black person. After all, to do other than concentrate on the negatives might mean that we have to engage in a struggle, where our individual psychology interacts with the group psychology. This generates a distorted sense of reality for a lot of black professionals, who find themselves continually involved in a series of confusions. The facilitators were asked to stress that we pay attention to hearing the questions (which are sources of information) and that the question was as important as the solution. The feedback would report the key points that were explored and the groups would present two or three new questions that they had generated in the course of their deliberations.

Finally, we agreed that, following the presentations to the whole group giving information about the project and its methodology, the participants would be divided into three groups, the managers, the practitioners and the educationalists. Although we felt that these were logical groupings, we also tested them out with the participants.

The outcome of the seminar

This first meeting was successful in that we were able to collect a vast amount of 'data', and the response to joining the subsequent groups was extremely positive. An outstanding feature of the day was that the participants stayed until the end because they were so engrossed in what was happening. Judi Marshall has spoken of 'a collecting space to which people come willing' (Marshall, 1998). This is exactly what it was. What made it so? After all, we might have issued the invitations and waited, and nobody came. I can think of three possible reasons.

- Timeliness: I fully believe that this was an idea whose time had come and people were in a state of readiness.
- The network: people either knew us or knew of us or had heard that we were OK. There was an implicit trust in us and in the process.
- Connection: the way in which the space was created meant that we were able to make connection in a way that allowed people to feel safe enough to respond.

The inquiry groups

The day ended with a request for volunteers to constitute the three inquiry groups (practitioners, managers, and educationalists/trainers), and there was no shortage of willing participants. My colleague and I were to facilitate these groups. We anticipated that they would function as follows.

Practitioners' group

This group was seen as the nucleus of the community of inquiry which should generate rich material in terms of testing ideas about the negative and positive experiences of being a student and/or practitioner. It would also:

- provide data on successes and explore the career trajectories of black workers in social work;

- explore whether there were differences between a public voice and a private voice;
- provide ideas about interactions between black practitioners and explore differences resulting from whether black people are seen to be the majority or the minority.

Managers' group

This group would offer data on the interactions between black managers and black practitioners. It would:

- explore how black people develop an identity as black managers and assess the impact this has on black practitioners;
- identify and analyse what they see in the workplace concerning the interactions between black practitioners and managers.

Educationalists'/lecturers' group

The purposes of this group would be:

- to tell the black lecturers' stories, i.e. find the black lecturers'/educationalists' voice, tracking our journeys;
- to provide analysis of the context, i.e. analyse the state of social work education from a black perspective;
- to analyse and review our roles in relation to black students;
- to explore how we are seen by black students, white students, black colleagues, white colleagues and the educational institution.

The groups then met for a period of approximately six months. Initiation and contracting represented a very structured stage of the work, to ensure that the process was appropriate and enabling. An example from this stage was the negotiation of the tape recording of the sessions. A clear decision was made that the sessions could be taped but that at any time a member could switch off the tape. There were questions to be asked about ownership of the material that were not made explicit then, but there was implicit permission for us as initiators and facilitators to go ahead and make sure that the stories became public. It is a difficult task to ensure that this trust is honoured in the most appropriate and useful way.

The emerging themes

What is now being described is only a small part of the outcome of a lengthy period of research. Three main themes emerged from the work of the project. These were: (1) encounter and trust; (2) identity/belonging; and (3) success.

Encounter and trust

The question 'What do we look for in a black person or a group of black people when we meet them for the first time?' (or one very similar) was asked by all the groups, and proved to be a fundamental question for all of us. It helped us to explore more widely the ways in which black people interact and seek meanings at all levels. This theme is referred to elsewhere in the chapter and provides its main theoretical perspective. Discussions on this theme helped us to identify and make attempts to repair some of the damage caused to black–black encounters. One participant pointed out:

'We are always looking at each other suspiciously when we meet each other, "checking" each other out until they prove themselves. How can we work out whether another black person is OK or not OK?'

Another speculated:

'I believe we have a fear of being open, honest and trusting of each other.'

Such thinking was important in helping us to examine our expectations of each other, to name the pain that was experienced because of suspicion and mistrust, and to understand how and why conflict could result from our encounters with each other. The focus was then to work out how to promote more healthy and productive encounters.

Belonging

The theme of belonging was not surprising as black people are often forced to consider how and whether they belong. The early sessions were taken up with questions about who we were, what we could become and how we could engage fully in our organisations. One participant was very clear:

'I am British and I like being British. There are countervailing forces that prevent us from being able to say that and we need to find out what they are. The common experience is that it is reinforced in all kinds of ways that we don't really have the right. Where do we get the confidence to assert this?'

This was seen as a crucial issue for British black people: we are very unsure about our sense of belonging. In many ways we are forced into taking on the ethnicity of our parents, into feeling that we don't really belong here, that this is just a temporary sojourn after which we will return home.

'Young people – suppose you ask them their nationality, they will say Caribbean, Asian, African. It hasn't been put across to them in a clear intellectual argument why this question has been posed.'

One of the participants reminded us that middle-class families in any society do well because there is a sense of them having the right to be there. There are role models, people have a place in the literature, and they have a strong sense of self from the culture. But the group was reminded that the Nationality Act, 1981, meant that black people lost their right to be citizens by virtue of being born in this country, and that this Act set out to exclude rather than to include. This was a legal method of trying to disenfranchise black people, notwithstanding that the requirements for patriality (i.e. that one's grandparents were British) will eradicate themselves in due course and black people will qualify automatically for full citizenship.

Many people spoke of the richness of our experiences and how it must be possible for us to take control, write our own experiences, write our own biographies and accept that these are valid. It was seen as refreshing although it was sometimes difficult to speak about the positive.

'It is refreshing to get a group of people together and it's not just about how awful it is – the experiences are similar.'

'James Baldwin said that to be black and conscious is to be in a constant state of rage. Social work courses expose people and make them more conscious about racism and inequality.'

The same could be said for black professionals in organisations.

'Compared to our white counterparts, how hard have we worked to get to the same place? Given our abilities we should be at a better place.'

People often felt isolated and therefore exposed in their own workplaces, and this could lead them to concentrate on all the negative things. This is why it can be so difficult to resolve conflict with each other when we work in a team setting. This was to be a recurring issue throughout the life of the groups.

Success

This theme was taken up by all groups but was particularly explored by the educationalists.

'What is the nature of success? Pre-Thatcher, people emigrated from the Caribbean, for instance, one brother comes to Britain and one goes to the United States. There were different outcomes in their life chances. This has changed. On any high street in Britain we can see the trappings of success for both black and white.'

There was much discussion about how we measure success and how we should define the variables. Ideas such as black self-concept and self-worth were discussed. It was thought that there would be a correlation between a strong self-concept and high view of success.

'Success depends on what is your notion of self. Success is not a single entity definition. There is the success that's about movement that you accredit yourself and there's success about movement that is accredited to you by society.'

This participant went on to point out that we have a framework in which to define success and a mindset that creates a framework. The very nature of asking the question helps us to change. As a means of illustrating this he asked the group to identify two areas in which they had been successful. However, the responses show that this was not so simple. One person said:

'It depends what you mean by success.'

But another made the comment:

'Overcoming obstacles. We cannot overestimate the barriers we have to overcome in order to name our successes.'

Once he had given illustrations people were able to record their successes such as passing a driving test, but first it was necessary to set the psychological space for this to happen.

There are different positions from which people approach the professional arena. Some started off naïve, some started with a measure of awareness, and others are firmly rooted in political awareness. They see their qualification as a means to an end and they have few illusions. Some became exhausted by the struggle; they are unable to live it every day, all day. Worst of all, the changing nature of the task they are asked to do means that the goalposts are moving, not fixed. The nature of discrimination itself is not fixed. However, we were reminded that going through the process of discrimination is part of growing up in white society: ideas about gender, class and social justice are clearly written down, taught and given credibility. We therefore need to continue to research, to contribute to a body of knowledge about race that people can have access to and intellectualise and integrate into social policy and other parts of the curriculum.

Making these sorts of connections was crucial in helping us to learn from the encounters we were having. One of the key lessons learnt relates to the nature of oppression. One aspect is that it helps us to develop strengths. These strengths are skewed in the direction of survival. We can use these strengths as a starting point. We should not claim that they are dysfunctional but we have to move them over and develop new skills for doing much more than survive in this country and in our workplaces.

Making sense: an example of the cycle of action and reflection

In the practitioners' group the action–reflection cycling was made formal. After one session the members set the following tasks for themselves.

Margaret would notice her reactions and responses when she listens to black people in order to reflect on how she 'hears' other black people. *Cathy* (facilitator) would focus on her own ambivalence in situations and notice how she deals with it. *Denise* would notice what happens when somebody pays her a compliment, to try to understand why she is so dismissive of her own successes. *Alice* would take note of how she joined a 'large group' of black people and reflect on the psychological moment when, for her, a 'group' of black people became 'large'. *Christine* wanted to think about her levels of self-confidence and asked herself a very painful question in relation to her black colleagues: why do they hate me? *Christopher* would notice when he was being judgemental about black people who presented themselves as super-confident in groups.

The reporting back at the next session was very poignant, illustrated by Denise's story. She had recently left the course and started a job.

> *Denise reported that the next day she was complimented by a friend. She paid no attention to this and told herself that she was just being modest. But at the graduation ceremony, her mother, who had never praised her before, told Denise how proud she was. Denise still could not respond. Gloria who had been absent at the last meeting intervened and said that she could not even attend her graduation: deep down she could not accept or acknowledge her success – she was not brought up like that. Why? She thought that whatever we do was not good enough. We have internalised so much negativity at an early age and were conditioned to believe that there was so much out there that is not ours to achieve. We can't believe it's legitimate to have it. Denise listened to all this and responded, 'My education seems to be just beginning.'*

This seemed to me like enlightenment. Her sense of awe at this insight with its mixture of delight and sadness gives an example of the transformational nature of the space that was created within the work of the groups. In such spaces knowledge is created. This is the essence of the sense-making journey on which the groups embarked, the process of getting to the inside of our meanings.

Conclusion: the educationalists' story

The educationalists' group explored the relationships between black students and black teachers, focusing particularly on the theme of 'encounter and trust'. At the first level of connectedness, when contact is made with another black person, there are certain unspoken expectations that we have of each other and the group explored these expectations. Often the white world expects us to have a black perspective (if not *the* black perspective), but this can be very confining and limiting, as we can leave ourselves with the inability to have an appropriate means of disagreeing with each other without this leading to a feeling of betrayal. Sometimes black students perceive us (black lecturers) as authentic, at other times they can be suspicious of us for having joined the white academy. Yet we can never be sure about what they have seen that has made them take their position. Black people in positions of authority are often faced with a 'no win' situation. There is an expectation that we will be role models for others to emulate but we can also experience the projections of anger and envy.

One important revelation in this group was the understanding that experiences of racism are wounding to the psyche and this can lead to damage and destructive interactions between black people. What was strong in the group was a belief that education has the property to limit the damage and transform experiences. We are often left with the dilemma, however, of whether, as educators, we are part of the problem or part of the solution for black people. For example, many students come to the profession with a high degree of unfocused rage, which they interpret as radicalism. How can a black educator enable black students to move beyond the victim position by transforming this rage into a politics as well as ensuring their psychic well-being? After all, they may well turn that rage against us. It would seem that, at both conscious and unconscious levels, interactions between black people are 'fiery' interactions. As educators we were conscious of the need to work to bring out the best in black students and prevent them from getting stuck in unhelpful and unhealthy positions. But in order for trust to be established between us we have to be aware of the types of 'transaction costs' that may be exacted and find ways to refuse to pay the 'social and emotional taxes'.

Social work practitioners, whether in higher education or social work agencies, come to know and theorise about their practice through knowing-in-action and reflecting on their practice. Schon's (1983) view of the reflective practitioner is of someone who examines, formulates and tests tacit knowledge and understanding of his/her practice. Our co-operative inquiry helped us to throw light on some of our initial concerns and led to new understandings of practice. It thus provides a warrant for doing this type of research.

Acknowledgement

I would like to acknowledge the contribution of all those people who were involved with this project, in particular the practitioners, educationalists and managers who entrusted their stories to us.

I would also particularly like to thank my colleague, Agnes Bryan, and the facilitators: Fauzia Ahmad, Carlis Douglass, Lorna Francis, Trevor Sinclair, Anthony Sobers and Lorna White.

References

Aymer, C. and Bryan, A. (1996) 'Black students' experience of higher education: accentuating the positive', *British Journal of Social Work*, 26: 1–16.

Fukuyama, F. (1996) *Trust: the Social Virtues and the Creation of Prosperity*, London: Hamish Hamilton.

Heron, J. (1996) *Co-operative Inquiry: Research into the Human Condition*, London: Sage.

Reason, P. (1988) *Human Inquiry in Action: Developments in New Paradigm Research*, London: Sage.

Schon, D. (1983) *The Reflective Practitioner: How Professionals Think in Action*, New York: Basic Books.

Chapter 10

Community involvement in a bid for urban regeneration funds

Richard Lawrence

Introduction: the concept of 'community involvement'

The following case study illustrates the utility and limits of the collaborative action research approach when applied to the development of 'community involvement' in urban regeneration. The context of the work is an attempt by a local authority to further democratic community involvement via community development and collaborative action research in formulating a bid for Single Regeneration Budget (SRB) funding from central government. This funding can only be bid for by 'partnerships' consisting of representatives from the public, private, voluntary and community sectors. There is, in effect, a competition for SRB funding which all bidders enter. As well as this, bids have got to show that there is 'community involvement'. But what exactly is meant by 'community involvement'?

Community involvement is now encouraged by central government owing to the lessons learned from previous urban regeneration schemes which merely concentrated on regenerating the physical environment and (purposely) did nothing to address social problems. Urban regeneration throughout the 1990s encouraged the involvement of people living in a geographical area – referred to as 'the community' but, initially, not necessarily with strong community attachments. Thus, such initiatives could (and possibly should) be based on 'communitarian' values of solidarity, participation and coherence, but this would depend on the values of the facilitators of the particular regeneration programme or those of central government. They certainly draw upon the notion of the active community but realise that there is always a need for building the capacity of communities (see for example Community Development Foundation, 1997, and Skinner, 1997).

In terms of 'community involvement', a number of authors have identified *levels* of involvement. For example, Burns *et al.* (1994: 164–77) identify three broad bands of participation – citizen non-participation; citizen participation; and citizen control – as follows.

- Citizen non-participation refers to 'civic hype' (manipulation of information and image to attract inward investment), 'cynical consultation' (decisions have already been made but 'the community' are 'consulted' in order to rubber-stamp those decisions), 'poor information' (dense and inaccessible), and 'customer care' (training front-line staff to be courteous, friendly and helpful to consumers of services).

- Citizen participation refers to 'informing and consulting' (providing significant information and the development of genuine consultation mechanisms), 'decentralised decision-making' (both limited and significant decision-making) and 'partnership and delegated control'.
- Citizen control: Burns *et al.* (1994: 179) argue that for 'citizen control' to be achieved there would need to be a 'fundamental transformation in the boundaries between state and market economy on the one hand, and civil society on the other'.

In the same vein, Willcox (cited in Taylor, 1995: 33) identifies five levels of involvement in ascending order of participation. At the bottom of the ladder (though not strictly 'participation') *information* is necessary before any other level of participation can be entered into. At this stage people are told what is planned or is to be done but the information flow is, on the whole, one way, from decision-makers to the community, with little or no opportunity for feedback from the community to influence decisions.

The next level, *consultation*, though offering residents a voice, offers residents the opportunity neither to develop their own ideas nor to participate in putting their plans into action. People are presented with a number of options and the comments received are taken into account in deciding what action is to be taken. Real decision-making still rests with the agency that is doing the consulting.

The third level, *deciding together*, offers opportunities for residents to contribute ideas and options and join in deciding the best way forward, but does not offer residents a chance for involvement in the implementation of the ideas. At this stage agencies work with the community to identify what is needed and decide in conjunction with the community (and other partners) what action is to be taken.

The fourth level, *acting together*, involves residents in putting plans into action. At this stage different interests decide what is needed, and then form a partnership to undertake the programme. The partnership may be short term or more permanent, and may involve the setting up of a new organisation.

The final level of this 'ladder of participation' is *supporting*. Here residents decide upon what needs doing and then the local authority and other agencies agree to support them with advice, finance or support in kind. In other words, various agencies support independent community initiatives.

In this particular case study, 'community involvement' began at the lowest of the Willcox levels and the action research process attempted gradually to 'move' it up the ladder to more substantial levels of involvement. The work took place over a period of almost two years, and is still on-going. It seems natural, therefore, to report the project in chronological order.

A minimalist approach to community involvement

The starting point must be the beginning of the preparation for the first bid for funding, which can be taken as February 1996. This is the point at which the Policy and Resources Committee gave the go-ahead for a feasibility study on the potential for a bid for 'Regeneration' funding to be made for the Carlisle South area, namely in the three areas known as Currock, Upperby and Petteril Bank.

The decision to prepare an actual bid for funding was made by the Policy and Resources Committee on 17 April 1996. I came into post as community development officer for the city council on 1 May 1996, and the first attempt to bring 'the community' on board as active participants was on 9 May 1996. This took the form of a hastily convened 'public' meeting to which were invited only the known community groups in the Carlisle South area, representatives from the local schools, and the city and county ward councillors. The meeting was held at very short notice due to the fact that the bid had to be handed in to Government Office Northwest (GONW) within twenty-eight days. There were approximately twenty residents at that particular public meeting, which was 'run' by five senior local authority officers, mainly from different departments within the city council, all seated at the head of the hall behind a line of tables. This immediately gave an impression of 'us' and 'them'.

The format of the meeting made it clear that certain decisions had already been taken by the local authority as to the nature of their spending priorities. The representatives of the local community groups were then asked their opinions on these decisions and whether there were other issues/problems that they could think of. Pro-formas were also distributed, to be returned to the civic centre. The city council spending decisions had been made at a series of meetings in the director of housing's office, open only to senior officers from within the city council, and one meeting which included representatives from Cumbria County Training and Enterprise Council, Cumbria police constabulary, 'Business Link', and Carlisle College of Further Education. Again, this latter meeting was run in the civic centre and did not include any residents of the Carlisle South area.

Those present at that initial 'public' meeting were then told that the city council were offering to be the lead organisation in putting the bid together and making the application. However, there was an official expectation that there would be community representation on any regeneration partnership. That being the case, the city council asked whether it could use the names of those groups in attendance at the meeting as potential partners. All agreed.

In terms of the 'ladder of involvement', information about this particular bid for funding had only been distributed to known community groups (not all residents in the area, and not all voluntary sector agencies operating in the area). There was a vague attempt at consultation of those given the information. This was clearly an example of what Burns *et al.* (1994) have called 'cynical consultation' and can be seen as a purely tokenistic attempt to further community involvement in the decision-making process. Community control over the decision-making process was almost non-existent. The 'community' only had control in terms of being able to endorse the bid or refuse to allow their names to go on the application form.

Setting up a 'community' working group to plan the way forward

Predictably, this first bid was not encouraged by the government, and at a debriefing by GONW (again, only attended by senior city council officers) it was suggested that the bid was 'a little premature' – coded government-speak for lack of preparation and lack of community involvement.

Over the next few months, from July to October 1996, I established a small working group of local residents, city council officers and ward councillors in order to look at the way forward. The working group decided that another bid should be prepared and decided that 'community involvement' could be encouraged through a series of small-scale public 'locality' meetings. I was given the task of organising and running these meetings with input from two community activists and other city council officers. Publicity for the locality meetings was via a newsletter (developed by a senior officer of the city council) and delivered as an insert in the local 'free' newspaper. Seven meetings in all were run, in November 1996, and specific regeneration issues were identified. However, attendance at the meetings was poor. It was at this stage of the process that I suggested a collaborative action research approach to further the development of 'community involvement', and wrote to all those residents attending the locality meetings inviting them to become participants.

Furthering community involvement and understanding via collaborative action research: re-planning the public consultation meetings

Over the next twelve months (2 December 1996 to 17 November 1997) a series of fifteen meetings took place, involving me and anywhere between five and seventeen interested residents. The purpose of these meetings was to adopt a collaborative action research approach to furthering community involvement and possible control of the regeneration initiative. The starting point for this work was to look at the previous locality meetings, what they had achieved, what they had not achieved, and how the community side of this regeneration initiative could be advanced. At a meeting that took place on 6 January 1997, work began on the evaluation and re-planning of the locality meetings. From a collaborative action research perspective, the initial *action* was the setting up and running of the public consultation meetings. The *observation* stage occurred during the action, the *reflection* stage was on-going and took place during the planning meetings, with *re-planning* taking place on the strength of that reflection. The first nine of these meetings focused on reflecting on the experiences of those attending the locality meetings – from the receipt of the initial invitations via a newsletter (delivered inside a free news-paper) through to the actual format of the meetings – and then on how to improve re-runs of the locality meetings, and how to widen the consultation process to include traditionally under-represented groups. In order to support this work I introduced ideas concerning different approaches to consultation – including public meetings, focus groups, questionnaires/surveys, and participatory type approaches. (The latter involved bringing in the consultants Scottish Participatory Initiatives, who ran a training session with the group.) I also decided to introduce some demographic statistics to give the group a greater understanding of the demography of the area, for example the numbers of lone parents, ethnic minorities, people with disabilities, young people and so on.

By the time of the meeting on 19 March 1997 the group had designed and produced a draft newsletter (advertising the re-runs of the locality meetings) which was vastly different from the original newsletter – the one designed by the senior officer of the city council. The group's complaints about the original had been (1) that its colour scheme made it look like an advertisement for a pizza parlour; (2) that it was full of jargon; (3) that the layout was not eye-catching; and (4) that it needed to include some form of 'artwork'. In the new version all these issues were addressed.

The group had also complained about the delivery of the original newsletters. They had been distributed as an insert in the local free paper along with quite a number of other glossy advertisements, and the general tendency for the majority of people was to take the advertisements from the inside of the newspaper *en bloc* and throw them in the bin. To address this problem the group had suggested alter-native forms of distribution, including Royal Mail postal delivery and a list of local shops and local authority decentralised housing offices and community centres, where the newsletters could be left on display.

Finally, the group decided to alter the format of the locality meetings, in the light of their experiences as participants in the original meetings. For example, they decided that, in response to the notion of equal opportunities (which I had introduced), the meetings should be run at different times of the day to suit those residents who work and those with childcare responsibilities. In effect, then, the group had reflected on the original locality meetings, and had totally planned the re-runs of the meetings, down to the last detail.

They had also been introduced to 'focus group' consultation, and had brain-stormed a list of ways of gaining access to various under-represented local groups. However, when asked if any member of the group wanted to assist in the running of focus groups, they all declined. A comment from one of the members of the group was that they hadn't the experience or confidence to do this, even with training.

The re-run of the public meetings did not occur, however. This was mainly due to the announcement of a general election in May, and the thought that if a Labour government was elected SRB bidding criteria might be changed. The group therefore decided to wait until after the general election. Word arrived shortly afterwards from GONW that the bidding timetable had been extended to October 1997 and that there had indeed been changes to the bidding criteria. The group were therefore asked if they wanted to re-run the locality meetings. However, by this time they had lost their enthusiasm for the re-runs. What they did discuss, on the other hand, was the idea of some form of questionnaire/survey to be administered to all households in the area.

The development of a community newsletter and questionnaire

From 23 June 1997 to early August 1997, the development of a questionnaire and newsletter was undertaken. Initially, the group asked whether a 'community survey' of the area might be undertaken by a 'professional' research organisation. The advice of a researcher working for the city council was sought. On the strength of this advice, the group decided that it would be too costly, given the limited resources available. In addition, the only organisation in the area capable of undertaking this research was so busy that they wouldn't be able to fit the survey into their schedule in time to meet the SRB bidding deadline.

At this point I suggested a 'community newsletter', incorporating a tear-off questionnaire, as a useful way of keeping all residents informed of what work had been undertaken by the group, and of further consulting with residents. The group suggested that if they wrote the text and developed the newsletter/questionnaire themselves, there wouldn't be the same problems as encountered with the newsletter which the city council senior officer had previously written and distributed.

One member of the group was aware that the city council had a public relations officer. He suggested to the group that the public relations officer be invited to their next meeting in order to give the group guidelines on how to write the newsletter, the layout, and some sort of timescale to work to. The meeting went ahead on 3 July 1997, resulting in a list of guidelines and a time-scaled action plan. One of the members of the group volunteered to take photographs of the area to use with the text, and it was agreed that articles should be written around a number of topics. These topics were: employment, education and skills, improving existing local businesses, encouraging new local businesses, improving the local environment, improving housing, racial awareness, tackling crime and community safety, health, and 'quality of life'.

On 16 July 1997 the first of four meetings took place which led to the development of the newsletter. One of the members had written the main article prior to the first meeting, which he thought could be used on the front page. All agreed that this article was good, and with minor changes suggested by the group, the article was used. Other articles were written by the group during the meetings, and at the same time photographs that another member had previously taken were selected to demonstrate the points being made. After each meeting the articles which had been written, along with any relevant photographs, were taken back to the civic centre to be 'desktop published' by an officer in the Economic Development Unit.

The draft newsletter was taken back to the group at their next meeting, or sometimes posted, in order for further comments to be made. When the group felt that there was a need for computer-based 'clipart' to be used to demonstrate a point, they would suggest the type of character they were thinking of so that the officer from Economic Development could select an appropriate character from the programme. Again this was then inserted into a draft and taken back to the group for comments. Finally, the back page of the newsletter was given over to a questionnaire. An important consideration here was that the business and employment manager of the city council had advised the group that GONW might ask them to reduce the programme by, for example, 20% or 50%. If that proved to be the case, then there would need to be some way of prioritising the projects/issues in order to save money by cutting those of lesser importance. The group decided that they would use the questionnaire to achieve this. It was also agreed that the questionnaire would ask residents to prioritise topics of concern, not projects, and that there would be space for further comments. (*A copy of the residents' newsletter is included as an Appendix on pp. 156–9.*)

The city council comes in for criticism

The group had worked hard at putting the newsletter together; they certainly felt that they owned it, and were justly proud of their achievement. Then a series of problems were encountered. First, there was a problem with getting the newsletter printed on time. This caused the delivery date for the newsletters to be moved back by a few weeks. Second, there was a problem with Royal Mail postal service, as the boundaries of their delivery areas did not fit with the local areas covered by the project. Third, somewhere along the line about half the newsletters went missing. This was only discovered when most of the newsletter working group did not receive their own copy through the post. Consequently, the business and employment manager who had been given responsibility for the printing and delivery was heavily criticised by the group.

At a meeting on 17 September, more general concerns were raised concerning the city council. First, the group were upset that the newsletters had not been distributed on 1 September when the group had worked hard to meet their own deadline. Second, the group were concerned by a report in the local newspaper which claimed that the city council had already made decisions at a committee meeting about how SRB money would be spent if the bid was successful. One member of the group brought the newspaper to the meeting to show the others. It was felt that this went counter to the notion of partnership between the city council and the community, and undermined their hard work over the past year. Third, the group were concerned that the business and employment manager had not been keeping them informed of the potential partner agencies with which he had been liaising. This led to more general concerns over the way that officers within the city council had been having meetings to discuss the progress of the bid from which community representatives were excluded. At this point I suggested that members of the group should be invited along to the next meeting of city council officers in the civic centre. Three of the group volunteered to attend, suggesting that the meetings should be arranged at a time when children were at school.

I had also been invited to update the Young People and Community Development Sub-committee of Councillors, on 22 September 1997, on the progress of community involvement in the SRB bid. I therefore asked the group if any of them would like to come along to provide this update, especially as the presentation was on community involvement. Three agreed, and gave that presentation.

So where were we, as regards the development of 'community involvement and control'? In order to communicate information about the funding bid and the group's progress to all residents in the Carlisle South area, the group had developed their newsletter. The questionnaire at the back of the newsletter had been an attempt to facilitate further consultation. And in terms of 'deciding together' as a model of partnership between the city council and the local community, decisions were certainly being made by the working group on how some parts of the initiative should be run.

However, it was clear that there had not been total commitment from all partners in the 'deciding together' process. There was concern that meetings of council officers were excluding community representatives from involvement in part of the decision-making process, even though it had been suggested to senior officers that there should be community representatives at their meetings and all had agreed that this should be facilitated. However, at the first meeting of officers which four community representatives attended, all senior officers sent apologies for absence. Those present – four community representatives, me and one other junior officer – had to adjourn the meeting. This reinforces the point made by Taylor (1995: 33) that *all* partners need to be clear as to where on the 'ladder of participation' they want to be. Taylor goes on to say that in most cases it is the 'professionals' who stop short of the 'deciding together' stage.

Beyond the newsletter

Three other developments occurred after the production of the newsletter/ questionnaire. First, I arranged for some members of the group to visit a nearby city, Blackburn. The purpose of the visit was to input information into our action–reflection cycle about successful types of regeneration partnership structures, as well as to look at a youthwork project that specifically targeted young people 'at risk' of drifting into crime. In preparation for the visit a group meeting was held to draft a series of questions which could be asked of the regeneration partnership and the youthwork project. The visit to Blackburn went ahead on 2 September 1997, and a further meeting was held on 17 September, back in Carlisle, to reflect on the visit, to look at their answers to our questions and the observations made. It was at this meeting that the group decided that they should now be looking to develop their own regeneration partnership. In terms of collaborative action research, this was an attempt to further community understanding of alternative forms of youthwork (alternative to the provision of youth clubs) and also an attempt to further understanding about community involvement in regeneration partnerships.

The second development began at the same meeting, partly in response to the Blackburn visit, with deeper reflection on what the group had (and had not) actually achieved, and the extent to which they had really been 'deciding together' with the city council (as well as other agencies). This led to the identification by the group of the need to become more organised as a community group. It was suggested that a constituted umbrella community organisation with elected community representatives be developed as soon as possible. Those elected would be expected to develop any regeneration partnership. To this end a public meeting took place on 17 November 1997 and the Carlisle South Regeneration Group was formed.

The third development began with notification from the government that our latest bid had been unsuccessful. The first meeting of the Carlisle South Regeneration Group occurred on 27 November 1997. The official feedback about the unsuccessful bid suggested that it had covered too large a geographical area and that future bids should be directed at a smaller area (Petteril Bank) suffering acute social and economic disadvantage. The group decided to do this. It was felt that alternative sources of funding could be sought for the other geographical areas (Currock and Upperby). One member of the group suggested that they adopt a similar approach to that of Blackburn, i.e. developing community associations for the different areas. It was pointed out the three areas already had residents' associations, which should be approached with the suggestion that they develop into self-controlled, self-running community associations. In effect, each group would develop into an umbrella community organisation specifically to deal with total regeneration of their respective areas. All individuals living in the groups' area could become members with a voice, and all community sector and voluntary sector groups could become affiliated members with a voice. Each community association could then look to forming a partnership with public sector and private sector organisations.

Conclusion

So what has been achieved? Was a collaborative action research approach useful, and did it have limits? Quite clearly, from the events narrated here, some of the decisions described were made by senior officers within the city council, and the community had little or no influence. However, it is equally clear that the community did gain control over some of the decision-making, in particular over decisions around how the community organises itself, how community consultation should develop, and how to publicise the development of the initiative. And this partial control was achieved through the action research process.

The regeneration initiative has also led to an extension of participatory democracy and the development of structures to facilitate this. There have been opportunities for individuals to come together and to organise collectively in order to promote the common good. And finally, there has been an element of 'community capacity building' (i.e. an element of education and training) and a change in professional practice on the part of the business and employment officer. Again, it was the collaborative action research process which enabled all this to happen.

In terms of my own professional development, the main issue arising from this attempt at collaborative action research was whether the work had facilitated community 'learning' and understanding, and thus enabled members of the communities of Carlisle South to move up the 'ladder of community involvement'. In other words, had the action research process actually facilitated 'community learning' in the Freirean sense?

What does this mean? Freire sees 'transformative education' as a community effort to acquire knowledge through which society can be reshaped. Transformation can be seen to operate at four levels: our own personal lives; our community; our environment; and the whole society (Hope *et al.*, 1984: 16). Freire argues that the role of the facilitator ('animator') in the 'transformative education' process is not to give answers to problems. Rather, it is one in which s/he sets up a process through which a group can search for the answers themselves in a systematic way (ibid.: 19). Freire calls this a 'problem-posing', as opposed to a 'banking', approach to group learning. The transformative process involves a cycle of action and reflection with a series of inputs which increase dialogue, leading to reflection and learning, and, ultimately, further action for social change (ibid.: 21). This Freirean approach to social transformation (based upon group learning, action and reflection) is not dissimilar to a collaborative action research approach to community development. The facilitator/'animator' (not necessarily a community development worker in the context of urban regeneration initiatives) is the crucial player in this process. Without a true understanding of the transformation process or with values which run counter to this way of working, there is a risk that a facilitator might achieve 'micro-change' at the neighbourhood level, without making links with the wider context.

In the light of this argument, then, our own approach to developing 'community involvement' has been useful in terms of both personal transformation and community transformation. The community activists within the project have developed personally in terms of their knowledge and understanding of:

* the ways in which the local authority works;
* the demographic make-up within their own communities and concomitant equal opportunities issues;
* different methods of engaging with the wider community;
* the inequalities between so-called partners within 'partnership working'.

There has also been personal transformation in terms of the confidence of group members in their ability to challenge the inequalities between partners.

Community transformation has also begun to occur, through the development of more organised structures within the three local neighbourhoods of Carlisle South.

As can be seen from this report, however, what has been achieved over something like a two-year period is limited, but the project is still on-going and still continues to adopt collaborative action research methodology. Transformation has occurred (and can continue to occur) at the personal (community activist) level and at the community level. Whether that can eventually lead to transformation within the structures of society remains to be seen. Transformation through collaborative action research process is a slow process.

References

Burns, D., Hambleton, R. and Hoggett, P. (1994) *The Politics of Decentralisation: Revitalising Local Democracy*, London: Macmillan.

Community Development Foundation (1997) *Regeneration and the Community: Guidelines to the Community Involvement Aspect of the SRB Challenge Fund* (1997 edn), London: Community Development Foundation.

Hope, A., Timmel, S. and Hodzi, C. (1984) *Training for Transformation: a Handbook for Community Workers*, Book 1 (revised edn), London: Community Development Foundation.

Skinner, S. (1997) *Building Community Strengths: a Resource Book on Capacity Building*, London: Community Development Foundation.

Taylor, M. (1995) *Unleashing the Potential: Bringing Residents to the Centre of Regeneration*, York: Joseph Rowntree Foundation.

APPENDIX: THE COMMUNITY NEWSLETTER

Regeneration News

Currock, Upperby & Petteril Bank
Written & edited by Community Residents

YOUR LAST CHANCE CAN YOU AFFORD TO LOSE £5 MILLION?

This newsletter and message is directed at every family living in Currock, Upperby and Petteril Bank.

Every resident, tenant, young person, lone parent, ethnic group member, unemployed person, person with a disability and disadvantaged people. That means everybody: YOU!

This is the final chance for you to have your say on how, if we're successful, the money from a Government's "Single Regeneration Budget" bid, should be used and managed.

A successful bid would bring improved employment prospects, housing conditions, community safety and security, education and skills, a better environment, recreation and leisure, a better deal for youths and children, health projects.

Your involvement and ideas could make all the difference. Make use of the tear-off questionnaire.

A successful bid could bring £5 million to this area over a five year period, £20,000 per week. *Don't let us throw it away.*

Is this you?

Regeneration News

SINGLE REGENERATION BUDGET - AN EXPLANANTION

SRB stands for Single Regeneration Budget.

It is a pot of money offered to us by the Government. We have to compete against other cities in the North West by proving that our need is greater and our proposed schemes are the best.

SRB is about improving in all ways the quality of life and the area in which we live - this means for everyone.

This money will only become available if YOU get involved.

SRB programmes are managed by a partnership which the Government says should be made up of local authorities (City and County Councils), the Training and Enterprise Council, voluntary and local community groups and representatives, as well as other organisations such as colleges, churches, health trusts, etc. This means that YOUR involvement is needed!!

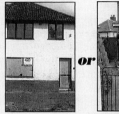 *or*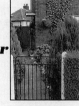

Which would you prefer?

WATCH YOUR STEP!!

Are you worried about the state of the area where your children play? SRB could provide funds to combat health hazards, to provide 'dog loo' areas, to make the area cleaner and safer for you and your family.

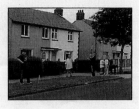 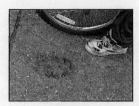

DO YOU FEEL SECURE IN YOUR HOME??

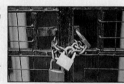

Do you have adequate door locks, window locks, security lighting, and so on?

Did you know that a home that has been burgled once is more than likely to be burgled again unless its security is improved. SRB money could assist those homes that are most at risk of being burgled to be made more secure. It could possibly be cheaper than feeding a Rottweiler for a year!!

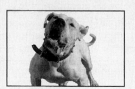

WOULD YOU LIKE PEACE OF MIND TO GO OUT AT NIGHT?

You could if we had better street lighting, a more effective Neighbourhood Watch Scheme, and a "safer transport/travel" project (such as more frequent buses, adequate lighting at bus stops, a shoppers' bus, and so on).

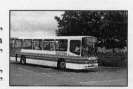

YOUNG PEOPLE DO LIKE HANGING AROUND ON STREET CORNERS! IS THIS BY CHOICE?

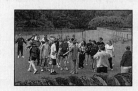

A successful SRB bid could bring much-needed money into Currock, Upperby and Petteril Bank to pay for youth workers, improved sports facilities and other opportunities for young people ranging from leisure and recreational opportunities through to learning.

Use the Questionnaire overleaf to make your choice.

Regeneration News

Regeneration News

PROPOSED CURROCK / UPPERBY / PETTERIL BANK SRB BID FOR 1997

Below are listed some areas of concern which have been expressed by residents in YOUR area through a series of public meetings. Please make any comments below each of the headings. In the right hand column, could you rank each area of concern using a number between 1 and 7 with 1 being the most important area of concern and 7 being the least important.

Employment

....

....

Rank Order

☐

Encouraging new local businesses

....

....

☐

Improving the local environment

....

....

☐

Improving housing

....

....

☐

Improving racial awareness

....

....

☐

Tackling crime /community safety

....

....

☐

Health / Quality of life / Sport / Art / Leisure

....

....

☐

If you want further information or want to be involved in the SRB bid please fill in your name and address below.

Name..

Address..

....

Please return this Questionnaire to either the Community Support Unit, Carlisle City Council, The Civic Centre, Carlisle; CA3 8QG or your local Community Centre/Neighbourhood Housing Office.

Chapter 11

The Citizens' Commission

A UK case study of service-user-controlled research

Peter Beresford and Michael Turner

Introduction

The UK 'Citizens' Commission on the Future of the Welfare State' was established to challenge an important contradiction in social policy. While recent policy changes have been associated with a more active role for 'welfare state service-users' in the creation and maintenance of their own welfare (with a much bigger role to play both in organising and paying for it directly), their role in the development of welfare policy and discussion has remained largely passive and limited.

This discrepancy is especially important because in recent years the emphasis in welfare internationally has been on radical reform and revision. This has been true for both political and academic discussions. The argument has been that traditional conditions for and assumptions about public welfare no longer hold, and that it must change to meet new demographic, social, cultural, economic and political trends. However, what has not significantly altered is the way in which welfare policy has been formulated and research to inform policy has been undertaken. These activities and their associated debates have continued to be dominated by traditional stakeholders: politicians, managers, academics and professionals.

The independent Citizens' Commission was set up in 1994 (supported by the Baring Foundation and *Community Care* magazine) to enable welfare state service-users to play a greater part in shaping their own welfare and to help gain the views, ideas and proposals of welfare state service-users about welfare nationally, at a time when fundamental reform is taking place in the UK welfare state. All the Commission's members are themselves welfare state service-users. They include disabled and older people, lone parents, people with learning difficulties, unemployed people and people living on benefits and low income. We were both involved, Peter Beresford as convener of the Commission and Michael Turner as the lead researcher.

The first task of the Commission was to undertake the first national UK inquiry into what welfare state service-users thought of the existing welfare system – both services and income maintenance – and what they wanted for the future. While the work of the Commission was framed in terms of an inquiry, it can also be seen as a research project, though very different in kind to traditional approaches to social research, and it is as such that we want to discuss it here. It is helpful to distinguish between the Commission's research 'methodology' (the philosophy on which it was based) and its 'methods' (how we carried out the work).

The Commission's research philosophy

The Citizens' Commission is linked with and develops three strands of research methodology: participatory, emancipatory and user-controlled research. All of these approaches are concerned with changing the relation between research, researchers and research subjects or participants. There has been growing pressure for a different, more equal and inclusive relationship between research and the subjects of research in recent years. In the context of social policy and 'social care' it can be traced to two developments. First is the increasing emphasis on the 'choice' and 'involvement' of service-users as welfare consumers through the strengthening influence of 'new right' political ideology both on right-wing and traditional left-of-centre politics and policy thinking. Second has been the emergence of movements of groups previously categorised as the passive subjects of social and 'care' policy, like the disabled people's, older people's and psychiatric system survivors' movements. These movements have developed their own philosophies, politics, ways of organising, cultures, arts, writings and research (Barnes and Mercer, 1997). While these movements have been particularly conspicuous and influential in the context of social and community care policy, their influence is also increasingly being felt on social and public policy more generally.

The three different strands of research methodology with which the work of the Citizens' Commission is linked have not so far been adequately related to each other. They have different histories and have developed in different contexts; for example, participatory research developed in the context of community development and education, and emancipatory research is most closely associated with the disabled people's movement. Nor is there any consensus about any one of them among its proponents and commentators. However, they do share similar concerns. These are to equalise relationships between the researcher and the subjects of research, to involve the subjects of research as researchers and in the research process more generally, and to make change which benefits the subjects of research. These shared concerns are also frequently highlighted as ideals of 'action research'.

Such an approach to research was adopted because it was consistent with the principles underpinning the Commission. These included:

- valuing the views, ideas and proposals of welfare state service-users;
- recognising the particular contribution which they can make because of the expertise they bring from their own experience;
- giving equal credibility to their perspective as to others;
- treating all welfare state service-users with respect;
- reflecting this in the Commission's own working, so that welfare state service-users involved in the Commission would always be treated and treat each other with respect (Beresford and Turner, 1997: 11).

Alan Stanton has identified some of the characteristics of participatory research, while making clear that there is no one rigid model. He says:

> Participatory research recognises that most research serves the powerful: government over the governed; management over workers. So its goal is democratic as well as collaborative inquiry. This means the core issue is empowerment; not only people's involvement, but their control. It challenges inequality by supporting people in the creation of their own knowledge; strengthening their abilities and resources. Its rationale is their right to participate actively in processes affecting their lives. Writers on participatory research often see this link between research and action as its characteristic feature. Investigation, analysis, learning and taking action, aren't separate and distinct, but an interrelated whole. Investigation may be initiated by outside researchers, but it should remain anchored in the issues of the community or workplace.
>
> (Stanton, 1989: 332)

According to Mike Oliver, the disability activist and writer, the two key fundamentals on which an emancipatory approach to research must be based

> are empowerment and reciprocity. These fundamentals can be built in by encouraging self-reflection and a deeper understanding of the research process by the research subjects themselves as well as by enabling researchers to identify with their research subjects.
>
> (Oliver, 1996: 141)

Clare Evans and Mike Fisher in their discussion of user-controlled research define it in the following terms:

> It must bring service users greater power to define their needs and the outcomes that matter to them. Service users must select the issues for research and acquire control over the funds to conduct it. We think that service users should wherever possible become researchers, so that their influence pervades the research: this includes responsibility for data analysis and for dissemination.
>
> (Evans and Fisher, 1999: 104)

By these criteria it becomes clear that the Citizens' Commission inquiry is an example of user-controlled research as well as embodying the commitments and priorities of participatory and emancipatory methodologies.

- Its aim was to offer welfare state service-users an opportunity to say what they wanted from welfare, both present and future.
- A small planning group of welfare state service-users appointed Commission members, to reflect the diversity of service-users according to age, 'race', gender, sexuality and disability, and identified the focus of the research.

- Members of the Commission were in control of the funding it received and decided as a group how to spend it.
- The Commission recruited and employed a welfare state service-user – a disabled person – who was accountable to them, to have lead responsibility for undertaking the research (i.e. Michael Turner).
- Most members of the Commission had not previously undertaken research, but with support all were involved in the research process, including identifying research issues and questions, analysing data and disseminating findings.

There is now a growing body of such participatory and emancipatory research, although the obstacles in the way of service-users mean that there have been fewer user-controlled research initiatives. There are examples of emancipatory research from organisations of disabled people, people with learning difficulties, psychiatric system survivors, people living with HIV/AIDS and other groups (Barnes and Mercer, 1997; March *et al.*, 1997; Whittaker, 1997; Stalker, 1998; Kiernan, 1999). This development represents a break with the tradition of one group of people studying and reporting on another to a system whereby people undertake their own research. It is used to find out what service-users want; to monitor and evaluate policy, practice and services. There is now more than enough experience to show that such participatory and emancipatory research is both possible and effective.

The Commission's research methods

Because the Commission had limited resources it could only reach some welfare state service-users, but it sought to reach as wide a range as possible. The aim was to enable both people who were and weren't actively involved in user groups and campaigns to offer their views; to include people who were familiar with debates about welfare and those who weren't; people who had formulated demands and people who hadn't; people with high and low expectations.

To achieve these objectives the Commission undertook a series of *group* discussions in different parts of the country and with different groups of service-users, and also encouraged groups and particularly *individuals* to send in evidence themselves. This widened the range of welfare state service-users who could contribute and also ensured that more isolated individuals, who might not be affiliated to organisations or involved in self-help or support groups, could take part. Each method has its strengths and limitations, but together they make possible a fuller, more inclusive picture from welfare state service-users. Evidence was received from individuals in letters, on tape, by telephone and through the short questionnaire leaflet that we distributed. Commission members and workers undertook twenty-eight group discussions and received evidence from sixty-seven individuals.

Commission members spent time at their second meeting working out what they would ask welfare state service-users; brainstorming and writing ideas up on a flip chart. These questions, with minor changes to ensure clarity and reliability and with some additions, were the basis for group discussions and the short questionnaires we produced for groups and individuals to give evidence.

The group discussions made up the largest part of the Commission's work of seeking evidence. They were carried out in two ways. First, members of the Commission organised and undertook discussions with groups they were in contact with or knew of in their areas, usually groups who shared the same experience as them, comprising, for example, people with learning difficulties or carers. We made a deliberate decision to do this, to make the most of people's shared experience and also to avoid situations where there might be competing interests, for example, if non-disabled carers were to meet with disabled people. Second, the Commission identified priority groups not represented by Commission members, and also made a special effort to talk to people in parts of the country not covered by members of the Commission. Priority groups were those whose views we thought it particularly important to obtain because they are often overlooked and experience particular exclusion. They included:

- young people aged 16–18 excluded from receiving benefits
- black and minority ethnic groups
- people working for low pay
- homeless people
- people living with HIV/AIDS
- drug users
- teenage mothers
- people with childcare responsibilities

Group discussions have particular strengths. They give participants the chance to develop their thoughts and ideas, bounce ideas off each other and take their discussion forward. They help give people the confidence to say what they want as a result of having each other's support. For these reasons this method of gaining people's views and ideas was particularly consistent with the participatory and emancipatory goals of the Commission, and with the general principles of action research.

To reach the different groups and areas we had prioritised required a more structured approach than when members of the Commission undertook their own discussions. We used a snowball approach, starting with existing networks which then led us to other national and local contacts. As well as identifying and contacting organisations linked specifically with our priority groups, we also contacted wider groups and projects like community and drop-in centres.

We discovered that while the voluntary sector is large, many provider organisations are not in direct contact with service-users or able to put people in touch with them. Also, while it was not difficult, for example, to reach groups of lone parents and disabled people, there seemed to be few groups organised around the welfare state or issues like unemployment.

Carrying out the group discussions highlighted the broader problems of reaching welfare state service-users and involving them in the discussion about welfare. It highlighted their isolation and frequently difficult circumstances. It took time, effort and determination. It required considerable skill and sensitivity. To reach the groups who took part in the inquiry, more than 100 were contacted by letter and phone. Thousands of leaflets and questionnaires were also produced and distributed.

We tried to support welfare state service-users' participation in the Commission by meeting all their expenses so that, for example, childcare responsibilities or lack of personal assistance or of accessible transport would not prevent them taking part or put them out of pocket. We went to see them rather than expecting them to come to us, and met the cost of meeting places and refreshments where necessary. But there were also other important obstacles in the way of welfare state service users' participation in the Commission. This was apparent from the reasons given by groups gave for *not* wanting to take part.

These reasons fell into three categories: they were too busy, they didn't see any point, or they weren't interested. The first two categories are of particular significance. The groups who *did* take part were often small, fragile, over-stretched and tied up with their own activities. This meant that frequently when they met with us, they were busy and had to break off from what they were doing. But the response of welfare state service-users and their organisations also seemed to be shaped by what they thought could be achieved. Many conveyed a strong sense of powerlessness. It was clear that they doubted that service-users or the Commission could make much impact on the future of welfare. Some asked us, 'What can it achieve?' 'What will happen with it?' This was not said in a dismissive way, but out of concern about what difference the Commission could make and whether it was just a paper exercise. Our response was that the Commission might achieve a little and that if we didn't participate, welfare state service-users wouldn't even have a chance to have a say. If they had that chance, it couldn't be claimed in the future that nobody knew what welfare service-users had to say and what they wanted. Similarly, some of the individuals and groups we contacted felt initially that they might not have anything to say or contribute, although, as we shall see, taking part in the Commission generally proved them wrong.

Motivating welfare state service-users to take part in the Commission was not always easy. The strong sense of disempowerment which many conveyed can be seen as part of a vicious circle which perpetuates and reinforces their exclusion. For example, we particularly wanted to include in the group discussions people who lived in residential homes and used day-care services. Sadly, when the Commission tried to arrange discussions in residential homes and day-centres, people were reluctant to get involved. Though probably those who are most reliant on the state, they appeared to believe that no importance would be attached to their views.

Carrying out the group discussions

Among the underpinning principles of the Commission were respect for each other's rights and wants, and ensuring that members had any support they needed to contribute fully and effectively, including the support they required to become researchers. As researchers, they had to be in a position to undertake group discussions successfully. These can be difficult and demanding to organise. However, the two-way nature of the process and the greater equality of the relationship compared to one-to-one research interviews encourages successful participation. Some members of the Commission had been involved in similar initiatives before. Others had not, and had not carried out any research themselves. The planning group had deliberately not made such experience a requirement of the 'person specification' for Commission members, as it felt that this would unnecessarily restrict membership. It believed instead that with support members could gain such skills. This is one of the lessons of user-led and user-controlled research, and it worked for the Commission. We put together information and support for people to carry out group discussions and spent time talking about it at one of our meetings. We also kept in touch with Commission members, offering information and guidance when they were needed. Members were able to gain new skills and new confidence from doing research. We also produced ground rules for the discussions to help ensure participants' confidentiality and a safe environment.

The discussions

In some cases, only some of the people present wanted to take part in discussions. One group of very young people seemed unwilling to say much. Some of those who did participate were initially reluctant to talk. Some were nervous about going on record; for example, one individual was concerned about the tape recorder. But once the discussion began, generally everyone present would contribute. Participants had a lot to say. They had ideas about how things could be improved as well as criticisms to make of existing arrangements. Members of the Commission who undertook group discussions emphasised the openness and honesty of participants. The discussions seemed to be a positive and empowering experience for both participants in the group discussions and the people who carried them out.

This relates to one of the principles underlying the Commission, namely that the trust, empathy, understanding and shared experience which comes from a 'user-led' approach to inquiry about welfare would generate fuller, more candid and reliable information. One member of the Commission, who had never undertaken any research before, said:

> It was important to the people that I spoke to that I was in the same boat as them. I wasn't just another academic or professional, that I wouldn't talk down to them, but I actually knew about their experience first hand and could understand it.

This may help to explain why people seemed to take us so much into their confidence. In contrast, one of the reasons why some people were reluctant to get involved was their negative experiences of conventional research. They said, for example: 'We've bloody been surveyed. We're fed up with it.' We don't believe that people would have shared with us some of the things which they said if our relationship with them had not been equal.

A frequent concern expressed about initiatives and studies which seek to involve service-users is that their participants are 'unrepresentative'. This is sometimes used to discredit or devalue their activities and findings (Beresford and Campbell, 1994). We do not claim that the Commission was a quantitative research project based on a random sample of people. It clearly wasn't, and it wasn't intended to be. But at the same time, we sought to include as wide a range of people and perspectives as possible and, with some exceptions (for example, travellers and deaf people), we succeeded. As we have said, we also sought to address issues of difference according to 'race', gender, sexual identity, disability, age and class. However, there seemed to be a significant degree of consistency in what people said. For example, groups of young people from different parts of the country and groups of much older people from the home counties all had similar proposals to offer for funding welfare for the future.

The groups ranged widely in size; there were thirty-five in one and just two in another. Mostly they ranged from about six to twelve people, which made a manageable and comfortable size for discussion. Mixed groups were generally balanced according to gender. In addition to the groups specifically of black and Asian people, some of the other groups also included black people. Discussions generally lasted between forty-five minutes and an hour.

Different groups had their own particular concerns and raised these in the discussions. For example, lone parents were worried about the Child Support Agency and people living with HIV/AIDS were concerned about the availability of treatment. The pressure on people in their day-to-day lives to focus on issues which specifically affected them meant that they often had had less time to think about broader welfare issues. The Commission both raised the issue of the need to connect particular issues affecting different groups of welfare state service-users with broader ones and began to address it. While some discriminatory comments were made, for example about drug users getting services and 'immigrants coming and getting benefits', these were uncommon.

Analysing and collating the evidence

If collecting information is a big job, then pulling it together is an even bigger one. When we had finished gathering evidence, we had a pile of transcriptions nearly half a metre high, a thick sheaf of completed questionnaires and three files of inquiries and submitted evidence.

We used a two-stage approach to analysing and collating the information we had gathered. This reflected the participatory goals of the project. First, the Commission worker (Michael Turner) began the process of analysing information. Then when he had identified key issues from it, these were used as the basis for discussion at the fourth and final meeting of the Commission. The aim was to enable members of the Commission collectively to offer their views and analysis of the findings. This discussion was tape recorded. Members of the Commission who could not be at the meeting contributed their views through telephone interviews, which were written down in full. These discussions also formed a basis for the Commission's proposals and recommendations. Thus, there was an important collaborative dimension to the collation and analysis of data in the Commission's work. To the best of our knowledge, this is the first time that this has been done.

Writing up the Commission's work

The Commission's worker (Michael Turner) had lead responsibility for writing up its findings, while the convenor (Peter Beresford), who had been involved from the beginning, was primarily responsible for the introductory chapters. The report of the findings from the Commission's work was published in the form of a book (Beresford and Turner, 1997) which went through a process of redrafting. We regretted that we did not send groups transcripts for them to correct and change or a first draft of the report. But we had neither time nor resources to do this. What we did do, however, was provide a copy of the final report for all groups who took part in the Commission.

In keeping with the participatory philosophy underpinning this project, in both analysing and collating information and writing the book we sought to reflect the issues and priorities raised by participants, rather than impose our own categories on what they said and group them together according to some system of our own. This is an approach which is known as 'grounded theory', one which builds on participants' own analysis and ideas rather than fitting them into some pattern pre-set by the analyst or researcher.

One consequence of this is that we organised the material according to policies and themes offered by welfare state service-users, rather than dividing them simply on the basis of their views about existing provision and their proposals for the future. While this might have been a simpler and more conventional way of presenting their views, it would not have corresponded to the way they were offered or reflected their trains of thought.

The Commission's findings

The Commission's first report (Beresford and Turner, 1997) sets out its findings in full. We can only headline them here, but some of the key issues that participants raised were:

- Welfare state service-users predominantly want to be independent rather than dependent on welfare.
- Good-quality, properly paid employment is the key route to achieving this – as a right rather than an obligation.
- Adequate, appropriate and good-quality support is essential for independence, whether for childcare or personal assistance.

- Welfare state services should receive greater political priority and be funded through taxation.
- Income maintenance and welfare services need to be integrated.
- Service-users' experience and views of existing welfare state services were generally very negative.
- They expressed strong feelings of being disenfranchised and disempowered.
- They saw education and training as the route out of welfare into decent employment.
- They identified lack of information as one of the key obstacles in the way of getting the support they needed.
- They felt that they generally had little say or control over welfare and its services and wanted more.
- They stressed the need for welfare state funding to be used more effectively and efficiently. They saw reforms which had been made on grounds of 'value for money' as resulting in further waste and inefficiency.
- They report that continuing political and media attacks on welfare state service-users had direct and destructive effects on them which made some people reluctant to seek support from welfare services, however desperate their circumstances.

This list of key findings can't really give a feel of the views and experience which people reported in group discussions and individual evidence. But, as the issues we have headlined make clear, participants were able to do much more than merely report their experience, which is what most conventional welfare and poverty research has confined itself to in seeking welfare service-users' views (Beresford *et al.*, 1999). They were also well able to offer their own critiques and make their own proposals for the future.

Making change

The usual approach to bringing about change after new knowledge or information has been obtained about a social issue or problem is to seek media coverage and try to influence politicians and policy-makers at local and central government levels. While we did not ignore this top-down approach and regarded it as important to gain mainstream media coverage and inform politicians and policy-makers, we did not see this as the main way in which we hoped to influence debates and developments about welfare.

We recognised at an early stage that the amount of interest we could expect following this route would be limited for an initiative like the Commission. We had little chance of bringing about change through conventional mass media/ parliamentary methods. Not only do large pressure groups and voluntary organisations have limited success in doing this but, as we have seen, reports on the future of welfare by other organisations much more powerful than ours can be lost without trace (for example, Transport and General Workers Union, 1994;

Yarrow, 1996). During the life of the Commission, we also saw the high-profile report of the Commission on Social Justice set aside by the Labour Party (Commission on Social Justice, 1994; Milne, 1995). We therefore could not assume that a conventional approach would work for us, whether or not it worked for others. At the same time, we did receive coverage in the national and specialist press, as well as in user and community newsletters, and in a House of Lords debate as well as frequent citation in academic social policy publications and discussions.

Our experience from involvement in service-users' community and disabled people's organisations and movements led us to another approach, which they have pioneered. This is one based much more on a model of 'bottom-up' than 'top-down' change. At the Commission's third meeting we said:

> It is possible for us to be different. It could be a good idea to seek the support of our different organisations. . . . We are not a powerful group in conventional terms, but the report could be useful and helpful for local and national campaigning if groups have access to it, to support what they want to do and the report has support from as many groups and organisations as possible. We agreed we would try and do this.
>
> (Notes of meeting, 20 June 1995, p. 3)

We therefore viewed the production of the Commission's report as part of a longer-term strategy of dissemination, particularly focused on grassroots organisations. We placed our priority on informing and supporting discussion and campaigning on the welfare state among and between welfare state service-users' groups, organisations and movements at local and national levels. Spreading the word among 'ourselves' seemed a feasible and achievable objective, which could provide a basis for wider action as well as accessing and exchanging ideas and information among welfare state service-users and their organisations. In this way we hoped that the efforts that individuals and groups of welfare state service-users who took part in the Commission would have a real chance of serving a positive purpose as a resource for others.

This process began with the public launch of the Citizens' Commission Report in 1997, attended by a wide range of delegates from grassroots, user and voluntary organisations as well as funding, policy, research and service agencies.

A second stage of work

Following the launch of our first report, our funder encouraged us to do more work. First, we responded to government proposals for welfare reform and, second, we spent more time thinking through our own priorities, concerns and agenda for welfare and for engaging with welfare reform. We received funding from the Baring Foundation and Joseph Rowntree Foundation which enabled us to do this.

The Citizens' Commission response to the 1998 Green Paper *New Ambitions for Our Country: a New Contract For Welfare* (Department of Social Security, 1998) was based on a further meeting of the Citizens' Commission and an initial survey of welfare state service-user organisations. The Commission received evidence from twenty-three user-controlled organisations in many parts of the UK, including organisations of older people, lone parents, disabled people, and low-income tenants and residents. The groups expressed concerns about the process of government consultation, its inadequacy and inaccessibility, and the need for genuine rather than tokenistic consultation reaching out to involve people when such major reform is at stake. Participants were generally wary of proposals for reform, feeling little ownership of them and worried by many of them. There were particular concerns about the failure to adopt a holistic approach integrating income maintenance, support and mainstream services, and about anti-discrimination measures and the emphasis of reforms on 'jobs at any price'.

With the removal of the Minister Frank Field, the 1998 Green Paper was sidelined and while the pace and scale of proposals for welfare reform accelerated, welfare service-users continued to be marginal in the process. This highlighted the need for the Citizens' Commission to be proactive rather than reactive in its discussions. In July 1999, members of the Commission met again and held a discussion which was tape recorded and transcribed to form part of its second report (Beresford and Turner, 2000). This focused on and highlighted the following issues:

- the importance of involving welfare state service-users in welfare reform and feedback on current developments;
- welfare service-users' views about the reforms so far – which emphasised their complex and ambiguous nature, as well as many service-users' increasing feelings of insecurity, anxiety and powerlessness in relation to them;
- the relationship between economic and welfare policies: members of the Commission thought this relationship was increasingly important but they felt they and many welfare service-users did not know enough about it and needed to be better informed, wanting to be more fully involved in discussion. The centrality of dominant political understandings of 'globalisation' for jobs, training and employment policy, as well as welfare policy and spending, all have massive implications for welfare state service-users;
- the importance of developing opportunities for different groups of welfare service-users to be able to link up and develop alliances. There are currently few chances or forums to do this. The Citizens' Commission has been unusual in working in this way. Different groups like disabled people, lone parents and mental health service-users have generally focused on their particular issues and campaigns, rather than being able to develop links and common activities with other groups. Government and business, highlighting globalisation, stress the need to make connections; meanwhile different groups of service-users are forced to compete with each other for inadequate resources and are divided and weakened in the process.

Taking the work forward: 'Our Voice in Our Future'

Members of the Commission tried to have realistic expectations about what it could achieve. We knew that it could only make a limited impact, and that this needed to be based on a different and more participatory approach to policy change. At the same time, we were anxious that the Commission should not be yet another ephemeral initiative which had little or no lasting effect. One of our concerns was to ensure that it could be the *start* of something, rather than just another participatory scheme which quickly fizzled out. Participatory developments tend to be short-lived, and are frequently characterised by insecurity and underfunding. Continuity is crucial if user-controlled developments, including user-controlled research, are to be helpful and effective. In the event, the Commission had a much longer life than we could have expected. It also provided a jumping-off point for further user-controlled work at both national and local levels.

This is being undertaken through a new parallel development, 'Our Voice in Our Future', which has built on and taken forward the work of the Citizens' Commission. We have both been involved in it. It is supported by the Joseph Rowntree Foundation and was established by the 'Shaping Our Lives' project, a user-controlled initiative and network, undertaking work on user involvement and issues around user-led outcomes. 'Our Voice in Our Future' grew out of a request from the Foundation to facilitate user involvement in its new 'Shaping Futures' programme. This programme aims to engage all stakeholders in the social care field in debates on issues about the long-term future of welfare, rights and entitlements (O'Neil, 1998). Part of the aim of the programme is to support service users and other stakeholders to have a voice in the process of policy development.

'Shaping Our Lives' was committed to ensuring that it would carry out this work in a way that put service-users in control and also build upon work that had already been done. To achieve this and to develop a proposal for the work, the project:

- sought views from the 300 user groups on its database on good practice in user involvement which should be incorporated in the work and bad practice which should be avoided;
- reviewed good and bad practice as recorded in current literature on user involvement;
- held a seminar with representatives of a wide range of service-user organisations to discuss general principles of user involvement and specific details about the shape and structure of a project to achieve the intended aims. This was followed up with one-to-one discussions by telephone and letter to enable participants at the seminar to have input into the proposals as they developed.

To carry out the work, 'Shaping Our Lives' is undertaking a one-year project (1999–2000), working intensely in two locations, with local service-user groups, to support and encourage discussion by service-users and their organisations about the long-term future of welfare. This is being backed up by work at a national level to ensure that these discussions are fully informed by the production by service-users of information on current debates on the future of welfare. These discussions will be both reactive – in terms of reacting to current political agendas – and proactive – in terms of developing a user-based agenda for the future. The aim is both to feed the results of these discussions into the 'Shaping Futures' programme, but also to disseminate them more widely. Key goals are to ensure that findings are disseminated around user groups as widely as possible, as well as seeking to reach politicians and the media.

Conclusion

The Citizens' Commission and 'Our Voice in Our Future' exemplify a new approach to social research, which radically revisits key relationships involved in research, notably relationships between:

- experience and knowledge;
- research and research participants;
- research, action and change.

We have been lucky. We have been involved in a user-controlled research initiative which, while modest in scale and funding, has had opportunities to develop and has encouraged and led to further initiatives. Not only have we been able to demonstrate the validity and legitimacy of such a research methodology, but we have also seen its methods vindicated. User-controlled research is possible – it works. Service-users can learn to be researchers. Service-users welcome *changed*, more equal research relationships. Important new findings do emerge from such research. It also offers confirmation from key but previously neglected user perspectives to complement existing findings.

The negative side, of course, is that there is still little user involvement in the radical programme of welfare reforms currently taking place in the UK. Initiatives like those we report, however, at least highlight the possibility and necessity of challenging this. They are impacting on mainstream social policy discourse and provide information for service-users and their organisations to use in their discussions and campaigns. So far, the disabled people's movement has been able to make some impact on New Labour's welfare reforms, making them one of the most contested and fraught policy areas which the UK government must address. However, this has been much less true for movements and organisations of other groups of people on the receiving end of social care and welfare policy and welfare reform. The government has publicly given its support to public debate about welfare reform, but so far done little if anything to make this happen (Lister and Beresford, 1999). By reframing and democratising research, service-users and their organisations are beginning to bring this about, while at the same time encouraging a radical rethinking of the process, aims and nature of research.

References

Barnes, C. and Mercer, G. (eds) (1997) *Doing Disability Research*, Leeds, The Disability Press.

Beresford, P. and Campbell, J. (1994) 'Disabled people, service users, user involvement and representation', *Disability and Society*, 9, 3: 315–25.

Beresford, P. and Turner, M. (1997) *It's Our Welfare: Report of the Citizens' Commission on the Future of the Welfare State*, London: National Institute for Social Work.

Beresford, P. and Turner, M. (2000) *Reclaiming Our Welfare: Second Report of the Citizens' Commission on the Future of the Welfare State*, London: National Institute for Social Work.

Beresford, P., Green, D., Lister, R. and Woodward, K. (1999) *Poverty First Hand: Poor People Speak Out for Themselves*, London: Child Poverty Action Group.

Citizens' Commission on the Future of the Welfare State (1998) *Response of the Citizens' Commission on the Future of the Welfare State to the Green Paper: New Ambitions for Our Country: a New Contract for Welfare*, London: Citizens' Commission on the Future of the Welfare State.

Commission on Social Justice (1994) *Social Justice: Strategies for National Renewal. The Report of the Commission on Social Justice*, London: Vintage.

Department of Social Security (1998) *New Ambitions for Our Country: a New Contract For Welfare* (The Welfare Green Paper, Cm 3805), London: Stationery Office.

Evans, C. and Fisher, F. (1999) 'Collaborative evaluation with service users: moving towards user-controlled research', in Ian Shaw and Joyce Lishman (eds) *Evaluation and Social Work Practice*, London: Sage, pp. 101–17.

Kiernan, C. (1999) 'Participation in research by people with learning difficulties: origins and issues', *British Journal of Learning Difficulties*, 27, 2: 43–7.

Lister, R. and Beresford, P. (1999), 'Poverty of Thinking', *Guardian* ('Society'), 28 July, p. 8.

March, J., Steingold, B., Justice, S. and Mitchell, P. (1997) 'Follow the yellow brick road! People with learning dfficulties as co-researchers', *British Journal of Learning Disabilities*, 25, 2: 77–9.

Milne, K. (1995) 'Welfare statement', *New Statesman and Society*, 27 January, pp. 20–1.

Oliver, M. (1996) *Understanding Disability: From Theory to Practice*, Basingstoke: Macmillan.

O'Neil, A. (1998) 'Taking forward consultations on the future of rights and welfare in social care and disability' (Briefing paper, unpublished), York: Joseph Rowntree Foundation, 24 February.

Stalker, K. (1998) 'Some ethical and methodological issues in research with people with learning difficulties', *Disability and Society*, 13, 1: 5–19.

Stanton, A. (1989) *Invitation to Self-Management*, Ruislip, Middlesex: Dab Hand Press.

Transport and General Workers Union (1994) *In Place of Fear: the Future of the Welfare State*, London: Transport and General Workers Union.

Whittaker, A. (ed.) (1997) *Looking at Our Services: Service Evaluation by People With Learning Difficulties*, London: King's Fund.

Yarrow, G. (1996) *Welfare, Mutuality and Self-Help*, London: The Association of Friendly Societies.

Chapter 12

The Camden 'Alternative Choices in Mental Health' project

Yan Weaver and Vicky Nicholls

Introduction

Examples of user-led research in mental health have been multiplying in the last few years, encouraged by the burgeoning survivor movement and demands not only for a voice in the planning and running of existing services, but also for choices and alternatives to traditional medical models of treatment (Lindow, 1994; Rogers *et al.*, 1993). In 1997 the Mental Health Foundation obtained funding from the UK lottery for a three-year service-user-led project, 'Strategies for Living', which was to undertake one of the largest ever pieces of UK-wide research devised, steered and carried out by people with experience of mental health problems (Faulkner and Layell, 2000). Beyond the national research, 'Strategies for Living' aimed to promote and support local user-led research through a 'research support network' involving grants, training and support for six local projects.

Based on evidence from an earlier survey (Faulkner, 1997), the main themes of 'Strategies for Living' included complementary therapies, self-help and religious and spiritual beliefs, and the local projects investigated a number of practical approaches related to these themes, arising from local interest. All the researchers had experience of using mental health services or of mental and emotional distress, and worked with other local service-users in various ways to refine and develop their research.

The six local projects looked into: the effect of attending places of worship on the well-being of Moslem men with mental health problems; the effects of regular ear acupuncture for women with long-term mental health problems; the benefits and drawbacks of peer support as experienced by attendants at a drop-in centre; how far involvement in a user-group affected ways of thinking about mental health and the sense of empowerment of its members; and the benefits of receiving and learning to give simple massage treatment in a group setting. The final project was based in the London borough of Camden and focused on 'alternative choices' in mental health; it forms the basis of the account which follows.

The Camden 'Alternative Choices' project was linked to the national initiative 'Strategies for Living', but it also grew out of existing local initiatives. In this account we describe the process involved, including some of the key issues of identity, power and responsibility in service-user-led research. The form of this report derives from its origin, as the transcript of a tape-recorded discussion. Yan Weaver was the facilitator of the Camden project and Vicky Nicholls works for the national project. (Breaks between our separate contributions and joint contributions are indicated by a row of asterisks.)

Identities

The first thing to say is that all of us involved in both the national 'Strategies for Living' project and the local (Camden) 'Alternative Choices' project are present or past service-users or would call ourselves 'survivors', either of the mental health system (perhaps statutory services, e.g. a psychiatric hospital) or of some sort of severe depression, distress or anxiety, even if we did not all become clients of statutory services.

* * * *

Yan: What first got me interested in alternative ideas about mental health was that I found myself in disagreement with the mainstream psychiatric/medical model of thinking. My first brush with the mental health system was after a period in my twenties of major ups and downs, when everything got too crazy for me and I got too crazy for the people around me. I ended up in a psychiatric hospital at that point. When I went into hospital I didn't want to take psychiatric drugs – I refused them and was allowed to do so. So my experience is probably quite unusual in that I went through what psychiatry would call 'psychosis' (in a word: 'madness') without psychiatric drugs. What I think I wanted most of all when I was going through the worst of it was someone who could be with me and listen to me, and take me seriously on my own terms. I was impressed by the idea – which I later found in the work of R.D. Laing, for example – that what people may need is someone who can stick by them and guide them through those times, to help them make some sense of it, not just throw drugs at them to suppress it all – although I know that for some people that's a choice they may decide to make.

I first got involved in service-user and survivor groups when I met some people from a national group called Survivors Speak Out and joined the group myself; and through that I got involved in our local service-user survivor group, Camden Mental Health Consortium, which is where the research project started out.

* * * *

Vicky: My experience of going through a time of distress about three years ago was that I felt very isolated and alienated, and I found it very difficult to get in touch with people who had been through similar experiences. I didn't really know how to open up about what was going on for me at the time. I was just very lucky that I stayed out of the mental health system. I got a lot of support from people close to me, even if they didn't really understand what I was going through.

Part of what brought me to the 'Strategies for Living' project was a belief in the potential for people to find new pathways through life through realising skills and being given opportunities to express the potential that they have. I had been working in the voluntary sector for many years, and I had worked on various projects that had an ethos of empowerment, working alongside people with learning difficulties for example. In these previous roles, however, I was coming from a different place, in that they didn't involve situations that had touched on my life so directly. So from that point of view the 'Strategies for Living' project has been an altogether different experience.

In carrying out and supporting service-user-led research, some important things have come up about disclosing the shared identities between researchers and participants. For example, if an interviewer is identifying her- or himself up front as someone who has experience of mental health problems (that's the term that has usually been used), some interviewees have said that that made them feel much safer, more able to open up and talk about their own experiences.

* * * *

Yan: I like the image of the 'round table'. We are meeting as fellow human beings on these things – all of us hearing and learning and swapping information. I struggled with the role of researcher at first. People in the groups that met wanted to know, for instance, what my experience of particular therapies had been. So I did say something but I didn't want to say too much about it, because it might colour the whole process. But then I just got to thinking, 'Well I'm part of this group as well, so I'll just share it. I don't have to be this neutral observer or chairperson.'

This research is essentially coming from people who have 'been there' rather than from people who are describing the experience of others. So the flyers for the Camden project, which were one of the main ways in which we got into contact with the people who took part in the group discussions, said something like: 'If you have experience of using mental health services, or coping with distress, come along to meet and share your ideas and find out more.' So people came along and said, for example, 'I'm paranoid schizophrenic and use general mental health services and I wanted to find out more about alternative and complementary therapies', or 'I've never used mental health services as such but I've suffered lots of traumas and distress for years and got involved in complementary therapies in order to work things through'. So there was quite a range of people, some with major mental illness diagnoses and others without. That in itself felt important: it was a kind of 'round table' involving people with very different experiences and different positions with respect to those experiences – some who had been through the worst of it and some who still felt they were pretty much in the thick of it.

The purpose of the work

The Camden project arose from two main sources. To begin with, there was my work with Diana Foley (another member of Camden Consortium) on a mental health handbook for Camden. This involved consultation and research, having meetings, and asking past and present service-users what they wanted included. Another aspect of this work was that we involved not only users of mainstream mental health services but also people coping with significant distress outside conventional services. (The fact that some people are using mental health services and some not doesn't necessarily reflect on the level of distress or difficulty they are in.) And another influence on the work was the document *Knowing Our Own Minds* (Faulkner, 1997), which is a national survey of how people in emotional distress take control of their lives, focusing on self-help, personal coping strategies and alternative therapies. What the Camden project tried to do was to give a local voice to this national initiative, to find out how people *here* do it, how *we* feel, how it is with *our* group of people.

The Camden project, then, was about discovering what people really want. We wanted to put together a report that we could put on the desks of social services and health authority officials, a report that they would have to take seriously, and that we could use as ammunition for campaigning and making people with power take notice. The important thing is that the ideas are not coming top-down from the professionals, but from people on the receiving end describing what they want, describing what works for them, and what goes wrong. We wanted the kinds of things that people were saying are relevant locally to be put in writing. It's about people exchanging information about what's around (services, ideas, groups and so on) and also what's not around. So people might be asking, for example, 'Why isn't there a crisis service that isn't based on the medical model, one that includes complementary therapies?' That's the sort of thing that people were asking about, the kind of thing that came up in the discussions.

This local research also ties in with the national initiative. It's a question of collecting the sort of evidence that can help to make a case for service planners to actually commit money to something new. At both levels the purpose is to gather evidence from people who have direct experience themselves, of what they would like and find helpful.

But, in retrospect, even if the powers that be don't take much notice, there has been another important purpose for the group meetings: the feedback, the sense of enjoyment and the exchange of ideas. So the whole thing was working on two levels. On the one hand it was providing campaigning evidence to be used later to influence people with official power, but it was also important to be expressing ourselves, having our say in a supportive atmosphere. The group felt accepting, like a good experience, and it was about exchanging ideas and information: so someone would talk about a support group that they went to and someone else would ask, 'How does it work?' 'How helpful do you find it?' 'What worked for you and what didn't?'

Getting started

The first groups we ran were to do with gathering information for the mental health handbook. They were open to whoever had an interest – health and social care practitioners, providers, service-users and others. We advertised through the Camden Consortium mail-out, and we also went through other channels, for example the mailing lists of providers who run day centres, and Voluntary Action Camden, which sends mail-outs to the whole of the voluntary sector. We tapped into all of these networks for both the handbook and the research.

For the research, we sent out a flyer that said, 'If you've had experience of using mental health services, of coping with "mental health problems", or distress, come along to a meeting to share your ideas and experiences or just to find out more.' First, we had a general meeting and split up into workshops, which we documented. We brainstormed ideas and collected them on a flip chart, and looked at three general themes: alternative and complementary therapies, self-help and support groups, and religious or spiritual beliefs and practices. Then, a while later, we mailed out to the people who had attended this first meeting, and to other people through the networks, saying that we were going to have a series of 'focus groups' or discussion meetings on these three themes. These groups then met, with an average of about ten people in each meeting. One focus group on each of the three different themes met separately, but people could choose: some came along to the meetings on all three themes, some came to one, and some people came to two. We also had some larger meetings concerned with the mental health handbook project. We held twelve meetings altogether, over a period of about fourteen months.

Some people would pick up one of the project flyers, ring up, talk about it and then come along to a meeting. But we also met people at local day centres and hospitals. For instance, Diana Foley and I (Yan) were invited to meetings at local psychiatric hospitals, such as depression support groups and a patients' council meeting.

* * * *

Vicky: Sometimes with projects like this (though not with the Camden project itself) enabling people to take part in the research can be quite a big issue. For example, on one occasion, when the research was going to be carried out in a local day centre, the manager of the centre wanted each person who was participating to have permission to be involved not only from their 'key worker' (the professional with direct responsibility for co-ordinating an individual's care) but also from their psychiatrist, before they were allowed to take part in the research – which was about giving and receiving massage! In the end, after some negotiation, a standard letter was drawn up describing the project; each person who wanted to participate was asked to check the letter, and if they were happy with what it said they had show it to their key worker and get permission like that. All this was necessary because in some settings the management take responsibility for the participants while they are on the premises. Perhaps one reason why there weren't these problems in Camden is that there were already so many local connections and contacts that 'the authorities' could simply be by-passed.

* * * *

Yan: *Where* the Camden project meetings took place was also important. The first meeting was at the Community Health Council premises. To some extent community health councils have a 'watchdog' role to play in relation to the mental health system, but the meeting room still felt a bit clinical. So we held the focus group meetings in a little community place up the road, which is really nice and cosy, a lovely little place. It's got a piano and a little stage and plants and posters, and people use it as a rehearsal space for plays, as well as the local Labour Party or a local anarchist group or a poetry group. So it felt very 'un-mental-health', which was deliberate. Also, we went out and bought some really tasty biscuits and water, fruit, and different sorts of tea and coffee. That felt like a way of valuing people, whereas when you go to some health authority or social services 'consultation' you can just sit in some horrible sparse room and get talked at.

Another way of making people feel that their contribution was valued was to let them know that they would be paid £5 to cover their costs. This was paid out of the Mental Health Foundation grant which helped to support the project. Payment is an important issue, and there's a lot of strong feeling about this within the survivor movement. People with experience of mental health problems or distress are quite often the *subjects* of research. We are asked to be part of surveys when mental health authorities come along and want to interview for this, that or the other, or we are asked to join consultation groups, or be on service-user committees. But the professionals are being highly paid for all that, while you as a service-user are having to watch out for your social security benefits. So, really, we felt that some sort of payment was essential. We wouldn't want to preclude people wanting to do this sort of work without any finances, and you don't need to have loads of money, but it can certainly help to oil the wheels.

* * * *

Vicky: Then, finally, in terms of 'getting started' there were the research training sessions for the local project facilitators. These concentrated on interviewing skills, questionnaire design, focus groups and data analysis. There was a series of detailed training days (see Mental Health Foundation, 1999). So, for example, during the interview skills session we watched a video of a 'bad' interview, and discussed where we thought the interviewer was going wrong. And we had a whole day on focus group training, where we all took part in a practice focus group during the day.

* * * *

The process, relationships and power

One important part of the research process in the Camden project was the use of 'topic guides'. Before the discussions, a list of ideas was drawn up by the facilitator for the group to cover. In some cases this list was built on a general topic guide developed in a research training session; in other cases the guides were developed from what had been said in a general 'brainstorm' meeting. We also asked people who came along to the meetings to fill out a brief questionnaire, asking them for personal details and their experience of, and opinions about, say, complementary therapies. Then they could write down what they wanted to say even if they didn't get around to speaking about these issues in the meeting. Here is an example of one of the topic guides.

1) **What experience do you have of complementary/alternative therapies?**

2) **Where did you have the therapy or treatment?**
   Was it privately/on the NHS/part of other mental health services, etc.?
   How was it paid for?

3) **Where did you find out about these therapies?**
   I.e. what was your route into these therapies?

4) **How did you start using complementary therapies?**
   What kinds of problems were you seeking help with, or what effects were
       you hoping for?

5) **What was/is your experience of these therapies?**
   If you've tried several, choose two or three which stand out in your memory.
   What were/are the advantages or disadvantages?
   What did/do you like or dislike about the therapies?
   What did you find most helpful or unhelpful?
   Good experiences/bad experiences
   What were/are the short-term or long-term effects?
   Any complaints? Bad practice?

6) **Additional:**
   a) **'Complementary' or 'Alternative'?**
      Have you used these therapies alongside or instead of conventional
          medical treatment?
      Are you still using complementary therapies?
      Are you still using conventional medical treatment?

   b) **What are your views about the use of complementary therapies in
       mental health?**

* * * *

Yan: I think there was a general feeling that during the discussions people were supportive of each other – emotionally supportive – and treated each other with respect. We talked about that as something to aim for in the introduction to each meeting. People were interested in hearing each other's opinions, and there was a lot of 'so what's that?' and 'so what happens there?' I felt there was something very cohesive about the group. Some people didn't say a lot at first, and sometimes when people were rather quiet I tried to 'bring them in'. So in the end it felt to me that everyone was a part of it. I felt that I had been part of a good group of people and the feedback on the meetings was really positive. One person, who knew me before anyway, said he thought everybody was given a space to speak, and no one was dominating the discussion. He felt that there was enough like-mindedness but also enough difference, so it wasn't bland and cosy. I was very conscious of the need to respect people's views. There were times when I intervened to say, 'Let's not argue this point too much, but respect that we do have different ideas.' I tried to be careful in the way I chaired the discussions, to make sure we didn't get too bogged down in the fine details of what someone meant by something.

Sometimes there were tensions, for example when someone said, 'I hate psychodynamic therapy' and somebody else was seeing a psychodynamic therapist. The focus group on religious and spiritual beliefs, in particular, were working in an area that for a lot of people is very personal and individual, and I was apprehensive about what might be very sensitive issues. At times this felt quite scary, because people had very different ideas about the way the world is and the way to approach it. So I felt I had to intervene gently: I was scared of religious wars breaking out! And also you have to remember that not everyone in the group was specifically involved with religion: they were kind of critical but didn't necessarily find it a problem. At times like that I was aware of the responsibilities of a group facilitator and the issue of how much you are changing what's going on. In a sense you are changing things, because you are focusing on something and trying to open up certain topics.

As the facilitator, I often felt very nervous. This relates back to the issue of identity, which we discussed at the beginning. I was nervous of the responsibility and I struggled with the idea of being the facilitator and therefore having a degree of power. I thought, 'God, this is all being tape-recorded, and part of a "research project" which may be circulated to lots of mental health organisations.' It felt like really big stuff for me, very grand, very big scale. But at the same time, I really wanted to do it, and thought, well, you know, perhaps it's going to be all right. And on the whole it was.

* * * *

Vicky: The power issue is very complicated. For example, as researchers we may not necessarily feel powerful in relation to the group of people we are working with, but to them we may *appear* powerful. Even though we may be feeling anxious and unskilful, to the other people in the group we're coming in with a 'researcher' hat on, and that may have connotations of power for some of them. So we had to acknowledge that, and acknowledge our own difficulties. Also, we were aware that we are trying to find different ways of working *with* one another, and that meant trying to make the process accessible. Because all of the researchers were new to doing research. That was one of the aims of the national project: to enable people with no previous formal research experience to carry out research. So we tried to demystify some of the language which is used in talking about research. For example, we wouldn't use alienating terms like 'quantitative methods' but instead talk about ways of measuring and describing things by using numbers.

* * * *

Yan: I don't think of myself as 'a researcher'. If I were to explain the project I wouldn't define it as 'research': as far as I am concerned we had 'discussion groups', 'meetings' and 'focus groups' – and even that sounds like jargon. If I had to describe what we have been doing, I would describe it not as 'research' but as 'sharing ideas' or 'seeking people's views'. That's how we described it to the people who came along, rather than inviting them to be part of 'a research project'.

* * * *

Vicky: And, thinking of another local project, I don't think that the people who are getting that off the ground have used the word 'research' once yet. Instead they've used phrases like 'sharing ideas' or 'meeting to discuss ideas that might influence services'.

* * * *

Responsibility, accountability

Another side of the power issue concerns our sense of accountability towards the participants and responsibility for supporting them through the process in an effective way, in a way that they find helpful. We also felt responsible for getting everyone's voices heard, for taking them seriously, for making them feel that their experiences and views *matter*.

* * * *

Yan: And this is why it was very important that the discussions were tape recorded and transcribed. Having the tape recorder there changes things: it makes people realise that they are being taken seriously. But there may be issues of confidentiality, of people not feeling safe, or it may be inhibiting or off-putting. Recording or documenting meetings makes a difference, and that's a kind of responsibility in itself. Often at official meetings, professionals set the agenda and then don't seem to listen to what service-users are coming up with. We all do this agenda-setting, of course, but at least in this project we were trying to look at *all* the things that were said. It's a matter of hearing the suppressed voice – not the voice of power – the voice that gets filtered out when service-commissioners and service-providers carry out conventional consultation exercises. So we used a tape recorder (the national project lent one out), just a little portable one, which cost about £300, including the microphone. We sat round quite close, with the machine on a chair in the middle.

As for confidentiality, in the Camden project we did talk about it. One thing we explained is that group members would have an opportunity to look at the material before it was published. This of course meant that we were asking them for yet more of their time and it was not clear that this was something that people were necessarily asking for; but we did feel that issues of confidentiality were an important area to address.

* * * *

Finally, there was the issue of how to manage the ending of the programme. There is an interesting distinction here, perhaps, between a national and a local project. At the national level it was important, when we were building up relationships during the programme, to recognise that the formal project would come to an end and that people would not necessarily continue those relationships after its ending. In a national project you really need to prepare people for losing contact. But locally things can be rather different. In Camden, for example, there has been quite a lot of contact since the end of the project between some of the people who were involved. Some people already knew one another, because the project was to some extent based in an existing network of service-users, and some people who met through the focus groups have continued to be involved in the work on the mental health handbook. And other people who met through the project have kept in contact with one another. So, if you have something really local like the Camden project, then one of the spin-offs is that you can generate supportive relationships which can more easily continue.

This links in with one of the key ideas about action research: the process itself is important, and if all goes well it doesn't need to come to an end, because it creates good relationships in a local place. It makes something else happen. There is a specific project, but as one phase comes to an end, another aspect opens up.

* * * *

Yan: So people found out about alternative therapy projects or counselling, or support groups, or spiritual approaches, and about non-medical crisis services. There has been an exchange of information, so that people have also started to think about what is missing locally, the kinds of projects we *could* have. There are all sorts of ideas around. And some people have said, 'When are you having another of those meetings?' Perhaps services should grow out of this sort of activity, out of supportive groups, 'round table' discussions, where people decide for themselves the kinds of services they want to see.

Project findings – a preliminary impression

As already mentioned, those involved in the work ranged from people who had never had contact with mental health services to others who had received a 'major' psychiatric diagnosis, such as schizophrenia or manic depression, and had used services over several years. Those who had received a diagnosis held a range of views about it, from those who accepted it or found it fairly correct to those who had quite alternative understandings of their experiences.

A full analysis of the questionnaires, notes and transcripts from the various meetings has yet to be completed. This section, therefore, merely summarises a general impression of the sort of insights which have arisen from the project. This preliminary stage has had to be based mainly on the work of the first of the three project themes (alternative and complementary therapies), although the ideas outlined below clearly have many links with ideas relating to the other two themes – self-help and support groups, and religious and spiritual beliefs and practices.

One general theme was that people seeking alternative and complementary therapies seemed to be looking for ways of becoming more relaxed and increasing their sense of well-being, other than through conventional drug treatments. Avoiding the negative side-effects of conventional treatments was a major concern. Thus, there was interest in practices such as meditation and in relaxation techniques, although some people found such direct attempts at relaxation very difficult, since they tended to increase anxiety. Some people thus preferred methods which approached relaxation through more active and indirect methods (e.g. regular exercise, walking, swimming). Some people suggested a combination of approaches, or practices such as yoga or Tai Chi, which in themselves combine both activity *and* relaxation, or therapies such as massage in which the therapist does more of the work.

Another theme was the importance of achieving a greater level of self-awareness, a greater understanding of how you respond to stress, in order to become better at looking after yourself. In other words, many people were seeking a greater level of control over their own well-being and their own treatment; they wanted to try alternative therapies as a form of self-help, rather than having to deal with yet another type of professional expert. One person said, 'I think you have to find your own way', and went on: 'I've followed other people's suggestions all my life, I'm just starting to really learn how to learn things for myself.' Even people who were not necessarily critical of conventional treatments were nevertheless interested in exploring complementary therapies, to see what these might *add* to their lives.

One important aspect of alternative or complementary therapies was that they involved a sense of being 'nurtured', whereas: 'Doctors don't have time for that type of thing: they just hand out medication, which doesn't really help but just suppresses everything'. This sense of being nurtured also seemed to arise from meeting like-minded people involved in these therapies, particularly through groups and classes.

A frequent complaint was that psychiatrists always seemed to 'just want to put you on medication'. However, a number of participants were interested in remedies such as St John's Wort and Chinese herbs, which seems to suggest the continued attraction of medicines as a form of treatment, as long as the side-effects of Western drugs could be avoided, for instance.

In many cases people were aware of issues surrounding conventional scientific evidence for the differential effectiveness of alternative therapies. Since there are so many choices available they wanted to know that treatments had been 'checked out', even though they recognised that it can be difficult to gather such evidence, given the problems of measuring such things as 'feeling better about yourself'. As one person said, 'The trouble with science is that it has a sort of blanketing effect; it says that something is only valid if it works for everybody', whereas, as many people emphasised, everyone is unique, so different things work for different people. Participants also recognised that it was difficult to know, in retrospect, after sampling a number of different treatments, what it was that had been beneficial, and thus most had an attitude of healthy scepticism concerning their experiences. Additionally, some people stressed the importance of social circumstances that they felt were too rarely taken into account by mainstream mental health services *and* alternative approaches – such as money, housing and discrimination.

Finally, one participant observed that when he had talked to his psychiatrist about his need for healing of his soul, she had wanted to know what proof he had for the soul, and said that as far as she was concerned the soul didn't exist: 'She didn't want to get involved in that aspect of things . . . kind of backed off the subject and went back to dealing with medication.' Someone else talked about having 'a damaged spirit'. This brings out a deep difference between the somewhat superficial, mechanical, professional emphasis on 'psyche' as simply 'the mind' and service-users' frequent attraction to the spiritual content of many alternative and complementary approaches. This emphasis on the spiritual and holistic dimension of mental health issues is one good example of the vital importance of service-users' contribution to improving mental health service provision.

References

Faulkner, A. (1997) *Knowing Our Own Minds*, London: Mental Health Foundation.

Faulkner, A. and Layell, S. (2000) *Strategies for Living: a Report of User-led Research into People's Strategies for Living with Mental Distress*, London: Mental Health Foundation.

Lindow, V. (1994) *Self-help Alternatives to Mental Health Services*, London: Mind Publications.

Mental Health Foundation (1999) *The DIY Guide to Survivor Research*, London: Mental Health Foundation.

Rogers, A., Pilgrim, D. and Lacey, R. (1993) *Experiencing Psychiatry: Users' Views of Services*, London: Mind Publications.

Chapter 13

A foot in the door

A collaborative action research project with cancer service-users

Jane Bradburn and Cherry Mackie

Introduction

The involvement of service-users in the National Health Service has been a prominent theme of health service policy in the UK since 1990. However, in spite of government policy to encourage user participation in the planning and implementation of healthcare services, the indications are that often where this does take place it is tokenistic rather than meaningful.

This chapter describes how a group of cancer service-users (all members of local cancer self-help groups) took part in a collaborative action research project with the aim of finding out how they could get their voices heard in discussions taking place on reorganising local cancer services (see Note on p. 197).

Background

A network of local cancer self-help groups was established in the early 1990s and met regularly at the Mount Vernon Hospital, a regional cancer centre in North London. The network offered an opportunity for members of the eighteen local cancer self-help groups to share issues and concerns and to learn from each other. Members identified specific concerns about the way in which cancer patients and their carers were treated, as well as drawing support from the network. For example, at one meeting members voiced their concern about the way in which cancer patients were given their cancer diagnosis, and about poor communication by staff when patients faced with what some considered 'a death sentence' were in many cases left feeling angry and isolated.

The local cancer self-help groups were located within the catchment area of the regional cancer centre. This centre treated cancer patients from a wide area who were referred for specialised treatment (for example radiotherapy and chemo-therapy) by the outlying local hospitals.

The network of groups developed largely because of the support of a local clinical oncologist who had a particular interest in the value of self-help groups, and this enabled the network to become part of a developing service, providing psychosocial support to cancer patients and families attending the hospital. The network facilitators (Jane Bradburn and Cherry Mackie) formed a link between the self-help group network and hospital staff. When issues were raised by the network about local cancer care these were relayed to staff. So when concerns about the way in which people were told they had cancer were raised, the centre responded by setting up a project with network members to investigate and address the problem (Walker et al., 1996).

The reason for explaining the background to this collaborative action research project is to illustrate that a relationship was already established between the service-user groups and hospital staff, in which group members felt confident in bringing their concerns to the attention of staff and having them acted upon. Unfortunately their previous experience had been often quite the reverse, self-help groups tending to be viewed by medical staff in a negative light, as groups of the angry and dissatisfied rather than as a source of first-hand knowledge and expertise about local cancer services. Research undertaken showed that relations between members of groups and health professionals in the local hospitals were often problematic, with groups feeling ignored and under-valued by busy health care staff (Bradburn et al., 1992).

It is against this background that in 1995 the government introduced a policy to reorganise local cancer services (the so-called *Calman–Hine Report*) aimed at improving the quality of services and ensuring more equitable standards of service throughout the country (Expert Advisory Group on Cancer to the Chief Medical Officers of England and Wales, 1995). Local cancer care professionals were charged, together with health authorities and cancer service-users, with implementing a strategy for reform in their areas. The initiative appeared to offer an opportunity for groups of service-users to become involved in decisions about local cancer services, from which they had previously been excluded.

At the time Jane was working as the self-help groups co-ordinator but with a research and development role. Though lacking experience of cancer and not a health professional, she had a background in community development, was well known to group members, and had achieved a measure of trust over the time that she had worked with them as an advocate. Cherry had had breast cancer and the experience led her to set up her own self-help group. She joined initially as a volunteer to assist in co-ordinating the network; then as a result of her enthusiasm and experience she was made a paid member of staff. These existing established relationships were important in carrying out the research collaboratively. Other action researchers have stressed the value of a special relationship of trust and acceptance between the group and the researcher (Whyte, 1991; Chesler, 1991).

Why we took a collaborative action research approach

A collaborative action research approach seemed to be the most appropriate to this study for a number of reasons; for example, it has been found to be a good way to work with self-help groups (Chesler, 1991; Borkman and Schubert, 1994).

This is because the collaborative process addresses many of the issues experienced by members of self-help groups, for example their perceived lack of power vis-à-vis the professional or expert. It allows for the inclusion of experiential knowledge and focuses on empowerment and power relations and the consciousness-raising of participants (Whitmore, 1994). The approach is also useful as it aims to find solutions to practical problems and to change practice.

The study took place over the period of a year and we have chosen to describe what took place during that period as a chronological sequence in order to demonstrate the 'process' of collaborative research. Three strands can be distinguished in the process (see Figure 13.1). One strand is the development of the policy programme, the timetable for implementing the *Calman–Hine Report*, which created the context within which the group was working. The report was published in April 1995 and in spring 1996 health authorities and hospitals were expected to have mapped existing local cancer services. In spring and summer 1996 they were to agree a preliminary plan for the organisation of services in their area. The group, however, had no knowledge of this information when it was formed.

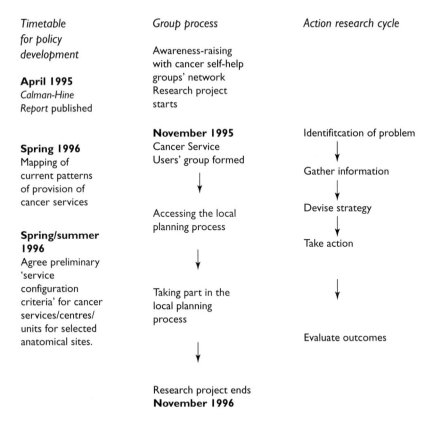

Figure 13.1   Chronology of the cancer service-users' network

The second strand is the group process. The group process is the way in which the group developed and changed over the year, from hearing of the opportunities for becoming involved and setting up the group in November 1995 to achieving the goal of taking part in that process and ending the project in November 1996.

The third strand was the action research cycle itself (shown in Figure 13.1 as linear in order to match the other processes, rather than as cyclical). This starts with the identification of the problem, in this case the cancer service-users wanting to be part of the local policy discussions. Next is the information-gathering stage, when group members gathered information about how they could do this, whom to approach and how to approach them. The next stage was devising a strategy (the 'thinking' phase – Stringer, 1996) about how to act on the information, and the final stage involved taking action and evaluating the effect of that action.

In practice the phases were not so clearly separated. For example, group members were individually applying the general approach to problems they came up against, as well as following this process in the group itself.

The process

In describing the chronological development of the group we have attempted to show how these three strands, context, group process and action research cycle, were interwoven. We also aim to reflect the process of development both in the participants as they became more confident and empowered and in the project itself as it unfolded, from raising awareness among the cancer self-help groups about the opportunities, to having their voices heard, and finally achieving their goal of participation in decision-making forums on local cancer service provision, with acknowledgement of the value of their knowledge and experience.

Informing users

The network members were not aware of the introduction of the government's new policy initiative. Even where copies of the policy document were available, group members' lack of understanding of the jargon used (e.g. 'purchasers' and 'providers') or of the organisational structure of the National Health Service, or of who was who in the local services meant that it was of little practical use.

Their first step as facilitators therefore was to raise awareness and inform members of the network about the new policy proposals contained in the *Calman–Hine Report* and about the opportunities for involvement in local discussions about cancer services. A meeting was held and a summarised version of the policy explained and discussed. As a result of that meeting seven members said they would like to get involved.

This process of raising awareness and informing at the outset meant that those who volunteered already understood what they were engaging in. Self-help groups usually exist to meet the support needs of their members (who may be ill or in need of support), so not everyone will want to engage in advocacy. In fact, as we describe later, those who did already had considerable experience of acting as advocates for their group members and enjoyed taking that role, reflecting a growing trend nationally (Bradburn *et al.*, 1992).

Setting up a Cancer Service-users' Group

Six cancer self-help group members who had expressed an interest in becoming involved in local discussions on the implementation of the changes laid out in the *Calman–Hine Report* came to a meeting at the cancer centre. In this way the collaborative action research project and the Cancer Service-users' Group had its beginnings. Each member came from a local cancer self-help group in a different part of the catchment area. This meant that as well as having an interest in the services provided by the regional cancer centre, they also wanted to see improvements in their local hospitals. A seventh member, a carer who was not associated with a local self-help group, joined later.

We decided that the aim of the project was to find ways of becoming involved in the local decision-making process. The joint agreement about the focus of the research was crucial, we believe, in leading to a shared purpose and commitment. Examples can be found of collaborative action research projects of which the aim has been largely (and sometimes unavoidably) determined by the researcher/facilitator or funders and this can lead to dissatisfaction by all with the outcomes of the project (Meyer, 1993).

We decided that we would meet together at regular intervals at the cancer centre. All the participants agreed to discussions being tape recorded and to keep papers and letters relating to the project.

Becoming informed

Our first task was to understand the local planning process to which we were trying to gain access. The user group only learnt about the policy changes as a result of the network meeting. Very little information was made available to cancer service-users. Such information as there was appeared in the newsletters of cancer charity organisations. The policy itself, though designed to be patient-focused, made no proposals about how patients might be involved in the planning stages. We felt left in the dark. Uninformed and unaware of the context within which we were trying to operate, we tried a number of different strategies in order to gain information about the local planning process.

To start with, the only information came through existing links with the local oncologist. We knew that discussions were being held in the local hospitals to consider how they might meet the criteria set for cancer centres and units by the *Calman–Hine Report*. As facilitator, Jane wrote to all the oncologists drawing attention to the Cancer Service-users' Group and its willingness to work with them in this planning process. The letter met with only one response, which was sympathetic but made no proposal for involvement. However, Cherry was asked to join her hospital committee where the lead clinician took a particular interest in promoting consumer involvement and employed Cherry as a patient adviser.

As a result of frustration at the lack of progress in gaining access to local hospital committees, a decision was made by the group to approach local health authorities as we learnt that consultation exercises were being carried out by some health authorities with cancer service-users. This only became apparent to the group as we gathered more information collectively and individually. The user group did not know whom to approach within the local health authority and had little knowledge of its structure or function. It was therefore agreed that we carry out a survey of all the local health authorities covered by the network to find out what activities they were undertaking to involve local people in decisions about the planning of local cancer services in the light of the *Calman–Hine Report.*

The survey had the additional benefit of informing health authority staff of the Cancer Service-users' Group's existence. It became apparent then that the health authority staff were unsure about how to access users for consultation exercises. Many of those contacted as a result of the survey were unaware of the existence of cancer self-help groups in the area. The group supplied contact details of local cancer self-help groups and helped to arrange discussions between users and health authorities.

Sharing fears and building confidence

Initially much of the discussion in the user group was around the barriers which members had experienced in working with health professionals in the past. Members anticipated difficulties in working on health committees as a result of their previous experiences. As patients, they were used to being in a subservient role: not only was the doctor a 'professional' but also in most cases a man in authority was treating a woman when she was at her most vulnerable.

'*It is getting the confidence to talk to other people about what I think is right and getting my point of view over. I find it very difficult to put over to them because of this barrier that I have built up about talking to doctors.*'

Cherry, who worked closely with health professionals to involve them in working alongside self-help groups, gave examples of ways she had found to be successful in making good communication links and involving staff in group meetings. Discussion also provided opportunities for reflection about how members saw their relationships developing with professionals on the committee.

'*It is going to be very much more a professional situation. With professionals you have got to be very careful because you do not want to alienate yourself. I think that is going to be my biggest problem, not saying things that I haven't thought through, being a bit more cautious perhaps in what I say.*'

Discussion meant that negative experiences were aired within a confiding environment and explored safely. Both positive and negative experiences were exchanged, and listening to the different stories gleaned from members of the self-help groups helped user-group members to gain a more complete view of the experiences of local cancer service-users.

Sharing experiences also meant that members gradually developed a confidence in their value as user representatives. Discussion of their role on committees led to discussions about why they had a place in healthcare decision-making, i.e. due to the legitimacy and authority of their experiential knowledge.

'I think people need to talk to other people about what is happening to them and share their experience because I think it is really important. But also maybe to share the fact that they are going to die like you are going to die. . . . I think this is what the professionals get upset about and what they find difficult. I have thought about that quite a bit. Having been around a lot of people who have died and seen the difficulties they have had with dying and not being able to share their problems.'

Later, as some members of the user group became representatives on health panels and committees, others learned in the discussion group about their experiences and discussed how they would react in similar situations. Through this interaction a form of shared learning took place, in which those who were already experiencing this new 'representative' role could reflect with those who had yet to experience it.

Problem-solving

A number of barriers to accessing the planning process were identified through the action research approach taken by the group. These included lack of information, attitudes of health professionals and the lack of procedures in place for user involvement.

The process of working together in the group enabled these to be explored and action to be taken either collectively or by individual members. Collective problem-solving within the group helped to overcome these barriers. Members learnt about how to access the discussions and gained through the mutual support and learning process.

'I come to this meeting because I learn from you all, I come to this meeting because I feel that I can give you information and you can give me information and everybody helps each other.'

The sharing of information and the development of strategies towards achieving the objectives of the group were intertwined. As researcher/facilitator, Jane provided a source of strategic analysis and information in order to help the group to move forward. To some extent this meant analysing power relationships and levers which might be useful to the group. For example, it emerged through contact with other organisations that the user group might be more successful in approaching health authorities than individual hospitals.

As part of her research role, Jane had scope for networking fairly extensively, both within the local area and further afield, and this was important. It meant that she was able to give information about the timetables for implementation of the policy, the activities of several of the health authorities, and key people to contact.

Members of the group were also given support and confidence, for example by being encouraged to go to a meeting with their regional health authority contact. They went with much trepidation but found that they were warmly welcomed and this led to links being established with other key contacts. One of them commented:

> *'You* [Jane Bradburn] *said, "Stop pussy-footing around at the bottom of the rung, go right to the top", because we weren't getting anywhere. Perhaps it might have happened anyway – who knows – but we felt good.'*

Group members contributed their experiences of linking with health professionals, indicating what worked and what did not work.

> *'I went to a meeting and all I did at this particular meeting was just to introduce myself to the committee. I had picked S.'s* [another group member's] *brains and asked her what she had said to her* [the consultant], *and one thing that really struck me was the fact that I was just there to be a patient representative and not to threaten them in any way which is what S. said to her guy. So I said exactly the same thing and it seemed to go down quite well – they seemed to sort of accept the fact that I was there.'*

There was a perception that professionals felt threatened by patient involvement. The frustration felt by members when they were ignored or felt that they were not being taken seriously by health professionals was defused through expression within the group, and (on the other hand) successes encouraged other members to continue their involvement.

There was not always agreement about the strategic decisions taken by the user group. One of the group members felt uncomfortable with the non-confrontational approach taken by the group and expressed anger at what she perceived as a failure of the group to take the initiative in a more proactive way. Her frustration at the pace of change was reinforced by the urgency she felt as someone who had experienced the disease.

> *'It is frustrating with this cancer issue because it is something that is death-defying, basically if it wasn't so terminal it wouldn't be so upsetting.'*

Eventually she decided to withdraw from the group, disillusioned by the failure of her local hospital to invite her to a committee meeting, in spite of apparently agreeing to her participation as a user representative. As facilitators, we felt that this was a failure on our part, but at the same time it showed the differences among group members in terms of personality, and their need to be acknowledged and accepted.

As a former cancer patient with experience of running a longstanding, successful self-help group, Cherry's role was to help the group make decisions grounded in their experiential knowledge. Because of her responsibility to the cancer self-help network, she was also concerned to ensure that the investment we were putting into influencing the local policy agenda would not draw resources away from the other important support work which the groups provided.

Taking part in the local planning process

Once members of the user group had been asked to sit on one of the local policy-making committees, they found themselves in what was, for most, quite a new situation, one which could be quite intimidating. Often they were the only cancer service-user representatives among a group of consultants, senior health managers and nurses. The group engaged in discussions about what their new role was, how to cope with it and how to communicate effectively with their fellow committee members.

'I am going in completely blind – I have no idea what is expected of me if anything for that matter. Am I there just as a token gesture or am I there as somebody who has got some input?'

In order to become effective committee members they had to reconstruct their identity in such a way that instead of feeling that they were 'the patient' they saw themselves as 'experts' in the experience of the disease.

'It is very difficult for me because at least three of the doctors on the panel that I am on treated me as a patient . . . and I find being treated as a patient and being on that panel are two different things. To me I am a patient still, whereas I don't want to be the patient when I'm talking to them; I want to be me as an individual, working as a representative.'

The group process helped members to develop that identity through discussions about the distinct contribution they could make:

'I think the thing to get past is the fact that you [as a user rep] *don't have to know as much as everybody else about the scientific side of it – that is their job – but what you have got is something that is quite individual that you have painfully gone through.'*

Group members found it difficult to overcome their feeling of lack of confidence and of effectiveness on committees, so we decided to invite a trainer who had developed a training programme for lay members of maternity liaison committees to provide the group with an adapted form of the National Childbirth Trust 'Voices' training (Fletcher *et al.* 1997). The training successfully addressed many of the problems they faced as user reps on committees, understanding the National Health Service system, confidence-building, making your case and building relationships.

At the end of the year, all seven participants had been involved in local planning forums and they decided that the need for the group had finished. In particular, the role of researcher/facilitator seemed to become less important as the group members became more involved in the policy process, shared their experiences about participation on the committees with each other, and achieved their goal of getting their voices heard.

Evaluation of the process

The development process was evaluated through semi-structured interviews with each of the participants in his or her own home, conducted two months after the start of the study and then again six months later. Analysis of the two interviews together with the tape recordings made during the meetings meant that a comparison could be made of language, attitude and perception. The emerging themes were taken to a group meeting for discussion to see if they matched the group member's own perceptions. Members also read and commented on the subsequent research report. One of the unexpected outcomes of this exercise was that they had an opportunity to reflect on the process which they had been part of and to realise how different they felt.

'The group was really important, because it enabled us to all speak together about different issues but each coming from the same sort of line if you like. How people have developed – seeing that has been very interesting. I have to be honest and say that without any of that back-up going in [to the committee] *on my own without previous knowledge, I don't think I would have lasted.'*

Conclusion

The collaborative action research approach described in this report successfully addressed some of the issues of inequality of power between the Cancer Service-users' Group members and health professionals, so that, in the end, group members spoke of 'getting a foot in the door'. From seeing others as the experts, they began to have a sense of their own 'expertness'. From feeling ignored by professional experts, they began to feel that they were taken seriously, and that their contribution to the discussion of policy was valued. Over the course of the project group members discovered how to exercise an effective advocacy role in supporting other cancer patients, in spite of the complexities that it entailed. On many occasions they succeeded in building effective collaborative relationships with healthcare professionals, overcoming resistance on the part of the latter, as well as their own initial lack of confidence. They began to experience their own identity in positive terms and to be able to project that positive identity effectively during formal policy discussions which would earlier have seemed highly intimidating. Most importantly, perhaps, they succeeded in establishing (for themselves and for others) the value of their own 'experiential knowledge' – as a substantial contribution to professional understanding, based not merely on individual experience but on *shared* experience, for which they could claim some degree of 'validity', if not 'representativeness'. In this sense, they came to see themselves as indeed possessing 'expertise'.

The most important 'conclusion' of the research project, therefore, is that it offered a means of empowerment to the members of the Cancer Service-users' Group. There is no doubt that most experienced a sense of achievement and of personal development, although this affected some more than others: tolerating dissension as a group was not easy, and the member who left dissatisfied by the process caused us much heart-searching.

In evaluating their part in the action research project, the group members might be expected to have focused on more tangible outcomes of their participation in the policy process. Indeed, more conventional research approaches would have focused on more objective and measurable outcomes, for example specific changes in cancer services and policy resulting from the service-users' involvement. However, the participants chose aspects of 'the process of participating' as their 'outcome measurements' because that is what they valued most. One might, of course, speculate that their perception of the outcomes of their work may change once they have got not only 'a foot in the door' but also 'their feet under the table', that is when the goal of their participation becomes more clearly a matter of making an identifiable impact on services.

Finally, it was crucial for the project that group members shared common practical goals. This meant that everyone could get something from the research for themselves, rather than just contributing to the researcher's agenda. For one of us, Jane, who was specifically acting in the role of 'researcher' for the project, the challenge of its collaborative, action research structure was to learn humility and generosity in both knowledge and emotions, in a way which is very different from the requirements of conventional research but which adds so much richness of understanding.

Note

We would like to acknowledge the contribution of all the members of the Cancer Services-users' Group as collaborators in this project and of Dr Jane Maher and staff at the Lynda Jackson–Macmillan Cancer Support and Information Centre, Mount Vernon Hospital; also the hospital staff and local and regional health authority staff who assisted us with this project.

References

Borkman, T. and Schubert, S. (1994) 'Participatory action research as a strategy for studying self-help groups internationally', *Prevention in Human Services*, 11, 1: 45–68.

Bradburn, J. and Maher, J. (1995) 'The growth of advocacy groups for cancer patients in Europe and the USA', *Oncology Today*, 12 July, pp. 14–17.

Bradburn, J., Maher, E.J., Young, J. and Young, T. (1992) 'Community-based cancer support groups: an undervalued resource?', *Clinical Oncology*, 4: 377–80.

Chesler, M. (1991) 'Participatory research with self-help groups: an alternative paradigm for inquiry and action', *American Journal of Community Psychology*, 19: 757–68.

Expert Advisory Group on Cancer to the Chief Medical Officers of England and Wales (1995) *A Policy Framework for Commissioning Cancer Services (The Calman–Hine Report)*, London: Department of Health/HMSO.

Fletcher, G., Buggins, E., Newburn, M., Gready, M., Draper, J. and Wang, M. (1997) *The Voices Project: Final Report*, London: National Childbirth Trust.

Meyer, J. (1993) 'Action research: stages in the process: a personal account', *Nurse Researcher*, 2, 3: 24–37.

Stringer, E. (1996) *Action Research: a Handbook for Practitioners*, London: Sage.

Walker, G., Bradburn, J. and Maher, J. (1996) *Breaking Bad News*, London: King's Fund.

Whitmore, E. (1994) 'To tell the truth: working with oppressed groups: participatory approaches to inquiry', in P. Reason (ed.) *Participation in Human Inquiry*, London: Sage, pp. 82–98.

Whyte, W.F. (1991) *Participatory Action Research*, Newbury Park, Calif.: Sage.

Chapter 14

Pauline and Alzheimer's

'Reflections' on caring

Philip Ingram

It started with my glasses. We were standing in the hallway, Pauline facing me with her back to the glass-panelled street door. I forget why we were there, but everything else is firmly implanted in my memory. She stared at my face in a curious but strangely concentrated way. Then a smile spread across her own lovely features, and she pointed.

I couldn't make out what she was on about. Had I got a dirty mark on my face? I turned to look at myself in the hall mirror. No, the same somewhat dishevelled and perpetually worried expression stared back at me – no dirty mark or anything unusual.

By this time Pauline was convulsed with laughter. It was good to hear her laugh. Life these days did not often promote such spontaneous hilarity. Her Alzheimer's had changed so many things – for both of us.

'Look.' Her speech was already reduced mainly to single words and sometimes even these needed a room full of interpreters to understand. But the 'Look' and the pointed finger actually touching my glasses now made quite clear that it had something to do with my spectacles. I took them off, inspected them myself and then found Pauline looking deeply into my eyes. Years ago intimate eye-to-eye contact like this would have brought all sorts of notions into my mind that were best not pursued in narrow hallways. But these things had long since disappeared from our repertoire of togetherness – Alzheimer's didn't encourage such things.

We both examined the glasses still held lightly in my hand. Pauline touched them again but then lost interest. As I raised them to my face, I saw the door panel reflected in their curved surface but, still none the wiser, I put them on again. With a lifetime of poor eyesight I felt very uncomfortable and vulnerable when not wearing them. The world becomes a blur, full of strange shapes that have little meaning unless I am in very familiar surroundings. It occurred to me that this was probably how Pauline's Alzheimer's brain perceived her surroundings too. But for Pauline, there were no magic spectacles to help her make sense of the strange new world she had entered.

Then Pauline pointed at my glasses again and laughed once more. 'Peoples,' she said. 'Little peoples.' Two words! Suddenly, I understood. She could see her own silhouette framed by the doorway and miniaturised on the reflective surface of my glasses. I laughed with her and tried to explain what she was seeing.

I always tried to explain the things that Alzheimer's prevented her from sorting out for herself. We held many a one-sided conversation. I had learned to construct short, simple, one-topic sentences which Pauline seemed to understand – some of the time anyway. But I could never be quite sure.

Pauline, like most people in the early stages of dementia, was a great actor and was able to put on a performance of which any RADA graduate would be proud. By acting the part of 'Pauline – a woman who had control of all her faculties', she had, so far, been able to hide from the casual observer most of the confusions that enveloped and tormented her. It was her defence, her means of getting on with life in spite of it all, her way of coping with the horrors that Alzheimer's forced upon her. She couldn't reject Alzheimer's impositions, only deal with them as best she could. The acting was obvious to me when the performance was directed at others, but it was more difficult to spot when we were alone. There was, in my mind, no need for her to pretend to me that she was more able than she actually was. I suspected, however, she had difficulties that even I, close as we were, didn't realise, let alone even begin to understand. The acting was for her own benefit – not mine.

Over the following days the reflections in my glasses stayed a source of amused fascination for her. We had many a giggle over them. We usually both tried to make light of the muddles in which Pauline increasingly found herself. Laughter is a great equaliser. If I could participate in the muddle or difficulty Alzheimer's had placed her in, so that we had joint ownership of it, then the pain of embarrassment and the hurt of failure became a shared experience and was all the lighter for it. Laughter healed the wound, and the memory of it was soon forgotten – in Pauline's mind at least. Painful memories seemed to last longer with her.

The reflections in my glasses continued to amuse for only those initial few days. Slowly, amusement changed to concern, concern to worry and then to fear. Sometimes this fear evolved into sheer unadulterated terror. If I came near her she became frightened, not of me, but of those reflections. Her hand shot out and she tore the glasses from my face and hurled them across the room. This happened not once but every time I went near her. I am lost without my glasses but I quickly learned to remove them every time she got within grabbing distance. At least we were then both in the same blurred and confusing surroundings.

I thought of non-reflective lenses. Were there such things? The optician told me over the telephone that there were coatings that would reduce reflections: come and see our samples. Not as easy as that. We lived in a village, a twenty-four-mile round trip away from the optician, and making arrangements for Pauline's care while I went took a few days to organise. I did eventually see the sample lenses but by this time Pauline's fear of reflections had transferred to other things. And life became more difficult – for both of us.

Mirrors caused panic, their surfaces and inner depths containing inexplicable terrors for her. I took them all down and stored them in the spare bedroom. I covered the mirror on the bathroom cabinet with paper. I stuck it down with masking tape which I planned to lift when I shaved. But as Pauline followed me everywhere, I was rarely in the bathroom alone, so I learned to shave 'blind' – less bother.

But all kinds of objects hold reflections. Framed photographs and paintings behind glass had to be removed and stored. The spare room quickly became an Aladdin's cave of glitter and glass, of things that sparkled and shone, each object competing for its share of reflected glory. A fun fair's hall of mirrors had nothing on this room. Fortunately, Pauline never attempted to go in there. She would have entered her own personalised torture chamber had she done so.

The big picture windows generated huge reflected images and produced horror on a similar scale. So I put up net curtains. The glass doors on the display cabinets in the lounge had to be covered with paper. In the kitchen, the black glass doors on the eye-level ovens were similarly camouflaged.

Pauline saw reflections everywhere. The TV screen, the shiny plastic of the toaster and the kettle held equal terrors for her. The light reflecting from the polished wood dining table caused apprehension. I caught her peering suspiciously at the far less shiny Formica surface of the kitchen table. It couldn't be trusted to stay that way. It was almost as though she found some masochistic pleasure in seeking out new reflective surfaces so that she could, first, get into a state about them, and then test my ingenuity in disguising the reflection in some way. Mercifully for me, as reflections multiplied around the home, her interest in my glasses subsided. At least I could see what I was doing as I experimented by coating objects with Windolene, allowing the resulting chalky surface to dull any chance of it becoming another object of terror.

Strangely, there was one source of reflection that didn't trouble her; in fact it became a friend. This was the large square mirror screwed to the wall between two wardrobes and above a chest of drawers in the run of fitted furniture in her bedroom. Pauline stood for hours in front of it talking to the person she saw reflected there. This person became her friend. The friend was constant, always there, looked at Pauline, talked with her when Pauline talked, but had the decency to keep her mouth shut when Pauline wanted silence. She could share a good joke too. She laughed when Pauline laughed but when Pauline was sad and cried, she shed a tear as well. She didn't threaten, she didn't get too near. When Pauline wanted to sit quietly on the end of her bed, her friend kept silent vigil with her too. If Pauline became animated, her friend reflected the mood but when this turned to rage at what was happening to her, her friend instinctively understood and they ranted in unison at this most cruel of life's inflictions. When Pauline wanted to get closer, to whisper feminine confidences, her friend responded and also leant forward for the intimate exchange. They touched. They held out their hands to each other, fingertip against fingertip. I was forever wiping the evidence of these physical intimacies from the mirror's surface.

They remained friends for two or three years, long after Pauline's fear of reflections had disappeared from her life. Regretfully, other horrors came to fill the spaces previously occupied by those of reflections, but these must remain untold, for the moment.

I should explain one apparent contradiction. Pauline could barely put two words together that made sense and yet she had these enormously long conversations with her friend. How was this? Fortunately her friend could understand what, to my undiscerning ear, appeared to be merely gobbledegook. But her friend not only understood it but also spoke it with great fluency. This was the mysterious language of those conversations. It was spoken with a full range of inflection, emotion and physical gesture. They stopped if I entered the room, so I often eavesdropped on the pair of them. The tone of voice and body language was quite explicit, but the words were in this foreign language known only to Pauline and her friend. Occasionally, just occasionally, the odd word in English was used, just as a source of emphasis, to make a point, or, perhaps, to fool an eavesdropper?

Commentary

It may be helpful to relay what motivated me to write *'Reflections' on caring*. The story form was deliberate. I wanted it to be understood and taken on board and used by the professionals. The bare facts could have been put more academically for their eyes. Nonetheless, I felt it important for the professional reader to have the 'clinical' observations exposed in the setting of their occurrence. I also knew that by relaying it as a story of a personal experience of caring for someone with dementia, it could also help other carers to relate and learn without being lectured – avoiding the aspect of yet another expert telling them what to do. That does get carers down.

I tried to make each paragraph not only advance the story element but contain an observation about dementia, or its effects, about caring or approaches to caring – to offer advice for the carer, information for the professional. Above all, I wanted it to remain human, to tell, as lightly as possible, about our lives, the imposition that illness brought to us and how we coped (or didn't), but also to record that our lives continued through it all by understanding, adaptation and revised expectations. Separating my life as a carer into little story sequences doesn't paint the reality of the whole by any means but it does allow me to make a few simple points.

All human life is just that, being human. People are put into groups, given labels – the elderly, the unemployed, the poor, the scroungers, carers, fat cats – in order to dehumanise them, so we can say things about them, do things to them, that we would have reservations about saying face to face or doing to any one individual. Another frequently used protective mechanism brought into play when hearing of individual experiences is to dismiss them as 'merely anecdotal'.

But I was dealing with actuality: a real live person in a real live, on-going situation. Pauline had an identity as a person, a complete human being, not just a set of symptoms or problems. She had a whole life history, her preferences, hates, foibles, sensitivities, beliefs and ideals. They were all part of her before illness struck and remained part of her even when Alzheimer's restricted and then dominated her relationship to the world around her. Knowing and recognising her characteristics were essential elements in my care of her. One could not expect professionals, dipping in and out of her life, to know the things that a near lifetime's association had given me, but they could draw on my knowledge of her whenever it had pertinence and could better inform their judgements and actions.

Apart from anything else, *'Reflections'* is a love story. In our marriage we shared much – we had joint interests but also individual ones. We operated as 'a couple' but also as individuals. The illness strengthened both aspects – the bonding becoming closer, tighter, a far greater and quite abnormal intimacy. For many things pertaining to service provision we were as one, inseparable: Pauline couldn't operate without me. In another sense we were two distinct 'clients', living in the same house but in very different circumstances and having differing, sometimes opposing needs. I continually tried to put myself in Pauline's shoes, sometimes with apparent success – *but I could never be quite sure.*

Pauline and I both learnt, together and separately. It also appears that, unknowingly, I used the principles of action research in much of my approach to Pauline's care. Certainly observation and 'reflection' played a great part in my own learning process.

Part III

Undertaking an action research project

A practical guide

INTRODUCTION

This part of the book is intended for readers currently engaged in (or about to undertake) an action research project. It provides practical guidance through the sequence of activities required in undertaking a project, including discussion of the issues and detailed advice concerning the methods of work involved in each stage. It contains a series of specific 'Supporting documents' on different aspects of the process (pp. 245–51) and suggestions on how the other parts of the book may be used at different stages of your work.

The Guide is intended for use by individual readers and as the basis for group meetings of two types: (1) meetings of the participants in an action research project, and (2) meetings where each member of the group is undertaking a separate action research project, e.g. an action research-based course, facilitated by a tutor. (It is assumed that all those taking part in an action research course will also be involved in establishing and facilitating meetings for project participants.) Where the term 'group meeting' is used below it can refer to either type of group or (more usually) to both. In either case, the material can be discussed either in a series of face-to-face meetings or through the medium of Email or a Website.

The Guide provides a framework for how to use the previous sections of the book – the general arguments and the examples – but if you have not yet looked at Parts I and II, it is recommended that you do so now, before proceeding further. The Guide contains frequent references to these previous sections, so it would be better if – as far as possible – all participants in the work have a copy of the book available as supporting material.

Suggestions for practical activities are indicated by bullet points in shaded boxes.

I CHOOSING A TOPIC

To some extent, you may feel that your topic doesn't have to be 'chosen' – that it is *there*, an issue that you know needs to be worked at: something of which you feel you need further understanding, and which clearly relates to an aspect of practice in need of development. But begin by checking a few things.

1   Remember that the work can start in one of two different ways. You can either start by carrying out an evaluation of some current state of affairs; or you can start by implementing a change in practice (with a view to evaluating it later).

2   Remember that in either case you will need to get together a group of people who are involved in the situation in different ways, and you will need to ensure that these people all feel that the work is something they would like to do *for their own purposes*. So the first step will almost certainly be to *negotiate* the topic; otherwise the work will risk losing its collective, collaborative dimension. Participants in the research should be, as far as possible, co-researchers, not subjects being researched, and the way you frame the topic needs to reflect this.

3   Apart from negotiating the topic with your participating co-researchers, you will need to make sure that the work you have in mind has the *support* of others, beyond the participant group. In a team or a working group, the support of *other members* is necessary. In an organisation, the support of *managers* is necessary. As you check this support you may find that, again, you need to redefine your first ideas about the focus of the work.

4   Above all, make sure that the work you have in mind is something for which *you* have some sort of responsibility, that you are going to investigate/develop *your* work and are not proposing an inquiry into matters which are clearly someone else's responsibility. Some forms of inquiry may certainly be useful but can't be carried out using an action research process.

- Read Chapters 4 and 6, by Noreen Kennedy and Philip Kemp respectively, and notice how in one case a specific topic is present from the outset whereas in the other case the focus only emerges gradually as the work progresses.
- Read Chapters 8 and 9, by Brenda Dennett and Cathy Aymer respectively, and notice how the focus of the work is negotiated as the work of a *group* of people, not just the author.

---

2   INTRODUCTION TO ACTION RESEARCH

Before planning your work it is important to have a clear conception of what action research is, so that you can start to imagine what sort of practical activities are necessary and also what is *not* necessary. Hence the importance of this section.

2.1   The nature of action research

- Begin by reading the section 'What is "action research"?' in Chapter 1. After you have read it, write down a list of five or six words or phrases which, for you, sum up the most important features of action research.
- Focusing on the general topic you have decided on, do the exercise presented on page 6 of Chapter 1.
- Make a list of the ways in which you hope that the *process* of initiating the work yourself in your own practice context might have a beneficial effect on relationships, and on your (and other participants') understanding of the issues.

2.2 How action research differs from other forms of research

- Read the section 'Action research and other models of social research' in Chapter 2, up to and including the paragraph beginning 'To sum up this stage of the argument' on page 19.
- Make a list of key points for discussion in your group and also a list of queries – things you feel need further discussion.
- Compare the points you have made with 'Supporting document 1: "Knowledge" – some key distinctions' (p. 245).

2.3 The various meanings of 'validity'

- Read the rest of the section 'Action research and other models of social research' in Chapter 2, dealing with data gathering, data analysis, theory, validity, generalisability, organisational politics and research ethics.
- From your reading, make your own list of 'criteria' for 'good' action research. (This is not intended to be final, just a way of clarifying your thinking so far.) Discuss your lists in the group and add to your list anyone else's ideas that you think are helpful but which you had omitted.
- Make a list of the different meanings of the word 'validity'. After you have made your own list, check in a dictionary and add any meanings you had not included. Then compare lists with the other members of your group and, using your lists as a starting point, discuss what we might mean when we say that an action research report needs to aim at 'validity'. (What senses of the word are most helpful and relevant?)
- Divide up the examples of action research reports in Part II among your group, with two of you reading each piece. As you read your example consider how far it illustrates your list of criteria and your ideas about action research validity. Share your ideas in the group, comparing your interpretation with the person who has read the same piece as you, and noting how the different examples raise different issues. (Remember that no single piece of work will be able to illustrate completely *all* the criteria you have listed (and this will also, eventually, be true of your own work!), so make sure that you fully appreciate the positive features of the example.)

2.4 The various contexts and dimensions of action research

- Re-read carefully Chapter 3 of this book. Whatever the context of your work, it is important to pay particular attention to Section 1 (on service-user research), Section 4 (on facilitation), Section 5 (on evaluation), Section 6 (on critical reflection) and Sections 7 and 8 (which both emphasise the political nature of action research).

- As you read, make notes on any *practical* points that strike you as relevant for your own particular study.

- Discuss your reading and your notes with the other members of your group.

3 CRITICAL REFLECTION

3.1 Introduction

This section is intended to help you to clarify in advance the sort of *learning process* at the heart of action research, to make it easier for you to plan the sequence of activities for your project proposal. It is intended to help you decide what sort of data to gather and what you might need to do in order to analyse it and learn from it.

- Begin by re-reading the first section of Chapter 2, 'Action research as an approach to inquiry and development'.

One of the most important purposes of 'research' is to learn something (from a situation, an event or a collection of data) that we didn't know before. This often poses something of a problem for action research because, as experienced 'insiders' to this sort of situation, we are already very familiar with data of this sort. Consequently, simply by counting and classifying the data under categories we are unlikely to learn anything new unless the categories themselves are different from the ones we would have used at the outset of the work.

Action research involves both a change in our understanding and also a direct preparation for changes in practice. This means that our approach to data collection, data analysis, etc. needs to contribute to the processes of collaborative negotiation, working across hierarchies of status and power, and establishing communication across boundaries.

The learning process within action research, therefore, needs to take account of the various issues raised in Chapter 3, e.g. being 'responsive' to different interests (Section 5), 'listening' to others and questioning our own assumptions (Section

4), empowerment as mutual learning (Section 8), and, generally, 'critical reflection' (Section 6).

3.2 Reviewing our 'resources' for critical reflection

- Study 'Supporting document 2: Practice-based learning through reflection – action research processes and resources' (p. 246).

- Consider each of the 'resources for learning' in the diagram and think of an occasion from your recent experience when you learned something significant from this source. In other words, think of a time when you learned something by working collaboratively with a colleague or a client, a time when you learned by becoming aware of your and others' emotions, when you learned about one situation by comparing it with a previous experience, a time when you had to interpret and combine (say) your knowledge of research findings and regulations or different theories to decide what to do in a situation, and a time when a situation made you think carefully about your different value commitments. Many of the incidents you think of will involve a combination of several of these 'resources', but perhaps it is possible for you to say that, on a particular occasion, one aspect ('resource') was particularly important, or that it was the starting point which led to the others.

- Discuss these experiences with each other.

3.3 The *need* for critical reflection: noting how our current knowledge can 'block' new understanding

One of the difficulties about doing research in an area with which we are very familiar is that we already know so much about it. As soon as we find a new piece of evidence it is always so easy to fit it into what we already know that it is hard to avoid doing so straight away. Of course, most of the time we *need* to do this (to 'make sense' of our experience). But if we are engaging in a 'research' project, our aim is to *change* our understandings, so that we can imagine *different* interpretations and ways of doing things. So our basic attitude towards the evidence we collect must be to *prolong* our sense of its 'newness', a sense of *not* (yet) understanding it. We need to ask ourselves such questions as: 'What ideas am I bringing to bear on this new experience *in order to* understand it?' 'What experiences am I comparing it with in order to *make* the experience seem familiar?' 'How can I understand this differently?' 'What other connections could I make?'

In other words, we need to work hard at re-creating a sense that this is indeed something we *don't* understand. The *easy* thing is to say, 'Here is a new experience and this (of course) is what it means.' The *hard* thing to say is, 'Here is a new experience and these are the various meanings it might have, but as yet I do not understand it.'

One useful example of this general point involves trying to avoid interpreting other people's perspectives in 'deficit' terms. When others 'do not understand' our concepts, values, etc., the obvious and inevitable first reaction is to explain this as a 'lack' in their understanding. But if we leave it there, that is the end of our own learning: we leave it as 'their problem', i.e. *their* need to learn something. But if *we* want to learn from the interaction, we need to ask ourselves the question, 'What is it that I do not understand about them that leads me to perceive them as "not understanding" something?' The interesting challenge here is to try to answer the question in a way that implies no deficit in someone else, only a limitation in our own understanding: spotting limitations in our own understanding is a step towards further learning, whereas spotting deficits in other people's understanding merely confirms what we knew before. Avoiding deficit interpretations is an important aspect of 'anti-oppressive', 'anti-racist' practice (see Chapter 3, Sections 7 and 8) and 'reflective' practice (Chapter 3, Section 6), and it is obviously very important for action research in which we are always trying to work *collaboratively* with people representing different interests from our own.

In this way, by emphasising what it is that we don't yet understand, our first interpretations become not 'conclusions' but *data*, which we (or others) can *analyse*, in order to identify things we now realise we need to go and find out about. And in this way we can try to go beyond our immediate, reassuring reactions, and to think thoughts which previously had been, as it were, 'blocked out' by the appeal and familiarity of our initial interpretation. The problem of learning from new experiences, then, is to try to *postpone* our *answers*, and to *preserve* our *questions*: 'What do these people mean?' 'Why do they say this?' 'What further questions can we put, what else do we need to do, to clarify this?'

Section 3.4 takes this discussion further.

3.4 Two principles of critical reflection – reflexivity and dialectics

3.4.1 Noting the 'reflexivity' of our judgements

Most of the time when we interact with other people or when we reflect on our experiences we are using language to *interpret* what is going on. In other words, we use language to 'judge' the meaning of events. For example, the way someone (let us call her 'Josie') responds during a conversation or an interview may lead us to make a judgement, after a few minutes, that she is 'anxious'. Once that judgement is made, it is easy to think of the word 'anxious' as a sort of label which refers directly to something objective ('out there') in the same way as the name 'Josie' refers to a clearly identifiable person, with an address and a national insurance number.

But this is misleading, because the two words 'Josie' and 'anxious' function quite differently. It is quite clear that there really is someone called Josie who lives at such and such an address, and it is not very helpful to ask the question, 'Is there *really* such a person or is she *really* someone else, or an illusion that I have imagined?' But what we are referring to as Josie's 'anxiety' is by no means clear-cut in this way. Certainly we are referring to *something*, but we are not *simply* referring to Josie's observable behaviour. Rather, we are also referring to *our own* conceptions of 'anxiety', what *we* mean by 'anxiety', how *we* think of the ways in which people behave differently when they are 'anxious' and when they are, say, 'relaxed' or 'calm', and how we ourselves behave when *we* are experiencing feelings that *we* would call 'anxiety'.

In this way, our judgement 'Josie is feeling anxious' is not simply a process of labelling an external event (external to us, that is). It is a 'reflexive' statement: we can only understand it by seeing how it is 'bent back' (re-flex-ed) into our own mental processes (assumptions, categories, feelings and experiences).

> • Look at 'Supporting document 3: The problem of making "reflexive" judgements' (p. 247) – which shows how a reflexive judgement easily creates the impression that it is a simple 'statement of fact'.

The importance of this principle for the learning process during an action research project is that it draws our attention to the fact that many of the judgements we make are not statements of external fact (and therefore 'final') but are open to question. By noting the reflexivity of our judgements we can ask ourselves (and join with others in asking) what we *mean* when we state them, and whether other people mean the same or something slightly different. Thus we can 'go beyond' our initial judgement and treat it as the start of a learning process.

> • Make a list of four or five judgements you have made recently and see which ones are 'reflexive' in the sense outlined above. Make some notes about how you might ask further questions arising from these judgements and discuss them with other members of the group to see if they suggest questions you had not thought of.

(For further discussion of reflexivity and suggestions for further reading, see Winter, 1989.)

3.4.2 Thinking 'dialectically'

> • Read 'Supporting document 4: Dialectics' (p. 248).

The principles of dialectical thinking provide three further suggestions about planning and learning from the work of an action research project, following the three aspects of dialectics listed in the 'Supporting document'.

First, we need to make sure that we interpret any particular experience or piece of data in relation to its *context* – personal, organisational, political, etc. But 'context' can be understood in various ways, and so there will be different interpretations as to what contextual factors are relevant for understanding any particular matter. These differences will need to be discussed, and this is another way in which we can learn from each other. We also need to think carefully about the range of different people we need to involve in the project in order to do justice to its contextual relevance – i.e. its 'scope' and significance. There is a link, in other words, between taking account of the 'context' and including 'relevant stakeholders'.

Second, it is useful to think carefully about how the situation you are working on has *changed* and how the changes you are considering are related to this 'history' of change. And it is important to remember that at the end of your work you will still be in a situation where practices will continue to change and where your (and other people's) understanding will continue to develop. A successful action research project does not simply 'stop'; it always looks forward to further developments. Action research is not about producing a *final* or complete description; even at the end, our learning is incomplete, and that is as it should be.

Third, one useful way of analysing data is to compare interpretations from different participants, through 'dialogue': *differences* of opinion will provide a useful starting point for deepening the analysis. Also, one person analysing data can begin by searching through them for *contradictions* – i.e. for dilemmas, disagreements, inconsistencies, tensions and conflicts of interest. This is a way of selecting the important elements from what can easily become an overwhelming mass of detailed evidence, without simply picking out those aspects which immediately link with our familiar thoughts and opinions. An analysis of 'contradictions' can also be useful in creating an agenda for discussing the next phase of the work, and in this way it feeds into the change process of the project. (See Section 7.5 below, on 'Dilemma analysis'.)

A practical exercise on dialectics

> • Write down at least one 'contradiction' which you think lies at the very centre of some of the items in the following list:
>
> Democracy
> Love
> Care
> Science
> Action research

continued

> An organisation you work in (or have worked in)
>
> Your role in this organisation
>
> Someone you know well 'professionally' (a colleague, a client or your care worker)
>
> A family you know well
>
> A close friend or relative
>
> Yourself
>
> • Discuss one or two of these in your group. (Some of your thoughts you may well wish to keep to yourself!)

3.5 Practical exercises on 'innovative thinking' in general

The term 'innovative thinking' is taken from Hart (2000: Chapter 2). It reminds us that the task in action research is to go beyond our current thinking, to interpret our experiences in *new* ways, i.e. to *learn*. The exercise is intended to help you bring together the various ideas on critical reflection presented so far.

> • Write a description of a recent 'critical incident' which seems important from the point of view of the topic of your action research project, i.e. a particular event from your own experience which in some way seems to sum up the nature of the issues you are concerned with. Make sure that you include the details of what happened, what you thought at the time and why it seems significant. Use the series of questions in 'Supporting document 5: Critical reflection as "innovative thinking"' (p. 249) to analyse your critical incident in such a way that you raise *new* issues. The list of questions is largely derived from the discussions in this section. Don't try to use all sections of the document, but you may wish to combine questions from different sections and /or to add your own questions. Discuss your analysis in your group.
>
> • Read Chapters 6, 7 and 14, by Philip Kemp, Valerie Childs and Philip Ingram respectively, and consider how they illustrate different ways of thinking 'innovatively'.

4 PREPARING AN ACTION RESEARCH PROPOSAL

Sometimes it is necessary to submit a formal proposal (e.g. if you are applying for permission to carry out the work or applying for resources). But even if no one is asking you for a formal proposal it is important to write out a detailed plan before you start work. Remember that you will be working with people with whom you need to preserve a good working relationship, so your planning of the initial phases of the work needs to be quite precisely thought out. On the other hand, an action research project proposal cannot include detailed plans for the whole of the work:

it needs to be open-ended, so that each phase can learn from the previous one. Also, it is important that as other people become involved they do so as full collaborators, as co-researchers, i.e. in such a way that they can influence the direction and methods of the work, perhaps quite radically. So the proposal needs to be drawn up from the outset as a process of collaborative negotiation with the other main participants, even if one person is acting as co-ordinator.

4.1 A preliminary checklist of questions

- Start to prepare your proposal by answering the following questions. Don't be surprised if your answers to some of the questions seem to overlap. By thinking through your answers to the questions you should find that (1) you are sufficiently clear about the work to be able to write a formal proposal, if necessary, and (2) that you will already have begun the practical process of negotiating the initial stages of the work.

1 What is the basic purpose of your work and why is it significant?

1 What is the practical problem that you think needs addressing? If there seem to be several, try to focus it down to just one. Make sure it is a matter on which you are in a position to take an initiative and for which you have some responsibility.
2 What makes you think this problem is important?
3 What sorts of practical changes do you have in mind?
4 What official or published writing also refers to this problem?
5 How does this problem relate to official policies?
6 How does this problem relate to professional values and theory?

2 Who else will be affected by the work you have in mind?

1 List the 'stakeholders'.
2 List those who have the right/power to affect the work.
3 Describe the basic purpose of the work from each of these points of view in turn.
4 How can you present the idea of the project to these people in such a way that it seems useful from *their* perspective?
5 How will you negotiate management support for the work?

3 What are your feelings and your initial assumptions concerning the issue?

Among the list of people in question 2 (above) make a note indicating who you think have similar feelings/assumptions, and whose are different.

4 How will you try to make the method of your work 'collaborative'?

1   How will you negotiate a *shared* purpose with the stakeholders? Note that this will not necessarily be easy, and you may need to be prepared to rethink your conception of 'the problem'. This process, if it occurs, will be an important and valuable part of the project.
2   How will you try to make sure that the process tests out your initial assumptions?
3   How will you try to make everyone feel that it is 'their' (collective) project, not just 'yours'?
4   How many people will you involve and what are you expecting them to do?
5   In what order will you approach them? (This can be an important political issue.)

5 Do you wish to involve someone in the role of 'critical friend'? If so, who?

A 'critical friend' is a person who is not involved in the project as a stakeholder or participant, and who is thus able to offer feedback, alternative interpretations or other advice from an 'independent' position. This can often be helpful, but if the group of participants is working effectively and harmoniously then the role is not essential, and you need to consider whether introducing a 'critical friend' may perhaps detract from the communication among the participants. Remember that the critical friend *must* be both an outsider and someone who can be fully trusted to be positive, honest and wholly discreet. The decision to involve a particular person in this role must be agreed by the project participants (see Bennett *et al.*, 1997).

NOTE: At this stage it is important to begin your negotiations with the other potential participants you have now identified, since the answers to the questions which follow really need to be agreed, in the end, by the project participants as group, even if you start by putting down, tentatively, your individual responses.

6 What forms of data will you collect?

1   What sorts of data illustrate the nature of the 'problem' on which the project is focused?
2   What sorts of data will illustrate the progress of the work as it develops?

3   What sorts of data will be important in order to evaluate the work?
4   What 'natural opportunities' are there for collecting data (i.e. those creating minimum extra work)?
5   How can you try to involve *all* participants in creating and collecting data?

7 How will you analyse the data?

1   Are the data such that quantitative methods may be appropriate? If so, which?
2   How will you include 'critical reflection' in the process of analysing the data?
3   How will you arrange for interpretations of participants' comments to be 'checked back' with their originators?
4   What 'natural opportunities' are there for sharing interpretations among participants?
5   How can you try to involve *all* participants in analysing the data?

8 How will you address the issue of 'validity'?

For example:
1   through the variety of data;
2   through the variety of different stakeholders' views included;
3   through procedures for establishing collective agreement on interpretations;
4   through procedures for evaluating practical changes;
5   through links with general theory.

9 How will you ensure that the pattern of your work has some form of the action research 'cycle' (as in the following diagram)?

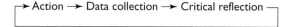

Action → Data collection → Critical reflection

Make a diagram of the *activities* of the work to show this, remembering that a meeting can be either a form of action (e.g. a practical negotiation) or a form of data collection, or both.

10 How will your plan allow for alternative lines of development?

It is, of course, not possible to plan exactly how the project will develop in its later stages, so include in the diagram you made in response to question 9 your ideas about how different possible lines of development may emerge at certain stages of the work.

11 How much time will be needed for the work?

1   Draw up an overall plan for the time span of the project as a whole, by trying to imagine how much time will be needed for each phase of the work.
2   Make sure that each participant is able to make the necessary time available. This may need to be worked out separately for different participants, depending on their role in the work.

12 What other resources will be needed?

Will you need, for example, any of the following, and if so are they available?

> Tape/video recorder
> Photocopying
> Typing
> Specific books, journals, documents

13 What ethical issues are raised by the work proposed?

1   How will you address the following issues?

   a)   Protecting the confidentiality of participants versus fully acknowledging their contribution;
   b)   Ensuring *informed* consent on the part of all involved and also the right *not* to participate;
   c)   Protecting the rights and well-being of colleagues/service-users and others – those who participate *and* those who don't;
   d)   Involving all stakeholders in defining issues, collecting/analysing data and drawing conclusions.

2   Do you need to seek the approval of a local Research Ethics Committee before undertaking your project? If you work in a UK healthcare organisation and intend to involve service-users you will probably need to do so. If so, try to make contact with the chairperson or your local representative in good time to obtain guidance, and show them a draft of your proposal for their comments before making a formal submission. (See Section 5 below for further discussion of ethical issues.)

14 What are the institutional politics surrounding the project?

1   Who are the important political 'players'?
2   Of these, which are likely, because of their position or their general opinions, to be supportive of the project? Consider carefully at what stage to approach them to enlist their support and how to present your proposal to them.

3   Are there people who are likely, because of their position or their general opinions, to be hostile? If so, what strategies can you adopt to minimise/avoid such hostility?

4   In general, think carefully about the *order* in which you contact different people, to make sure that no one gets irritated because they feel they should have been involved earlier. (A lot of empathy and imagination are needed here.)

5 ETHICAL ISSUES AND PRINCIPLES OF PROCEDURE

5.1 Introduction

The guiding impulse of action research is the 'improvement' of situations involving a practical responsibility for others' well-being. So, immediately, its ethical basis is different from, and in some respects simpler than, the ethical basis for conventional research, where an ethical basis needs to be provided for 'purely experimental' activities which contrast sharply with responsibility for practical care. For example, conventional medical researchers may need to justify ethically involving service-users in a situation where, unknowingly, they do not receive a 'real' treatment but a 'dummy', so that the process is one in which they are being 'experimented on' rather than 'cared for'. In action research, however, this contrast should not exist. All aspects of an action research process are intended to be directly beneficial *for the participants themselves*, because action research is an elaboration, an intensification, of the care process itself (or the management process or the educational process, etc.), *not* a temporary interruption or suspension of it.

Hence, there are three different sources for the ethics of an action research project. First, the initial ethical principles of action research include those of the 'professional' relationship itself, often elaborated in codes of practice. This means that action research (like nursing, social work, teaching and management, for example) operates under such principles as:

1   the duty of care (over-riding merely personal interests);
2   respect for the individual irrespective of race, gender, age, disability, etc.;
3   respect for cultural diversity;
4   respect for individual dignity;
5   protection from harm.

Second, there are also the ethical rules guiding social research generally (see Section 5.2), and third, there are essential procedures derived from the basic principles of action research (see Section 5.3).

5.2 Ethical considerations common to all social research

Irrespective of the difference between action research and conventional research, many of the ethical principles drawn up to guide social research in general are of the utmost importance and relevance for action research, and should be carefully considered. It is particularly important to ensure that the issues below are fully dealt with in any formal proposal submitted to a Research Ethics Committee, such as those established for UK healthcare organisations. The following list of points is drawn from a variety of sources, including the UK government Department of Health (1992), Neuberger (1992), British Sociological Association (1992), Ayer (1994) and Prendergast (1997).

5.2.1 The value of the project

The value of the project is an ethical issue, since one is asking people to devote their time to it. For an action research project this should not be a problem since its purpose is, in principle, to improve the experience of practice, the understanding of practice, and practice-related relationships for *all* participants. The 'ethical danger' here lies in initiating a project for individual motives such as getting a qualification or otherwise advancing one's career. So one ought to be able to give an honestly positive answer to *any* potential participant who asks, in some way or other, 'What's in this for *me*?' Such a question must be seen as raising a genuine ethical issue, and the project should be planned so that its value for all participants is immediate and obvious.

5.2.2 Informed consent

There are a number of different aspects here.

1   All participation must be voluntary, of course, and it is important to ensure that no one feels any pressure to take part. For example, service-users being 'invited' to participate by professional staff may feel that choosing not to take part might have negative consequences for them. They will need to be reassured that this is not the case both by explicit statements and (if possible) by specific procedures.
2   Participants must be clearly informed that they have the right to withdraw from the project at any stage.
3   Particular issues are raised where participants are children or people with a physical or a mental health disability, and may have difficulty in understanding the project. Consent in such cases may need also to be negotiated through people who have some sort of 'guardian' role and status.
4   Official permission must always be sought to use confidential documents or information for any purpose different from that for which it was originally collected.

5   Permission must always be sought before making tape recordings and before including participants' data in material to be published or circulated to others.

6   An information sheet must be prepared which must be given to potential participants when their involvement is being negotiated. As more people are drawn in to the project this information sheet itself may need to be progressively refined, but the individual or small group initiating the work needs to draw up a preliminary draft. Remember that the *tone* of this document should be accessible and user-friendly rather than legalistic or bureaucratic. The information sheet should indicate:

a)   the aims of the project and how the project report(s) will be disseminated;

b)   contact names, addresses and telephone numbers in case of queries or concerns;

c)   the nature of participants' contributions and some indication of the time involved;

d)   an explicit statement of the right not to become involved and to withdraw later;

e)   the nature of possible risks (see Section 5.2.3) and how these will be avoided;

f)   procedures for checking and 'releasing' data from project participants;

g)   how participants' data will be stored and used;

h)   the extent to which confidentiality can be guaranteed and how this will be managed.

5.2.3 Protection from harm

As indicated in Section 5.1, this should be less of an issue in action research than in other forms of research. But it must be remembered that involvement in the project may involve participants in talking about emotionally difficult issues, or taking part in discussions with people representing roles of which they feel suspicious and where conflicting opinions may be voiced. In principle, therefore, participants *might* experience some parts of the process as quite painful emotionally; and they have a right to expect the process to have been planned in such a way that such pain is minimised and that support is available should it occur.

The process of the project and the publication of the project report could also affect participants' 'reputation'. In general this is more likely to be a positive than a negative outcome, but there is a risk involved, especially in a small locally based project where the anonymity of all participants cannot be absolutely guaranteed, and this needs to be recognised and explained.

5.2.4 Honesty

Conventional researchers have an ethical duty to be honest in their explanations to participants 'as far as is consistent with the research aims and methods'. In action research this principle is absolute and cannot allow of any exceptions, since participants are co-researchers rather than objects *of* research. There is also, of course, an ethical duty to be honest in the reporting of data and in analysing and drawing conclusions from it.

5.3 Principles of procedure for action research

Over and above the general ethical considerations outlined above, there are a number of procedures which derive from the basic principles of action research, i.e. from its specific concern to ensure that all stakeholders are treated as co-researchers and are thus fully involved in defining issues, collecting/analysing data and drawing conclusions. The following list is loosely based on Kemmis and McTaggart (1988: 106–8), omitting points already covered in Section 5.2.

1 Make sure that discussions are fully documented, so that the process can be made available to those who were not present. (This needs to be agreed and procedures negotiated for recording or taking notes.)
2 Procedures for taking joint decisions need to be negotiated, ensuring that the voices of *all* participants are fully taken into account.
3 Make sure that the work of the project is distributed as widely as possible among all participants. In other words, circulate regular progress reports, so that the work remains fully 'visible' to all participants.
4 This requires the prior agreement by participants that (1) their contributions have been accurately described and that (2) they are in a form that can be shared with others by general consent. So all 'interpretations' need to be 'checked back' and 'authorised' before being circulated.
5 This in turn means that a participant must be enabled to amend her/his contribution before it is circulated to others.
6 Make sure that progress reports clearly invite participants to make suggestions concerning future developments. In other words, ensure that all participants know that they can suggest changes to the focus and the methods of the project at every stage where a new cycle of decision-making is about to begin. This is an important reason why participants need to know the plan of the project activities.
7 Differentiate clearly between documents which are confidential to project participants and reports intended for wider publication.
8 Negotiate rules of confidentiality which are acceptable to all participants, for which all agree to accept responsibility, and which are appropriate for the different uses to be made of the various project documents.
9 Make clear that reports intended for an audience beyond the group of participants will be circulated in advance, and that individual participants will have the right to withdraw any material containing a reference which may identify them.
10 Negotiate the right of the group of participants as a whole to publish a project

report more widely if they wish. In other words, negotiate in advance how possible disagreements concerning publication will be resolved in a way which preserves a balance between individual, minority and majority rights.

11 If one (or more) of the participants wishes to write up their work as part of an assignment for an academic qualification this also needs to be negotiated beforehand. (Note that in such cases it is possible to ensure that the work is only seen by academic examiners under strict conditions of confidentiality.)

12 Finally, make sure that these various principles of procedure are drawn up early in the work, so that they are available in the form of a clear statement which can guide potential participants when making their decision on their involvement or otherwise.

5.4 Drawing up a project information sheet

'Supporting document 6: "Pattern for a project information sheet"' (p. 250) indicates the sort of information sheet which you will need to have available when you invite people to participate in your project. It is based on the ideas presented in this section on ethical considerations and action research principles of procedure.

- Use this document as a basis for drafting your own information sheet. Remember that at this stage you are only drawing up a *draft* information sheet, which you are prepared to change if participants suggest their own ideas as they agree to join the project.
- Discuss this work with the other members of your working group.

5.5 A practical exercise

- Select one or two of the examples from Part II and consider how they address the ethical issues and the action research 'principles of procedure'. Make a list of their strengths and limitations.

6 GATHERING 'DATA'

6.1 Introduction

In order to *extend* our current understanding of a situation, it is important to gather fresh 'data' to give us something new and precise to reflect on. But first the notion of 'data' within an action research project needs to be reconsidered. For example, since all participants must be considered as 'co-researchers', the creation of data needs to be, in some sense, a collaborative process. And for action research even the way the project was initially formulated is itself already part of the 'data': it is not simply a defining framework which anticipates and 'contains' the whole process, but an 'interesting document' to be placed alongside subsequent interpretations as they develop, and to be subjected to critical review.

The main problem about data-gathering is always how to arrange exposure of our initial thinking to evidence which will *test* it, i.e. ensure that we explore it further. One simple and familiar method here is what is called 'triangulation' – gathering different sorts of data so that one sort will act as check on the others (questionnaires compared with interviews, for example). But action research always has the added dimension that data-gathering takes place within a situation where we are, to some extent, *known* to the others involved. It cannot, therefore, be conducted 'impersonally' – the conventional scientific ideal – because existing roles, responsibilities and expectations are always present. However, this in itself can create useful opportunities. For example, Ana Nwichi, a health visitor, was wondering how to 'interview' mothers about their experiences as they were just beginning to breast-feed their babies without thereby adding to their anxieties. One solution was to ask the mothers to make notes of the questions they wished to ask her as their health visitor, in preparation for her visits. Ana thought she could then collect these notes, which would document the mothers' thinking. And this would be not only 'data-gathering' for her action research project but also, she thought, 'good practice' in her role as health visitor.

Perhaps the most common form of data-gathering consists of 'asking questions', but this can easily cast the respondent in a rather passive role, and considerable care is needed, therefore, to try to make the process of asking questions feel like an *invitation* rather than an *interrogation*. Moreover, it is very easy to phrase questions in a way which is either too general (so that they don't help to *focus* on the issues of the project) or too specific (so that they *lead* participants in a predetermined direction). So, face-to-face data-gathering may need to take a form which is more like facilitating a group meeting or a 'workshop' session than simply 'asking questions'. Here are some examples.

John Brown Lee undertook an action research project while acting as a senior social worker with responsibility for setting up contracts with providers of care for clients in their own homes and for checking their 'quality assurance' procedures. In the first stage of his project he wanted to find out from the managers of these agencies their understanding of the term 'quality', so that he could establish official guidelines which would be realistic and effective. But he was in a position of power with respect to these managers: how, therefore, could he avoid asking questions which would signal obviously 'correct' (expected) answers and, instead, get responses which would be both honest and sufficiently detailed for him to *learn* from them? His solution was to write a number of brief fictional scenarios and to ask each manager to describe how that particular agency might respond to such a situation. John was able to *focus* each fictional scenario by its detailed content, and yet he was also able to keep the scenarios open and ambiguous enough to allow for a variety of responses and thus, crucially, to enable himself to be surprised by some *unexpected* responses.

Tom Mason was carrying out a project in a hospital for psychiatric patients with a record of dangerous behaviour. He wanted to help a group of staff (to whom he was well known, as a former colleague) to address aspects of violence and machismo in their professional culture, in order to help them try to change their culture from a largely 'custodial' to a more 'caring' emphasis. As part of his project he asked each of them to write a fictional story about their work (and did so himself). The stories were then circulated (anonymously) and discussed, leading, again, to quite unexpected themes and group dynamics (Mason, 1995).

The general point, in other words, is the action research principle of involving others as *creative* partners in one's own thinking about shared experience, rather than as 'subjects' to be interrogated. (Chapter 14, by Philip Ingram, is a particularly revealing example here.) With this in mind, some suggestions are given below concerning some typical data-gathering activities.

> • Before you go any further, however, this might be a good time to re-read some of the various examples in Part II, bearing in mind that they are only examples 'for consideration', not 'perfect models'. Make a note of the different forms of data they include.

6.2 Observation

Remember that our 'observations' of a situation are never purely objective, but are carried out from our own perspective, consisting of our values, beliefs and assumptions. So record your observations in a way that leaves open the possibility that other observations of the same situation may differ. For example, try to arrange for more than one person to observe and to compare their observations in order to agree a 'joint interpretation', and recognise that this jointly agreed interpretation is *still* not 'objective'. Always feed back the interpretation you have made to those who have been observed, and be prepared to alter your interpretation in the light of their comments and suggestions.

6.3 Keeping a research diary

The previous section emphasised the importance of making sure that data-gathering is a process which encourages participants to engage creatively rather than passively. This section emphasises (in accordance with the principle of reflexivity) that our *own* thinking is treated as data, and is made available for re-interpretation. From this point of view, keeping a research diary is most important. (See Chapter 6, by Philip Kemp.)

6.3.1 The different purposes of a research diary

Creating a data-base of events, experiences and thoughts

It is important to make detailed notes as things occur and as ideas 'strike' you, without waiting for them to fall into a clearly significant pattern. This is especially important for matters that seem 'significant' but one is not sure how or why. Unless you note these down *at the time* you will forget them, and it is precisely those experiences and thoughts that don't immediately fit into what we are expecting that are the growth points for new thinking. And unless you note them down *in detail* at the time, you will afterwards only remember them selectively in a way that fits them into familiar lines of thought and neglects those aspects that were unexpected. So the research diary is a way of encouraging and facilitating one's own personal learning, by enabling us to use our earlier thoughts and experiences as 'data' which can be re-interpreted in the light of later developments and ideas.

Creating a collaborative basis for reflection

Ideally, it is a good idea to avoid a situation in which just one person is keeping a research diary. If only one person keeps a diary undue prominence will gradually be given to that person's ideas, which goes against the collaborative spirit of action research. So encourage as many participants as possible to keep a diary, or at least to keep their own notes on the events of the project. In this way, several differing perspectives will be created and documented, and these can be compared as part of the reflective process.

In practice it may be difficult to persuade most participants to keep a continuous diary. But the important underlying point is that ideas are often created through the process of writing (as well as through discussion, of course). So, at least, encourage all participants to write by, for example, asking them to make notes in preparation for a discussion and to circulate their own notes on a meeting.

A way of keeping a train of thought 'alive'

By setting aside a regular time for making entries in your research diary and for reading over its contents so far, you will find that potentially useful ideas 'pop up' unexpectedly, at odd times, as if from nowhere. Make sure that you note them down as soon as they occur. The diary is a convenient way of keeping one part of one's mind creatively occupied with the research, without necessarily being aware of it. So keep the diary (or at least a few spare pieces of paper) with you at all times, so that you can take full advantage of this helpfully creative 'unconscious' level of your mind. Keeping a diary is thus also an *economical* use of *time*. If you allow two weeks to go by without doing any work on, or thinking about, the project, you will find that when you do sit down you will need at least half an hour just to remind yourself of where you were when you last thought about it. In contrast, by spending just half an hour twice a week working with your diary you will avoid needing to spend precious time just getting back into it.

A source of documents you can share with others

If you feel that your own thinking has become 'stuck' in rather familiar lines, then one way of starting a new line of thought is to show some extracts from your diary (e.g. a detailed description of an event and your comments on it) to other participants or your 'critical friend'. This can be a useful way of gaining new perspectives, i.e. other possible ways of thinking about the event in question.

Notes for any final report

The final report will in some respects be a sort of narrative of the work that took place (see Section 8 below). And it is comforting to know that when you come to put together the report you will not need to start from scratch because you will already have lots of the material there, in your diary.

6.3.2 Some suggestions on keeping a research diary

* Use a loose-leaf binder, so that you can add other comments later and so that you can easily arrange and rearrange your diary entries under different headings.
* Leave a wide margin, so that you can later add other comments and cross-references to other entries.
* For every entry indicate the date and any other relevant details (e.g. the place, the occasion, who was present) so that you can refer to the entry precisely.
* Set aside specific times at frequent intervals (say twice a week at least) for reading through the diary and adding comments and cross-references. Stick to this even if you think that nothing significant has happened recently. You will be surprised at what springs to mind once you begin writing.
* Keep separate (on different sheets):

    detailed descriptive reports of events and verbatim notes of conversations
    your interpretive comments
    other people's comments
    quotations from your reading

* Keep the diary in a very secure place and never leave it lying around. It is essentially quite private and may contain some things that you do not yet wish to share with others without further consideration. If these early thoughts fall into the wrong hands at the wrong time it could be very embarrassing.

6.3.3 Practical work based on research diaries

- After you have been keeping your diary for two or three weeks, have a discussion with other members of the group about how it is going, how you are arranging it, any problems in managing it and any useful ideas that have emerged from the process.

- When you have agreed that several (or all) participants in your project will each keep a research diary, set aside some time to talk about your different experiences. Check whether everyone has a clear perception of its value and discuss whether further guidance on the process is needed by some participants.

- Agree that on a certain day you will each bring in some extracts from your diary on which you would welcome others' comments – e.g. a detailed description of an event or conversation which seems 'somehow' important but you are not yet sure how or why.

6.4 Questionnaires

6.4.1 Limitations of the questionnaire survey method

In many forms of social research the central activity is concentrated on designing a questionnaire survey and then processing the replies to produce the results of the study. In general terms, there are two inherent limitations on the questionnaire method. First, the validity of the results depends on a high response rate, which is very rarely achievable, partly because people often do not see how taking the time to reply will be of benefit to them personally. With a typical response rate of between 20% and 30% one cannot know how far the replies are *representative*, and so the generalisability of the findings is always in doubt. Second, the validity of the results depends on knowing what people 'mean' by their replies, but we can always only guess at this, or make assumptions. So the significance of the findings is always open to question.

For an action research project the questionnaire survey method of data-gathering creates a further set of problems, as indicated below.

1   Questionnaires create a very clear distinction between researchers taking initiatives and respondents who merely *receive and reply*; action research, however, is concerned to involve *all* participants as *creative contributors*.

2   Designing a questionnaire involves *anticipating* possible responses, so that they can be processed easily, even mechanically (e.g. using a computer programme); but action research tries to collect data that are genuinely new and surprising, so that we can *learn* from them in ways we had *not* anticipated.

3   Questionnaires create material for writing a *description* of a state of affairs (how many people think this/have had this experience, etc.); and this can divert attention from the main focus of action research, which is to negotiate a *practical* intervention.

4   Questionnaires create an expectation that the analysis of data will mainly take the form of *counting similar* replies; whereas the analytical work of action research is much more to do with *critical reflection* on *particular* experiences.

Nevertheless, it can often be useful to incorporate a questionnaire into an action research process, as a convenient means for expanding the range of people consulted. The question is: how can we do this in such a way that we do not breach the essential action research principle of collaborative empowerment of *all* participants? Some advice on this is given below.

6.4.2 Incorporating a questionnaire within an action research process

*   Remember that the questionnaire process needs to be conducted in such a way that you learn something new and it feeds directly into the negotiation of practical developments.

*   There is more chance of learning something new from reflecting on the detail of individual replies than from *counting* the replies as a group. So make sure that you include some very open questions which allow respondents to give you ideas that you have not already thought of, i.e. questions which simply invite respondents to outline their thoughts or experiences. Leave plenty of space for elaborate and detailed replies to such questions.

*   Always include a final question which asks respondents to make any other comments which they think are relevant but which they have not so far mentioned.

*   Don't ask for any more information than you really need. In other words, respect the preciousness of the respondent's own time. Keep the questionnaire document *short*.

*   Bear in mind that you will probably gain many genuinely new ideas from discussing what questions to ask. So treat the process of consulting with different participants on the form of the questionnaire as an important phase of the project, not as a mere preliminary to the 'main business' of analysing the completed replies.

*   (Consequently) keep a careful note of how the questionnaire sheet changed as you consulted with different people. This will be useful for the project as a whole, documenting an important aspect of your collective learning process.

*   Plan carefully from the outset how the questionnaire phase of the project will link with other processes; e.g. either (a) as building on the earlier learning of the project, as a sort of 'check', or (b) as a preliminary gathering of ideas to be followed up in more detail through a further process, e.g. a sequence of group interviews.

*   Think carefully about the wording of your covering letter and your introductory notes to the questions. Make sure that the style casts the recipient not in the role of a passive respondent but as someone whose special expertise and

knowledge are appreciated, and whose potential contribution to the project is valued.

- Re-read Chapters 4, 5 and 10, by Noreen Kennedy, Fergal Searson and Richard Lawrence respectively, and notice the different ways in which they incorporate questionnaires as part of their projects.

6.4.3 A practical exercise on developing a questionnaire sheet

---

- Draft a preliminary set of questions and add notes on how the questionnaire is linked to the rest of the process of your project. Check that your draft questions are as open and inviting as possible, that the question sheet is not too long or in any way 'off-putting', and that you have addressed the respondent in a tone of invitation and respect. Bring this material to your group for discussion. Before the discussion re-read carefully the suggestions in Section 6.4.2.

6.5 Interviewing/questioning

Interviews take up a lot of time, so it is important that they are conducted in such a way that we *learn* from the interaction: i.e., we want others to bring out ideas, experiences and perspectives that we haven't yet thought of as being important for the investigation. This is not easily achieved. How can an interview be a *collaborative* interaction, rather than simply an 'interrogation' in which interviewees merely respond to the interviewer's initiatives? How can an interviewer maintain a focus on a set of issues without 'leading' respondents towards ideas which the interviewer has already anticipated? (See the comments on this by Yan Weaver and Vicky Nicholls in Chapter 12.) Here are some suggestions.

6.5.1 The value of group interviews

In a one-to-one interview it can be difficult for the interviewer to avoid leading and steering the conversation, especially if s/he has a higher status than the interviewee, for example if a care worker is interviewing a service-user, or a manager is interviewing a member of her/his staff. In a *group* interview, however, the interviewer can respond to what one person has said by asking others to comment and encouraging discussion *between* interviewees. In other words, the interviewer can concentrate on acting as a 'neutral chairperson', and thus avoid falling into the 'interrogator' role. (The 'group interview' is another name for what has recently become well known as a 'focus group' – see Morgan, 1997: 52–3.) One must remember, however, that under some circumstances people may feel anxious about revealing their ideas to others, so it is important to give individuals the option of being interviewed separately, to consider carefully the membership of group interviews, and to allow plenty of time for introductions and preliminary discussion of the process and issues of mutual 'trust'. Another important point to be considered is whether to form interview groups from representatives of the same 'stakeholder' interests or to form 'mixed' groups. You may well wish to do both at different stages of the work, but the dynamics of these two sorts of groups will obviously be different, and the role of chair will thus be different as well.

6.5.2 The value of distributing questions beforehand

Since interviewees are 'co-researchers' we want them to have plenty of time to consider their views, collect their thoughts and remember their relevant experiences before the interview. So we need to enable them to *prepare* for the interview by letting them know the key issues in advance. This preparatory letter needs to be carefully worded, so that it indicates the topics without seeming to anticipate any particular views; it must read like a friendly invitation to share experiences. (See, for example, in Chapter 12, the 'topic sheets', used by Yan Weaver and Vicky Nicholls.)

Distributing a preparatory document in this way also helps us to manage the development of the work: the reflections and conclusions from one series of interviews can be 'fed into' the preparatory document for the next series. In this way the project can become progressively more 'focused' through a process which is nevertheless essentially collaborative.

6.5.3 Questioning as inviting and listening

Irrespective of the format of the questions and issues which have been distributed in advance, it is important that the interview starts by a signal that it is an opportunity for all to share their experiences and views. Thus, it is a good idea to start with a very open, *inviting* question (e.g. 'Could you tell me about an occasion when you ...?'. It is important also that the interviewer frequently responds by 'reflecting back' what the interviewee has said and asking for further elaboration on particular aspects. Thus, instead of always asking precise 'questions' ('How' or 'Why?' or 'What do you think of ...?'), one needs also to use 'prompts', such as: 'Could you give me a few details of that?', 'Can you remember an example of that?' The interviewer thus needs to signal that they are *listening carefully* to all the contributions. Another important point here is to ensure that everyone is allowed time to *think* during the discussion. Silent pauses should not always be 'filled up' immediately, either by the interviewer or by other participants. Make sure that 'thinking time' is protected.

The purpose of all this is to try to ensure that the data include the *details* of individuals' experiences and perspectives, since it is those details which will be new and different and open to various interpretations. The problem with too *general* a discussion is that all the interpretation has 'already happened', and it is easy to feel – on reading through the notes – that not much more can be said about it. With a discussion centred on *detail* (of points of view, of experience) there will always be details that can point in a number of different directions and that one can 'pick up' either at the time or later.

6.5.4 Recording and making notes

The advantage of tape recording an interview is that it captures the detail of everything that is said, and that you can listen to the tape afterwards and pick up things that you did not notice at the time. So, as a *resource* for critical reflection a tape recording is valuable. (See also the comments on tape recording in Chapter 12, by Yan Weaver and Vicky Nicholls.) Another use of a tape recording is that it will enable you to listen critically to your own interviewing skills – those indicated in Section 6.5.3 in particular. Unless you are already highly skilled in counselling methods, you will almost certainly find that there is a lot of room for improvement, that your interview was much more directive and less 'accepting' than you intended it to be. On the other hand, many people are made nervous by a tape recorder, and even if it is easily forgotten during the actual discussion, people may feel anxious at the end about issues of confidentiality and security. So precise reassurances will need to be given. A tape recording takes a long time to transcribe exactly, and so it is probably more practical to use a tape as a basis for making detailed notes (with just a few passages transcribed exactly); otherwise the burden of work becomes quite excessive. (But do keep the tapes after you have made your notes in case some other issue emerges later in the project, which makes you want to transcribe another passage.)

However, there is a lot to be said for using note-taking as a method of recording. First, you don't necessarily have to do all the note-taking yourself. For example, you could ask a colleague to do it. You can also ask all the participants to make their own notes and give them to you at the end, which is a nice way of emphasising the collaborative dimension of the process and also a neat way of immediately generating *different* perspectives, as a basis for further discussion and analysis. Second, you can build your own note-taking into the interview process in such a way that you use it to emphasise your careful listening and the *value* being attached to contributions: 'Can I just check that I have got down the point you are making here? I've written ". . .". Is that right?' This also a way of ensuring plenty of 'thinking time'.

6.5.5 Practical work on interviewing

> • Bring along for discussion in the group your plans for conducting your first interview and the draft of your preparatory document. Re-read Section 6.5.3 before you begin your discussion.

continued

- Work in groups of five or six to prepare and evaluate a 'mock' group interview. One person, acting as interviewer, distributes a preparatory document and conducts a group interview lasting about twenty minutes, with three or four people acting as interviewees. The remaining member of the group acts as observer, paying particular attention to the issues raised in Section 6.5.3. Tape record the interview. Afterwards, listen to the tape, discuss your feelings about it, and discuss the preparatory document and observer's comments. Repeat the exercise, with a different observer and interviewer.

- After your first interview, bring along your notes and comments and share them with the group. Focus the discussion on what you have learned which will affect how you conduct your next interview.

6.6 A general exercise on data-gathering

- Make a list of the different ways in which you will be gathering 'data' within the project, remembering to include your research diary. Then ask yourself the following questions:

  * Are there some useful and accessible sources of relevant data which you could easily add (for example, case notes, minutes of meetings, letters, policy documents)?
  * Are there ways in which your methods of data-gathering could give more opportunity to allow other participants to play a greater part, and to take more responsibility?
  * Could some (at least) of your data-gathering methods be made more like developmental 'workshops' rather than simply situations where information is requested (see 6.1 above)?

- Bring your list of data-gathering methods to the group for discussion based on the above questions.

7 ANALYSING AND REFLECTING ON DATA

7.1 Introduction

- Look again at 'Supporting document 1: "Knowledge" – some key distinctions' (p. 245) and then re-read in Chapter 2, the section 'How action research transforms some key aspects of social inquiry', pp. 19–22.

The main point that we need to remember in considering the process of 'analysing' data within an action research project is that the focus of action research is concerned with *learning* and *implementing change*, whereas the focus of other forms of research is on description or *constructing an interpretation*. This key distinction explains why much of the general literature on data analysis can, unless one is very careful, be somewhat misleading (or at least impractical) when applied within an action research process. So in considering the process of 'data analysis' we need to bear in mind the following general points.

First, we are not necessarily concerned to create a comprehensive interpretation of all the data which been collected, but to think about them in ways that reveal or stimulate *new* possibilities for *action*. The *problem* about data analysis is how to use the data we have collected to develop ideas that we didn't have before we started. Clearly, some of the data we collect will merely 'confirm' our original thoughts, but in an action research process this is less helpful than in conventional ('outsider') research, for two main reasons: (1) we only have time to collect a relatively small amount of data, so our 'results' will not have a very firm *statistical* base; (2) as action researchers (unlike outsider researchers), we start off as experienced participants in the situation, and so any new data which confirm our initial thoughts only add to what was already a fairly substantial stock of evidence. In other words, if an action research project is really going to be worth all the effort we put into it, 'data analysis' needs to be a process of learning through 'critical reflection' on the data, rather simply describing or classifying it according to categories we had before we started.

Second, we need to ensure that as many participants as possible are involved in the process, so that data analysis, like the other aspects of the work, becomes a collaborative process of negotiation. Thus, if one person carries out an analysis, it is important that the interpretation is then fed back to other participants for their contribution and amendment. In this way, *different* interpretations are created, and these differences stimulate debate about alternative interpretations and new practical implications.

Third, the process of data analysis must not be so time-consuming and elaborate that it distracts us from the collaborative and action-oriented progress of the work. Action research is a developmental process moving through time in a sequence of action, data collection, reflection, further action and further reflection. In contrast, most of the literature on 'data analysis' describes procedures established for conventional social research, in which a single but very elaborate process of collecting data is followed by a single but very elaborate process of overall interpretation. For conventional social research, this single comprehensive 'analysis' sums up the findings and conclusions of the whole piece of work. In action research, on the other hand, reflections on the data collected at one stage of the work become the data informing the next stage. It is the *sequence* of *several phases* of critical reflection within an action research project which carries forward its development. And it is the narrative of this development which the project report needs to describe, not a single, final analysis of 'results' (see Section 8 below).

In the following sections, more specific guidance is given with respect to particular methods of data analysis.

7.2 Statistical analysis

The main thing to remember is that in an action research project one will rarely be able to claim that statistical results are 'significant generalisations', since our samples will always be relatively small. Instead, they are either a *guide* in deciding on the next action step or a *check* on what has been done so far. So keep the statistics simple. Try to set up the questions in such a way that the practical implications can be 'read off' as simple percentages. If nothing interesting, new or helpful emerges at this level, it might be better simply to accept that the exercise has not been very illuminating and go on to something else. Or perhaps the really interesting point that has emerged is that the results are unexpected, in which case you have a starting point for reflection. (What were you expecting, and why?) But if you try to force the data to 'say something' by engaging in complex statistical procedures, you risk spending a lot of time reaching conclusions which are *still* not very strongly based or very informative, and also being distracted from the developmental aims of the project.

Remember that the 'closed' questions which create easily counted answers are a way of *imposing* your categories on the respondents, whereas in action research your aim always is to *learn* from them. So don't frame your questionnaire in such a way that respondents are forced to accept and use your categories even if they don't want to. Thus, if you ask respondents to answer 'Yes' or 'No', also allow the reply 'I don't know'. And if you ask them to 'Agree' or 'Disagree' with a statement, always allow them a neutral reply ('I find it hard to say one way or the other'). This goes against the advice in textbooks on statistics, but that is because such works assume that the statistics will be the main 'result' of the work, and are therefore seeking ways to *make* the results significant. In action research the situation is different: statistical analysis will always only be a *phase* of the project – an initial exploration or a final evaluative check – and our statistical methods must be compatible with our overall attempt to find collaborative, 'non-impositional' ways of working.

It is also possible to derive quantitative data from verbal responses to open-ended questions and from interview transcripts. The process is called 'content analysis'; it simply entails going through the responses and picking out key phrases or words, and counting the number of times they have been used in the whole set of responses (see Weber, 1985). This can be quite a useful way of finding a pattern, but, again, it requires the person analysing the data to impose her/his own pre-defined concepts. Within an action research project, therefore, it is important to consult as widely as possible before deciding which are the key words and phrases you will be looking for, and to use this technique only as a starting point or as a final check: it is *not* a way of avoiding the basic strategies for critical reflection (outlined above in Section 3 of this chapter and below in Section 7.4).

7.3 'Coding' qualitative data

The most common approach to analysing verbal data (notes or transcripts from interviews and meetings, letters, extracts from diaries, etc.) is to 'code' the material, i.e. to categorise it in terms derived from the key concepts and concerns of the project. The process involves repeated re-readings of the data collected in order to find a good 'fit' between the variety of the data and our conceptual framework as it gradually emerges. The 'conceptual framework' for the project is stated in a preliminary way as soon as the project has a theme and a purpose, i.e. the initial understanding of the 'problem', the set of anticipated theoretical issues, alternative practical possibilities, etc. Then, when the data starts to 'come in', from partici-pants' responses, diaries and so on, we need to go through it and collect particular comments to be grouped together under headings, as throwing light on this or that aspect. At the same time, of course, we will start to change the initial framework of ideas, as respondents begin to contribute concepts and lines of thought which we had not considered. This is obviously a lengthy process, whether we use a computer programme, such as NUD*IST (see Gahan and Hannibal, 1998) or undertake it manually (by, for example, colour-coding passages in the texts and then cutting out extracts and sorting them in boxes or envelopes).

The basic process of 'coding' data is important, since – in general terms – we are always trying to learn from what various respondents have said in the light of our overall framework of ideas. (See, for example, the three 'themes' of Cathy Aymer's project, Chapter 9.) But some of the specific methods used in conventional qualitative research do not fit very well with the relationships and the overall structure of action research. There are two reasons for this.

First, the more comprehensively we try to accommodate all the data, the more the analysis will inevitably become the work of one person, whose accumulating expertise on the 'meaning' of the data will prevent others (who have not had time to engage in such a lengthy process) from offering their suggestions. In other words, a 'full' coding of the data fed back to respondents will not seem to offer much scope for alternative interpretations, and is thus likely to meet with a fairly passive acceptance. Producing a highly elaborate analysis can therefore reduce the collaborative dimension of the work. One way forward here is to treat our first coding of the data as further data, to be circulated to others for comment and suggestions.

Second, there is the following dilemma. The more we try to reduce the data to manageable proportions, the more we tend to use our original set of concepts as a criterion of relevance, and thus exclude respondents' ideas. But, on the other hand, the more we try to include ideas from respondents which were not part of our original framework, the more unwieldy becomes our analysis, so that it becomes almost a 're-description' of what everyone said. ('Dilemma analysis' is one solution to this issue: see Section 7.5 below.)

7.4 Data analysis and critical reflection

Given the problems outlined in the preceding paragraphs, it is suggested that the basic approach to data collection within an action research project should be based on the ideas concerning 'critical reflection' already referred to.

> • Re-read 'Supporting document 5: Critical reflection as "innovative thinking"' (p. 249) and look back also at your analysis of a 'critical incident' using that document.

In general terms, these questions can be used to 'analyse' the data you have collected by starting a discussion among project participants about what is most 'significant' about the data. The questions are intended to encourage an approach to the data analysis phase of the work which (1) focuses on what you can learn from the new data; (2) can be undertaken collaboratively; and (3) is concerned with how the data can be used to inform the next stage of the work.

7.4.1 Reflecting on your data: a practical exercise

> • Select a piece of data you have collected (e.g. a set of notes from an interview or a set of replies to a questionnaire, your account of a significant event) and use some of the questions in 'Supporting document 5' to develop a line of argument about the implications of this piece of data for your project.
>
> • Ask other participants in your project to comment on your analysis.
>
> • Bring the data and the various commentaries to a group meeting, and share your ideas.
>
> • What does your combined analysis suggest might be a useful next step in your project? (This might be a suggestion about further data to be analysed, further data to be collected or the next practical development.)

Clearly, this is not simply a 'one-off' exercise, but a pattern to be repeated as one of the main processes of the project work.

7.5 'Dilemma analysis': a way of using qualitative data in action research projects

The procedure described below is a direct application of 'dialectics' (see Section 3.4.2 above). It is based on the fundamental idea that most events, situations, states of mind, etc. contain or consist of *contradictions*, and thus pose 'dilemmas' as to how we should interpret them or respond to them.

7.5.1 The problem which dilemma analysis is designed to solve

The total amount of communication even within a small action research process is so enormous that we can't possibly use *all* the data we collect. We must *reduce* it in some way, in order to focus on those elements in the data which seem particularly 'significant', i.e. the ideas from which we can most easily learn, and those which can help us to decide what to do next. But if we just read through them and pick out 'what seems interesting', there is a danger that we will be struck by the ideas that already fit into our familiar lines of thought. Thus we may not develop any new *ideas* even from a large amount of new material.

The participants in an action research project are co-researchers. Their interpretations are therefore (in an important sense which is essential to the basic theory of action research) 'at the same level' as those of the research initiator/ facilitator. If we simply *classify* participants' words (using 'content analysis' or a 'coding' procedure) then we are putting our co-researchers' ideas into 'boxes' which we have created from our own initial theories. And in this way we fail to learn anything new or unexpected from their responses.

What then can we do? In reducing the data to manageable proportions, how can we *select* the most 'significant' data in such a way that we *learn* from the new and surprising aspects of our co-researchers' thinking? How can we avoid simply using our own pre-existing theories as the criterion of what is to count as relevant?

7.5.2 Dilemma analysis as a method

Dilemma analysis is a way of selecting out certain parts of the data as being particularly significant.

The first step is simply to go through the data and select out those statements which are in some way in contradiction with one another. It may be that one person says two things which don't quite fit or that one person says something which doesn't fit with what someone else says or goes against a statement from a key policy document, etc. Statements which are contradicted in any way are thus picked out from the rest of the data as indicating *issues* in the situation about which participants may disagree. Such issues are potentially 'interesting', not only as a way of creating an interpretation of the situation but also for the practical development of the project, in that they indicate areas where further discussion will be needed in order to create agreement on the next step to be taken.

An example

Philip Kemp used this method in 'Supporting the supporters' (1997). He gathered data from residents and support workers in a housing development for people with mental health problems, and reduced the themes of what they said to a set of 'dilemmas', as follows.

On the one hand, involving residents in shared accommodation was beneficial but, on the other hand, it also created the stress of excessive intimacy.

On the one hand involving residents in decision-making was seen as valuable, but, on the other hand, it often precipitated anxiety in residents by giving them increased responsibility.

On the one hand, residents desired independence but, on the other hand, they wished to be looked after.

On the one hand, the staff wanted to be supportive of residents but, on the other hand, they wanted to allow residents the freedom to take risks.

The second step is as follows. When we have selected (or constructed) from the data a set of 'dilemmas' (like those above), then we may assume that we have identified from the data a set of issues which are experienced by the participants as complex and thus 'interesting'. (Note that these issues have emerged from what the participants have said, *not* from the initiator's themes, theories or classification 'boxes'.) These issues can then be taken back to the participants as a brief paper outlining an agenda for discussion. The questions for the meeting at which the dilemma analysis is discussed might have the general form:

Where do you, individually, stand on these issues? (i.e. more on one side or the other?)
Are there ways in which we might try to resolve these issues?
Which ones are most important?
Which ones should we tackle first?

NOTE 1

For examples of the 'practical effect' of this approach, see Philip Kemp's discussion at the end of 'Mary's scenario' in Chapter 6 and Brenda Dennett's discussion of 'A key incident' in Chapter 8.

NOTE 2

Earlier references to and presentations of the method of dilemma analysis are to be found in Winter (1982; 1989: Chapter 7); Altrichter *et al.* (1993: 146–52); and McKernan (1996: 141–5). These presentations contain more detail and examples, but they are also more complex in ways which are, I now think, not very helpful. The account given here contains the essence of the approach and clarifies its practical use within the process of a project.

7.6 A final note on data analysis

Although the main emphasis has been on the importance of critical reflection as a way of learning from data, it is important to remember that there will also be occasions when all that is needed is a simple collection of responses as a form of direct feedback. (See, for example, Chapter 5 by Fergal Searson.) The work of data analysis in itself doesn't *always* have to be complicated because the value of the project is also based in its sequence of innovative *actions*.

8 WRITING AN ACTION RESEARCH REPORT

8.1 General considerations

At this point, it would be useful to re-read the examples in Part II. They have been selected to illustrate the different 'styles' of writing in which a report may be presented, and also the many different 'shapes' that an action research project can have. For example, it can start off from an evaluation of current practice, or a process of gathering participants' perspectives on a general issue, or some form of innovative *action*. The shape of the project will affect the structure of the report, but in some way it will probably follow this sequence:

1 a brief statement of the basic issue;
2 the background – including a description of the context, the roles of the participants in the context, and the relevant literature which defines the state of current understanding in relation to the issue, i.e. why this issue is 'interesting', both practically and theoretically;
3 An explanation of the method of the project, including: a *general* theory of action research and how the methods in your specific context relate to the general theory; ethical and political issues and how you attempted to resolve them;
4 an overview of the sequence of activities you undertook;
5 examples of the data you collected at different times, and how you analysed it;
6 a description of changes introduced and/or other practical impacts of the work;
7 an explanation of how these changes/impacts were evaluated;
8 'Conclusions': the current state of affairs, how far it is an improvement on the previous state of affairs, and how you know it is; what you learned that you didn't know before; your current understanding of the problem; the next steps in the work, as you currently anticipate them.

(NB If your work included more than one 'cycle', then 5, 6, and 7 will be repeated.)

The report is likely to have the general form of a *narrative*, but a narrative which explains itself as it goes along. (This is where we started (and why); this is what we did (and why); this is where we ended, and what I/we think it signifies). You will need to explain the initial problem, and explain the *reasons* for your various practical decisions, i.e. who were involved as participants, how you worked together, what data you collected, how it was analysed, etc. In other words your report will need to combine narrative, description and analysis. (For contrasting examples, see Chapter 7 by Valerie Childs, Chapter 10 by Richard Lawrence, and Chapter 11 by Peter Beresford and Michael Turner.)

Your report should combine description, narrative and the detail of events and different perspectives in such a way that it brings the situation to life. So make sure that you quote plenty of *details* – from your data, from your research notes, and from what others have said (including published sources). An action research report should enable readers to learn from what the writers have learned from their work: it should present the inquiry in a form that others can learn from.

Even if after a lot of effort you were finally unable to do what you intended (e.g. if the change you tried out did not have anything like the effect you hoped for), you will still have the basis for a report which others would find interesting, in which you describe a sequence of experiences, your interpretation of these experiences, and what you have learned from the overall process. We can learn very effectively from our 'mistakes', and/or from finding problems that we had not at first anticipated (see Chapter 7 by Valerie Childs).

8.2 Some more particular suggestions

8.2.1

Think carefully about the audience for your writing. It is most useful, in many ways, to imagine that you are writing for well-informed colleagues (whether staff, managers or service-users) in the same area of practice. Thus, your readers are well informed about the practice area in general, but they do not know about your project (yet) and may not share all your assumptions. If you are undertaking the work in the context of a course in an educational institution do *not* think mainly of your tutor, who already knows about what you are doing. Instead think of an external examiner who is sympathetic to action research in general but may have a slightly different conception of it and thus may need to be convinced of the soundness of the particular approach you have adopted. She/he will be on the look-out for such obvious matters as clarity of structure and presentation, correct referencing, the carefulness of your arguments and the accuracy and 'up-to-date-ness' of your specialist/'professional' knowledge. These are also important matters to bear in mind even if you are not writing for an examiner but for an audience of colleagues, because they concern the *clarity* and the *persuasiveness* of your report.

8.2.2

Readers will need to be *persuaded* by your writing, so you need to write in a way that takes into account their possible *sceptical* stances, anticipating their questions and trying to answer them.

8.2.3

Readers always need *help* in following your argument, so you need to: (1) make quite clear at the outset your starting point, your initial 'problem' and your aims;

and (2) use headings and linking statements to help your various readers move with you through the argument. You could think of your argument as a very twisting road, because your project is complex and so is the argument of your report. In order to help the reader to negotiate the twists and turns successfully you need a series of signposts indicating where the road (the argument) is going next. Otherwise they will miss the road and feel 'lost', and they will then (of course) blame you for not giving them proper assistance.

8.2.4

Think very carefully about what makes a piece of writing persuasive. What makes you take someone's line of thinking seriously even if, first, you don't initially agree with it and, second, the writer has no particular official authority? One might answer:

1   The authors seem to be knowledgeable.
2   The authors seem to be aware of a variety of possible lines of thought and to have selected this one only after considering others.
3   The authors seem to be thinking self-critically about their own assumptions; they seem to have changed their ideas in response to their work (i.e. they seem open-minded).
4   The authors seem to be 'honest', i.e. they don't seem to be concealing or glossing over things.

You could extend this list for yourself. The point is: your writing needs to make your readers feel that they are in 'safe hands', that they can trust you; and you need to keep them sufficiently interested to follow you along your argument and find out where you wish to take them.

8.2.5

An action research report (like any other research report) should explain how data was selected, collected and analysed. But in action research it is also important to bring out the way in which you attempted to do all this using (as far as possible) a *collaborative* method of working. So ensure that you explain clearly how you attempted to make the process collaborative, and allow the various participants to speak in their own voices, rather than always in the words of a single narrator speaking on their behalf. (See, for example, Chapter 13 by Jane Bradburn and Cherry Mackie.)

8.2.6

If you use signposts and links carefully, you can easily include different types of writing in your report: quotations from transcripts, extracts from official guidelines, extracts from practical documents used in your work, including notes circulated to participants, etc. You can use the your narrative/argument to 'string them together'

– like beads on a thread. You might also think of your text as a drama, in which there are a number of different 'characters' speaking.

8.2.7

Don't forget that some supporting material can be placed in an appendix, in order to keep the main text of the report as 'readable' as possible.

8.2.8

Although your report is an account of your own practical experience, this does not mean to say that references to others' work is not important. It is, of course, particularly important to provide a sound, up-to-date account of current thinking in the area of your topic. (Notice how most of the examples start by doing this.) Also, because action research cannot simply use the pre-defined techniques of 'scientific' investigation as a 'guarantee' of its validity, an action research report needs, all the more, to show how the work has nevertheless drawn critically upon a *range of resources*. This does not just mean citing people or books which you agree with, but indicating how, through discussion of the various resources cited, your ideas, categories, interpretations, etc. have been explored and developed through the work of the project. These resources may include other experiences and general reading as well as the professional and methodological literature.

8.2.9

Remember that the essence of the action research approach is the on-going movement between: actions undertaken, data produced by the actions, reflections on the significance of these data, and decisions as to what to do next, based on these reflections. So try to make sure that the pattern of your writing embodies this 'dialectical' to-and-fro.

8.2.10

Remember that, in some respects, an action research project does not simply end. There will usually be an important sense in which you are reporting merely on how far you have got 'so far'. So there is nothing wrong with ending your report with new data, new thoughts, new practical proposals, together with brief notes as to their possible significance, rather than a presentation of 'results'. In other words, your report can be quite open-ended.

8.2.11

Finally, share your report with the project participants and with at least one independent reader before you 'publish' it or otherwise treat it as 'finished'. You will be surprised how many things are 'not clear' to them and thus need a little more explanation.

APPENDIX: PRACTICAL GUIDE SUPPORTING DOCUMENTS

Supporting document 1: 'Knowledge' – some key distinctions

Positivist/Natural Science Research   Action Research

Type of Knowledge:

Abstract (generalisations, statistics)	Experiential (details, quotations)
Referring to a wide range of situations	Referring to a single situation
Product ('findings')	Process ('outcomes', 'spin-offs')

Origin of Knowledge:

Observation (+ analysis)	Action (+ analysis)
Detachment	Involvement, collaboration
Outsider objectivity	Insider sensitivity
Social power, authority and high status	Experience of exclusion and low social status

Criteria for Validity:

Is it generalisable?	Was it effectively implemented?
Is it replicable?	'Political' feasibility
Statistical significance	Can a variety of others 'relate' to it?
Comprehensive data and analysis	Innovative reflection on data
Outsider authority	Insider (Collective) ownership

Note

In a very crude way, the left-hand column expresses the positivist/natural science model of research and the right-hand column expresses the action research model. In some ways, 'qualititative/descriptive' research combines elements of both. However, these are not hard-and-fast distinctions but relative *shifts of emphasis*.

The main point is that there is not just one ideal of knowledge that all forms of inquiry aspire to (and achieve in different degrees). Rather, there are two equally important ideals which form a continuum on which different forms of inquiry are placed at different points.

Supporting document 2: Practice-based learning through reflection – action research processes and resources

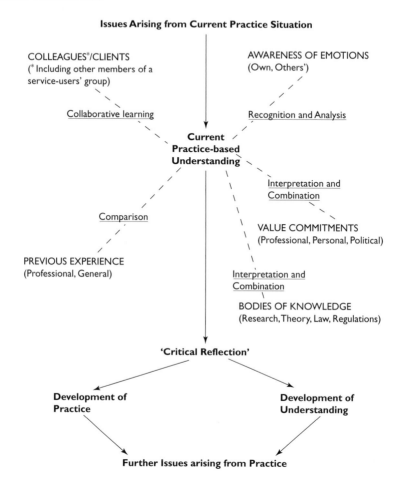

Issues Arising from Current Practice Situation

COLLEAGUES*/CLIENTS
(* Including other members of a
service-users' group)

AWARENESS OF EMOTIONS
(Own, Others')

Collaborative learning

Recognition and Analysis

**Current
Practice-based
Understanding**

Interpretation and
Combination

Comparison

VALUE COMMITMENTS
(Professional, Personal, Political)

PREVIOUS EXPERIENCE
(Professional, General)

Interpretation and
Combination

BODIES OF KNOWLEDGE
(Research, Theory, Law, Regulations)

'Critical Reflection'

**Development of
Practice**

**Development of
Understanding**

Further Issues arising from Practice

Explanation

When issues arise in our current practical experience we become aware of the need to review our current understanding. The different 'resources' for our understanding are indicated by the phrases in capitals and the different 'processes' through which we draw on each of these resources are underlined. (For example, we learn collaboratively from our colleagues, fellow group members and/or clients; we make comparisons between this experience and previous experiences, and we interpret and combine our various value commitments and the different bodies of knowledge we are aware of in the context of this particular situation.) The whole of this process is what one might term 'critical reflection' and leads to the development of our practice and our understanding.

Supporting document 3: The problem of making 'reflexive' judgements

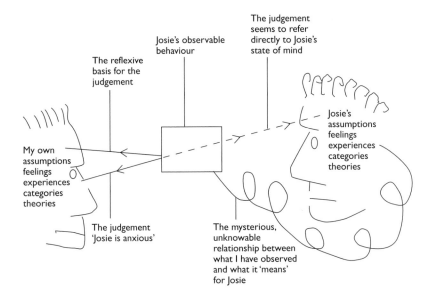

The judgement seems to refer directly to Josie's state of mind

Josie's observable behaviour

The reflexive basis for the judgement

Josie's
assumptions
feelings
experiences
categories
theories

My own
assumptions
feelings
experiences
categories
theories

The judgement
'Josie is anxious'

The mysterious, unknowable relationship between what I have observed and what it 'means' for Josie

Explanation

When I make a judgement, such as 'Josie is anxious', based on how I observe her respond during a conversation, I am actually and inevitably referring in part to my own assumptions, feelings, experiences, categories and theories. In other words, it is a 'reflexive' statement (the continuous line in the diagram, which is 'bent back' ['re'-'flex'-ed] into my own mind). But it is very easy to forget this and to be misled (by the broken line in the diagram) into thinking that we have made a statement that refers directly to Josie's experience. But the principle of reflexivity (as a general theory of language) suggests that the relationship between what we observe other people do and say and those people's own experience is fundamentally unknowable (the looped line in the diagram).

This is only a 'problem' if we think that our judgement about other people ought to aim at being objective, accurate and final. But the principle of reflexivity suggests that we don't need to aim at this, and indeed that it is a quite mistaken aim. Instead, as soon as we recognise that our judgements are indeed reflexive, then we need to make our judgements in a tentative, exploratory fashion that leaves them open to question and revision. In this way, when we compare our judgements with other people's judgements of the same events, they do not need to become the basis for disputes but opportunities for learning from each other.

Supporting document 4: Dialectics

'Dialectics' is a general theory (with a long tradition) about the nature of the social world and how we understand it by means of language. Dialectical thinking rests on three basic arguments:

1   All things (people, situations, ideas, feelings, organisations, etc.) are *connected* with one another in a system or network of mutual influences, *not* separate from one another or linked in a simple chain of single causes producing single effects.

2   All things (people, situations, . . . etc.) are *changing*, rather than static. The one thing which we know for certain already is that the present is different from the past, and therefore the one safe prediction we can make is that the future will be different from the present. So unless we understand how things are changing, we can be sure that we don't yet understand them properly.

3   All things (people, situations, . . . etc.) are complex, are made up of *contradictions*, rather than simple and unified. Hence the term 'dialectics'. 'Dia' means 'separated into two parts', as in 'diameter', which divides a circle into two halves. 'Legein' is the Greek verb 'to speak', from which we get 'lexis' ('word'), as in 'lexicon' or dictionary – a collection of words. Hence 'dialectics' is a form of understanding which is achieved through *dialogue* and, in particular, through argument between two (or more) people holding opposing (i.e. 'contradictory') points of view. As a general principle, this point may seem initially somewhat unexpected, but it fits quite neatly into a model of the action research process and in some ways it is quite familiar. For example: we are aware of the contradictions in our own characters and those of the people we know well – only when you don't know someone well do they seem to be easily summed up by a single term; we know that 'love' and 'hate' are supposed to be closely linked, that people may say that they are 'only being cruel to be kind', and that religions advocating universal love cause horrendous wars. So the dialectical principle here is: we don't understand something fully until we can see its contradictory elements.

Note
This account of dialectics is based on Israel (1979), Fisk (1979) and Markovic (1984). The tradition goes back through Marx to Hegel and to the ancient Greeks – see Bertrand Russell's account of Heraclitus in his *History of Western Philosophy*. There are also deep analogies between dialectics and the ways in which we understand religion, history, spirituality, art and ecology (see Reason, 1994: Chapters 2 and 3). For a more detailed account of dialectics in relation to action research, see Carr and Kemmis (1986: 180–7), Winter (1987: 11–16; 1989: 46–55).

Supporting document 5: Critical reflection as 'innovative thinking'

The term 'innovative thinking' is taken from Hart (2000). The purpose of the following sets of questions is to help in analysing incidents, events and various types of data in such a way that we learn from them something that we didn't know beforehand. You may find it helpful to combine questions from the different groups below and/or to add your own questions, along similar lines.

1 Welcoming Surprise
- What is there in this (incident, data, etc.) which I find surprising?
- Why am I surprised?
- What was I expecting different?
- What does this tell me?

2 Analysing the Reflexivity of Interpretive Judgements
Given my first interpretation of this (incident, data, etc.):

- What are its origins in:

   my values (general/political/professional)?
   my feelings?
   my general theories about this sort of incident, situation, etc.?

- What personal experiences lie behind these values, feelings, theories?
- If someone else had had quite different personal experiences, they might bring different but equally relevant values, feelings and theories to interpreting this incident, data, etc. So what alternative interpretations might be made?
- Imagine an interpretation from the perspective of another actor within this situation.

3 Thinking Dialectically
Given this situation/event/data:

- What is the *relevant* context, and *how* is it relevant?
- What are the tensions/dilemmas/conflicts of interest/disagreements?
- What is the origin of these tensions, dilemmas, conflicts, etc.?
- What possible lines for future development do these tensions etc. suggest?

4 Five Key Questions for Going Beyond Initial Interpretations
The following series of linked questions (adapted from Hart, 1995) is designed to help in *re-interpreting* events, situations, data, etc., in order to take our thinking forward. In some respects they include and sum up both the reflexive and the dialectical principles.

- What other things are influencing this event, situation, data, etc.?
- How might this event, situation, data, etc. be understood in a contrasting way?
- How might this be understood by the other person/people involved?
- What are my feelings about this and what do these feelings tell me about my original interpretation?
- What else do I need to do/find out about in order to reach an adequate understanding of this?

Supporting document 6: Pattern for a project information sheet

Heading (1) Name of the organisation from which the project is being initiated.
Heading (2) Project title, e.g. 'Developing the Service-User's Forum Project'.
Heading (3) Project information sheet.

This information sheet provides an outline of the Project, in order to help you decide whether you are interested in taking part as a participant in the work.

The main aim of the Project is to. . . . The value of the Project is as follows. For staff it should enable . . . For service users, it will be an opportunity to. . . . And for managers it will . . .

The project is being initiated by [*Name, Position, Address, Contact phone number*].

The other participants in the project will include [*List intended 'stakeholder' groups*].

All participants will be involved in decisions concerning the focus of the work, the methods to be used, and the form and content of any project reports.

Participation is entirely voluntary. You have the right to decide *not* to take part, and if you *do* decide to take part you have the right to withdraw at any stage. Involvement in the project will not affect any other care relationships or organisational relationships, and if you have concerns about this, please raise this issue with [*Name of project initiator*] or with anyone else you wish.

The work of the project will take place over a period of (*e.g. five months*) and will consist of, for example:

1   *an initial interview of participants to establish their views*;
2   *a series of group discussions between . . .*;
3   *a further series of interviews bringing together . . . in order to decide . . .*;
4   *a two-month trial of the new . . .*;
5   *a final series of discussions to evaluate the . . .*;
6   *circulation of a draft report for suggestions.*

This will probably involve a minimum of about (*e.g. ten hours*) work for each participant over the whole period of the project.

No recordings will be made without permission from those involved, and notes made from discussions and interviews will be checked for accuracy with those present.

The data created by the work will be circulated to other participants for their comments, but you will have the right to check and amend any record or interpretation of your own ideas before they are circulated to others.

Permission will be obtained before any data are used for purposes other than those for which they were originally collected. All material concerning the project will be treated as confidential by all participants throughout the period of the project, and all written material concerning the project will be kept securely locked. Detailed rules for confidentiality will be discussed in relation to each stage of the work.

Interviews and meetings will be carefully conducted in such a way as to ensure that any tensions or anxieties are resolved harmoniously, and the project co-ordinators accept responsibility to provide whatever support they can, should this become necessary.

Any reports of the project work intended for publication outside the group of participants will be written in such a way as to preserve the anonymity of participants, if they wish, and to acknowledge the contribution of all who wish to be named. Reports intended for publication will be circulated beforehand for comments and suggestions. At this stage all participants will have the right to delete any material which they feel may damage their own reputation, but the project initiators retain the right to publish an account of the project.

The above points are only a first draft, indicating generally how the project will be conducted, and your comments and suggestions concerning all aspects of the project are most welcome.

Part IV

Action research as a form of social inquiry

A 'theoretical' justification

Introduction

Action research is controversial. At a commonsense level, we know perfectly well that different forms of knowledge are expected and recognised as valid in different social situations. In some contexts (e.g. making policy decisions within large organisations) those responsible generally expect quantitative data drawn from questionnaire surveys of large population samples; in other contexts (e.g. conveying our opinions and beliefs to friends and colleagues) we expect the testimony of personal experience. However, we live in a society where *politically influential* knowledge conventionally takes the form of statistically or theoretically based generalisations, established by academic or professional experts and promoted through organisational power hierarchies. In contrast, as we have seen, action research tries to create *non*-hierarchical relationships as a key aspect of the inquiry process. And action research reports tend to present knowledge in the form of narratives of personal experience, giving a voice to those who are (relatively at least) culturally and politically silenced by the conventional structures of social inquiry. Thus, action research emphasises the importance of practitioners' knowledge (vis-à-vis academics), service-users' knowledge (vis-à-vis professionals), and community members' knowledge (vis-à-vis government officials). And it prides itself on producing specific practical changes and 'empowerment effects', at least as much as on any generalised 'findings'.

These contrasts between action research and conventional social inquiry create real and practical problems for action research. Action research reports risk being marginalised, or even rejected, by senior managers, academics or officials in charge of allocating research funds, as merely partisan or sentimentally idealistic, as mere voices of dissent or exercises in raising morale, as simply lacking the validity and reliability of 'proper research'. Such reservations on the part of those with political and professional influence have to be taken seriously, not least because of action research's own practical responsibilities. 'Good practice' in action research is about *justifiable* decision-making in situations directly involving human well-being.

Action research projects, therefore, if they are to be influential, must seem convincing and professionally 'sound', and consequently they must be clearly seen to be justifiable as expressions of our *best current understanding* of the nature and processes of inquiry. Various justifications of action research were presented in Chapter 2: as an ideal of reflective practice, and as a 'culture of inquiry' in the workplace. But Chapter 2 focused on the way in which action research is *different* from conventional forms of social inquiry.

In contrast, the purpose of this final chapter is to show that action research is not a way of 'ignoring the challenges' of conventional social inquiry but, on the contrary, a way of addressing real philosophical difficulties which are widely recognised as being inherent in the task of undertaking *any* form of social inquiry – large-scale surveys, theoretical analyses, randomised control trials or local development projects. Thus, we return briefly once again to the philosophical basis for action research, in order to demonstrate that the characteristic features of action research presented so far can be justified in terms of the general theoretical considerations underlying any social inquiry. The argument focuses first on the issue of relativism and then on the concept of 'critical realism'.

Action research and relativism

Let us start with a general criticism of action research, which might be articulated by a sceptical senior manager or fund-holder, or indeed by anyone conscious of the doubts outlined above.

> Action research seems to accept that the 'validity' of its outcomes resides in the formulation of *consensus* among a particular group of participating stakeholders (see, for example, Chapter 2, 'Organisational politics', p. 22; Chapter 3, Section 5, p. 48). Similarly, action research seems to accept that its findings are limited by *what can be effectively implemented in a specific context* (see for example, Chapter 2, p. 22). But, surely, this is to admit that the value and the validity of an action research project may be entirely limited to the specific context in which it is undertaken. Moreover, some contexts may be 'backward': what can be implemented may be distorted by oppressive power relations, and participants may form a consensus around an understanding which is not properly informed by recent 'advances' in the published research literature.

How might we, as action researchers, counter such criticisms? Our first response might be, indeed, to emphasise the value of 'local' advances in practice, no matter how limited, and to stress that action research in no way condones not being up to date in one's professional field of knowledge.

More generally, we might also point out that notions such as 'backward' and 'up-to-date' states of knowledge are theoretically problematic. Knowledge in the social sciences (e.g. theories concerning ethnic identity, models of nursing care, policies concerning child protection) does not simply 'advance': it *changes* along with social and political *values* and even 'climates of opinion'. A substantial body of currently influential philosophy, therefore, emphasises that human knowledge is always situated within, and thus limited by, the discourse of a particular culture and that there is no single 'universal' language which can adjudicate between the discourses of differing groups (Wittgenstein, 1968). Consequently (it is argued), philosophical inquiry can never be more than a 'conversation' motivated by the 'hope' for mutual understanding and dependent on the recognition of inevitable differences between individuals and between groups (Rorty, 1979: 315–19). 'Truth' can have no universal foundation, no 'common ground' (ibid.).

Two aspects of this philosophical emphasis – that all truth is culturally relative – seem to provide strong theoretical grounds for the context-bound, action-oriented work of action research (see Stringer, 1996: 151–6). The first is frequently summed up in the postmodernist doctrine that there is no longer a single 'Grand Narrative' of the advancement of Truth, but only 'little narratives', i.e. 'local determinism' (Lyotard, 1984: 60, xxiv). The second is the 'pragmatist' tradition, which stresses *practically effective* knowledge and inquiry as a *communal* enterprise (Peirce, 1992: 52–5, 131).

An important element in both postmodernist and pragmatist arguments is the rejection of a 'correspondence' theory of truth. Statements made in a particular language cannot be claimed to be true because they 'correspond to' an objective reality external to the language, since we have no way of referring to such a reality except through the language itself; so such claims are circular. Instead, it is argued, the truth of each statement in a language depends on its 'coherence' with other statements (Ramberg, 1989: 44; Murphy, 1990: 108, 116). In the case of statements such as 'There is a flower in the garden', the significance of this theoretical point is fairly trivial. But in the case of statements like 'Adopted children need to maintain contact with their birth parents', rejecting the correspondence theory of truth raises crucial practical questions. Does it imply that the validity of such statements can never be established by theoretical clarification and empirical evidence? Are such statements culturally circumscribed as merely 'what some people currently believe'? Can there never be any firm foundations for a *general* policy or for guidance protocols requiring us to act in a particular way?

There are two rather different responses to this crucial question. On the one hand, we might easily agree that scientific findings are never 'proved' but are always 'so far not refuted' in the on-going 'conversation' of inquiry within a scientific community (Popper, 1959, 1963). The current state of our knowledge is therefore always open to question as part of an always incomplete (*communal*) narrative of inquiry, and the presentation of knowledge must therefore always include the (*individual*) narrative of its production (its 'method') to enable others to continue the process of questioning, refinement or rejection. From this point of view the difference between an action research report and the report of a conventional piece of scientific inquiry is but a shift in emphasis.

Alternatively, we might go further, and argue that 'hypotheses' can never be properly refuted, since the facts required for refutation of an experimental hypothesis do not exist separately in the world of our experience; they are always conceptualised in advance and 'produced' by the experimental conditions themselves (Habermas, 1974: 201). Once this is admitted, the way is clear for the argument that the knowledge created by scientific method draws not simply on the *rationality* of scientific method itself but also on the *political power* of scientific and professional institutions (Lyotard, 1984: 45–7). The creation of knowledge is therefore always influenced by political, practical *motives*, including solidarity within a professional culture, for example (Kuhn, 1970: 151–2), and by value judgements which, in a secular and culturally divided society, are always open to dispute.

But although this line of argument – that truth is entirely relative – may be presented as a form of philosophical 'rigour', many would say that it is not only theoretically problematic but also politically dangerous: it threatens 'a wholesale levelling of value distinctions between truth and falsehood [and] a generalised scepticism with regard to issues of truth and justice' (Norris, 1996: ix–x). In particular, a relativist conception of social inquiry does not address the practical problems of those who are responsible for making and justifying specific decisions in which the well-being of human beings is at stake.

To agree that our knowledge is incomplete, socially constructed and fallible does not mean that we can never have rational empirical grounds for making judgements that have a genuine purchase on the reality we experience (Bhaskar, 1989: 24). Indeed, human discourse is founded on the assumption that we can discriminate between well-founded and less well-founded judgements concerning reality. Otherwise, most human interactions would be unintelligible, not only decisions about when it is safe to cross a road but also philosophical arguments in favour of relativism, which always include the selection of 'supporting evidence' (Bridges, 1999). And if truth is wholly relative, then inquiry can play no part in helping us to contest injustice, lies and oppression (see Norris, 1996: 61–5).

This means that, for action research at least (with its concern for the improvement of human well-being), the debate about the validity of the outcomes of social inquiry needs to be moved away from a simple opposition between 'absolute, objective truth' and total relativism in which each local 'reality' has its own 'subjective' or culturally determined truth criteria. Instead, we might, for example, follow Hilary Putnam and start by accepting that 'empirically established' general statements about the world we experience are always only true 'under normal conditions' (Putnam, 1987: 24). We can then move on to acknowledge that agreeing a description of the 'normal conditions' under which 'water boils at 100 degrees centigrade' involves a different (and rather simpler) process from agreeing the normal conditions under which 'chemotherapy successfully eradicates cancer' or 'adopted children need contact with their birth parents'. Thus, instead of simply using a dichotomy between 'objective' and 'culturally relative' statements, we can redefine the issue in terms of a 'continuum' (ibid.: 27–32) on which different types of statements can be placed at different points. In this way we can differentiate statements according to what sort of process is needed to create a consensus as to the conditions needed to verify them.

From this perspective, the value and purpose of the 'local narratives' of action research are not dependent on the theory that there are multiple realities and that truth is contextually relative. Indeed, the relativist argument leaves action research dangerously exposed to the sort of criticisms previously indicated. Action research inquiries are closely bound up with criteria for 'good practice', and this obviously entails a strong link between the rationale for the inquiry process and 'a reality' that is fully (officially and intensively) *shared* between practitioners, service-users and accountable managers at local and national level (even though values and priorities may be contested). Instead of claiming, therefore, that action research can (or should or does) simply operate with truth criteria that are entirely local, we might suggest that action research reports describe the *local process* (of challenge and negotiation) whereby eventual agreement is reached concerning the *generally shared truth criteria* implicit in their various conclusions and outcomes. This would certainly be one way of describing most of the action research projects presented in this book.

In the light of the problems of relativism outlined above, the rest of this analysis tries to establish a link between the principles and procedures of action research and a sophisticated 'realist' model of social inquiry. Such a model of inquiry needs to avoid the crude assumptions of positivism, i.e. that the methods of social inquiry can achieve some form of absolute objectivity for its results (see Chapter 2). But it also needs to accept that social action always presupposes the existence of an external reality which provides a final constraint upon (and a source of criteria for) interpretation. To keep the argument brief and focused, it concentrates mainly on the example of Roy Bhaskar's influential work on 'critical realism'. (Bhaskar's work is a philosophical analysis of the basis for *all* scientific inquiry, including the natural sciences, but the following summary focuses on his account of the theoretical foundations of *social* science.)

Critical realism

Realism and the limits of human knowledge

According to Bhaskar, our *experiences* are not to be equated with objective reality (the doctrine of 'empiricism'), because they are always structured by our concepts. But this does not mean that our concepts are the only reality to which we have access (the doctrine of 'idealism'): we do not simply *construct* our reality (Bhaskar, 1986: 102). In contrast to both of these, the doctrine of 'realism' asserts that the existence of an objective reality is 'implied' in all our actions (ibid.: 33) and that we must *assume* the existence of an objective reality insofar as our knowledge makes any claims concerning cause and effect relationships (ibid.: 102). 'For realism, it is the nature of the world that determines its cognitive possibilities for us' (ibid.). In other words, although we are free to conceptualise many different interpretations of the world, events and structures independent of our concepts can show us that some of our interpretations were wrong.

But critical realism asserts that while we have no option but to assume the existence of an objective reality, our knowledge of it is destined to be forever 'fallible' (Collier, 1994: 16, 50) for two main reasons.

First, our inquiries can never be undertaken from an independent standpoint (Bhaskar, 1986: 160). There are no 'foundations of knowledge', no pure data: we experience the world in terms of the 'stories' we tell about it – we are members of 'a story-telling species', and we 'produce' our experience in the form of our narratives and concepts (ibid.). Inquiry, therefore, must be seen as an ongoing and never completed process of practical *work* (Bhaskar, 1989: 22), of checking our narratives and concepts against events, using whatever cognitive resources (theories, evidence) we may happen to have available at a given point in history (Bhaskar, 1986: 107–8; 1989: 120). Thus, in some respects, any existing state of knowledge may be seen as a historical 'accident' (Bhaskar, 1986: 102). We have to accept that social inquiry is always situated within, and part of, the historical development of the social world it seeks to explain. It is therefore necessarily 'self-reflexive' (Bhaskar, 1989: 24): it will always need to explain *itself* and to recognise explicitly its limits. In other words, it must give up any claim to have 'permanent, neutral, a-historical . . . foundations' (ibid.: 179) and recognise that it is inherently value-laden (Bhaskar, 1986: 169).

Second, our knowledge of objective reality is limited because the phenomena of real-world experience constitute an 'open' set of variables, unlike the 'closed' systems of experiments; the experimental conditions from which 'laws' are derived are not found in naturally occurring situations (Bhaskar, 1989: 148–9). For any given event, therefore, there are always many 'causes' (Bhaskar, 1986: 107) and experiments never produce results which are only consistent with a single interpretation (ibid.: 36). Hence, *finally decisive* tests of our hypotheses are not possible (Bhaskar, 1989: 185). In other words, conventional social science can only *explain* (Bhaskar, 1986: 107); it can help us decide between alternatives (Bhaskar, 1989: 186) but it cannot tell us what to do for the best in a particular situation (Bhaskar, 1986: 187).

Realism, transformation, critique

But although critical realism emphasises the limitations of social science, it also emphasises its practical function. The work of inquiry, it is argued, should attempt to identify the objective structures which generate the form of the events we subjectively experience, in order to *change* the social world we inhabit (Bhaskar, 1989: 2). This is the reason why social researchers must keep themselves 'in touch with' the external world, seeing themselves not (as is sometimes suggested) as passive observers but as engaged in an active process of 'work', i.e. as engaged in a 'causal exchange with nature' (ibid.: 22).

For critical realism, therefore, social inquiry is, like any other form of social action, necessarily a 'transformative' process (ibid.: 3–4). We each find ourselves involved in social relationships and sets of ideas which were in existence before our involvement, but these pre-existent structures (patterns of relationships, modes of thinking, etc.) never wholly constrain us. All human activity and thinking have an interpretative, creative dimension, so that the structures we (as it were) 'inherit' are always, to some extent, *transformed* through our own activity (ibid.: 173–4). In this sense, social inquiry must be seen as always 'intrinsically critical and . . . evaluative' of existing 'vocabularies and social practices' (Bhaskar, 1986: 183; 1989: 175).

Dialectics, emancipation

Evaluation and critique, of course, never yield a final truth, only historically situated conjectures, which in turn require further practical work of evaluation and critique, in a continuous 'dialectic' (ibid.: 20). Dialectics is a key aspect of critical realism.

It is both a model of social reality and a model of inquiry. It starts from the recognition that our current understandings are determined by, among other things, the social world we inhabit, but it goes on to identify the specific *freedom* inherent in the form of our understanding (Bhaskar, 1993: 378), which enables us to engage in transforming both the world and our understanding.

The basic principles of dialectics are:

1   that societies (and social relationships) consist of opposing forces;
2   that social change is created by the practical struggle between these opposing forces;
3   that adequate understanding must involve a grasp of these contradictions and the processes of social change through which they are temporarily resolved and continuously transformed;
4   that adequate understanding thus includes both critique and causal explanation of social events, in order to establish the possibilities and limits of change;
5   that the growth of knowledge is a self-emancipatory process based on practical action (Bhaskar, 1989: 124–5).

The need for an 'emancipatory' dynamic at the heart of the social inquiry process has its origin in the obvious point that we frequently do not fully understand the events in which we are caught up. Our actions frequently have unintended consequences because they are affected by motives, tacit skills or external conditions of which we are unaware (ibid.: 4). Critical realism asserts that the fundamental purpose of social inquiry is to explain the forces at work within a situation by seeing them in terms of 'structures' underlying immediate experiences (ibid.: 2). But the point of such an 'explanation' is to improve our understanding of how to change the situation in such a way that it is no longer determined by forces we experience as unjust or oppressive but by those we accept or desire (ibid.: 178). The critical realist model of social inquiry thus aims to enhance social justice and human 'autonomy', by enabling participants to 'see themselves under a new description which they have helped to create' (ibid.).

In this way, social science is *not* value neutral. Whereas the positivist model of social science *can* be used as an instrument for political domination, for critical realism, social science must always be conceived as a means of increasing the autonomy of human action (Bhaskar, 1986: 182). For Bhaskar, the *values* of justice and equality are implicit in our relationships and transactions, just as the values of truth and rationality are implicit in our use of language (Bhaskar, 1989: 114). (Liars make the assumption that others mean what they say and have good grounds for their assertions, and oppressors anticipate respect from their colleagues and care from their doctors.)

'Ideology' and 'critique'

Any account of a *critical* model of social inquiry, through which we 'emancipate' ourselves from politically powerful ideas that serve the interests of others, needs a theory of 'ideology', i.e. of how ideas are related to social interests (Bhaskar, 1986: 242–3; McLellan, 1995: 83). This is particularly important if we are to clarify the relationship between freedom of thought and the constraints within which it always operates, since it is within this relationship that we need to explain the crucial processes of 'reflexive' analysis, critique and evaluation.

Let us begin with the notion of 'critique'. This does not simply mean being 'critical' in the sense of stating that one disagrees with something, or putting an opposite point of view. Rather it means taking a set of ideas and *questioning* them, making them 'problematic' by subjecting them to 'analysis'. The concept of ideology explains why this is necessary, why it is difficult, and how it is possible.

In one sense 'ideo-logy' means the science of ideas, discourse about ideas (McLellan, 1995: 5). As an extension of this, the term is usually used to suggest that our ideas do not come from nowhere, they are not 'independent', but have causes and motives. In other words, the concept of ideology gives us our sense of cultural *identity*, and it also suggests that it will be difficult for us to *change* our thinking, because it is powerfully influenced by forces beyond our direct control. It therefore also suggests that our ideas (including our beliefs, our concerns and the way we interpret events) cannot be taken 'at face value', that they need to be *examined*, as interesting 'data'. But how can we do this? If our ideas have causes and motives and are part of our sense of identity, how can we stand 'outside' them in order to subject them to examination ('critique')?

Ricoeur (1981) argues that the term 'ideology' refers to the way in which ideas and beliefs can be understood as part of the 'culture' of a *social group*, i.e. the way in which the members of different groups gain their sense of *identity* through seeing the world from a particular perspective (ibid.: 225). Thus, there are political ideologies, religious ideologies, racial ideologies, class ideologies, gender ideologies and ideologies of age groups (e.g. teenagers, pensioners). There are also managerial ideologies, professional staff ideologies and service-user ideologies. Indeed, *any* clearly identified and organised social role or activity will have its supporting ideology, e.g. academic research, cookery, gardening, football, mountaineering, parenting, community activism, slimming, etc.

However, the important point about Ricoeur's argument is that each of us belongs to a variety of different groups, so our ideas, beliefs and concerns are influenced from several directions at once. In other words, our identity is complex and 'multiple'. (One may be a political Conservative *and* a Buddhist *and* a manager *and* a gardener *and* a parent *and* middle class *and* a keen mountaineer.) This in turn means that our 'ideology' is not a single force which traps our thinking within a narrow set of constraints but a rather loose structure, containing tensions, gaps and contradictions. It is not like an enclosing prison wall, but an entangling mesh, with holes in it. Thus, we might think of our 'critical' self as standing at the centre of a sort of Venn diagram, and thus able to survey and examine the 'components' of our ideology. The shaded area at the centre of Figure IV.1 is the point from which we can *pose questions*, i.e. conduct a 'reflexive critique' of our ideologies – and thus obtain, for a moment, some notion of a 'reality' that lies 'behind' them. The 'critical self' here can refer not simply to an individual seeking to clarify her or his own self-understanding. It also describes the 'collective self' of a community of researchers as they seek to clarify the basis for their critical, evaluative interpretation of a social situation in relation to the various ideological/political forces tending to influence their interpretation in various and often contradictory ways.

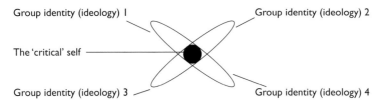

Group identity (ideology) 1

Group identity (ideology) 2

The 'critical' self

Group identity (ideology) 3

Group identity (ideology) 4

But if we can, in principle, achieve this 'critical' understanding of our social 'reality', as critical realism claims, what are the processes involved? One of the methods we have available is, precisely, action research, which brings us to our concluding section.

Action research and critical realism

The argument of this section is that action research is a way of attempting to realise in practice the theoretical ideal of social inquiry proposed by critical realism. In many respects, there is nothing very surprising about critical realism: it can be seen simply as an attempt to avoid the naïve claims of positivism and the exaggeratedly destructive doubts of relativism in order to synthesise a 'middle path' for human knowledge, combining both scepticism and hope. Furthermore, although critical realism is a model for inquiry in general, it also seems to be generally compatible with the values and processes of action research. Indeed, as indicated below, in some respects the model of action research described in the early chapters of this book offers a way of addressing certain aspects of critical realism which remain highly problematic within the framework of conventional 'academic' social science. In the following analysis, each paragraph begins with a restatement of one or two key elements of critical realism, from the account in the previous section. It then draws a parallel with corresponding aspects (ideals, values, procedures) of action research, with key phrases, drawn from the presentation of action research in Chapters 2 and 3, presented in italics.

1. Critical realism asserts that the complexity of social situations is such that no general laws can prescribe action for particular instances. Hence the value of – indeed, the necessity for – the *contextually specific* inquiries of action research, as *narratives* of our attempts to *interpret the here-and-now implications* of bodies of generalised knowledge.

2. Critical realism asserts that social inquiry is always a part of the social world it describes. (Hence the action research principle of *reflexivity*, which emphasises that the *process* of research is always also a topic for inquiry.) It therefore follows that social inquiry does not have an external 'platform' from which researchers can conduct 'objective' observations of 'those being researched'. Hence the significance of the action research ideal of research as a *participatory, collaborative* process, in which participants are encouraged to take a *creative* part in *negotiating* the focus and the conceptual framework for interpreting data.

3. Critical realism asserts that any current state of knowledge is fallible, incomplete and influenced by historical factors such as the ideologies, values and interests of particular groups. Hence the important emphasis, within action research, that 'analysis' (of data, events, situations) is always *a mutual process of critical, evaluative reflection.*

4. Critical realism asserts that the purpose of social inquiry is to understand situations in such a way that we are able to bring about *change*. This, of course, is explicitly one of the central, defining principles of action research.

5. Critical realism asserts that social activity does not simply reproduce situations; it transforms them: there is always a 'space of freedom' between, on the one hand, initial conditions and contextual constraints and, on the other hand, what we actually, finally do. This is what makes it realistic to propose that inquiry *can* bring about change (point 4). If, in principle, structures of power do not wholly or finally determine individual action, there are theoretical grounds for optimism on the part of action research participants in their pursuit of *change in particular contexts.*

6. Critical realism asserts that inquiry is a process of 'work'; our understanding develops through a continuous process of 'causal exchange' with objective reality. This is the 'dialectic' whereby knowledge develops through an interaction between creative conjecture and the 'test' of experience. For academic social science this is problematic: its methods (surveys, controlled experiments, ethnographic observation, etc.) always interpose a pre-defined conceptual framework between any hypothesis and the experiential world in which (supposedly) it is tested, so that the 'reality' of any 'findings' is always in question. For action research, however, the dialectic between conceptualisation and reality is considerably clearer. In seeking *practical change* action research necessarily places a primary focus on the 'real world' of participants' experience. Action research includes the *experiential realities* of professional practices, clients' situations, institutional structures and social relationships, as essential elements of the *dialectic between action and reflection* which constitutes the inquiry process.

7. Critical realism asserts that social inquiry seeks to identify objective 'structures' and 'forces' underlying subjective experiences. For academic social science this is problematic, because researchers' conceptual frameworks for interpreting a situation are not necessarily derived from the experiences of those involved in the situation to be interpreted. For action research, however, the objective structures and forces at work in the situation are identified as the basic shape of the inquiry, i.e. as the set of '*stakeholders*' who need to be involved as *participants in the research*. The form of an action research inquiry is thus directly derived from the 'objective structure' of the situation in which it takes place, since it consists of *dialogue and negotiation between the potentially conflicting forces which make up the situation*, as an attempt to identify and resolve contradictions among a variety of interest groups, both at the level of theory ('ideology') and practice.

8. Critical realism asserts that social inquiry is not value neutral; it must assume and seek to enhance the values of justice, rationality and truth. Its purpose is to increase the autonomy of citizens, to enable them to re-describe their experience in terms which they themselves have helped to create, and to re-create that experience in the form of a collectively desired state of affairs. For academic social science such values normally remain a set of criteria for evaluating the purpose and the impact of an inquiry. Action research, however, seeks also to *embody these values in its processes*, i.e. in the attempt (never fully successful, of course) to carry out inquiry through suspending hierarchical role relationships in favour of a *free and collaborative interchange of critical analysis among all interested parties*.

Conclusion

The analysis presented here has attempted to reply to the criticism that action research is not 'proper research', that action research simply *lacks* the formal characteristics that give other types of research their theoretical authority.

In reply to such criticisms, it is important to compare action research not with the naïve claims of positivism but with a sophisticated account of the philosophical basis of social inquiry, one which recognises, on the one hand, its fallibility and inconclusiveness and, at the same time, its responsibility to contribute to human well-being in a real world of practical action.

When such a comparison is undertaken, the various characteristics of action research emerge as having a clear theoretical basis. Action research (with its narratives of reflexive critical evaluation of current practices and theories, describing collaborative negotiations among stakeholders with differing interests in order to agree and implement practical changes) may not be the only way of contributing to the progress of human knowledge and certainly not the easiest. But, speaking philosophically as well as practically, it has much to recommend it. In other words, as the argument presented above has tried to suggest, it represents a coherent response to theoretical issues which have been identified, in contemporary philosophy, as raising important questions of purpose, methodology and validity for social inquiry in general.

Bibliography

This bibliography covers references in Parts I, III and IV. References in Part II are covered by sections at the end of the individual chapters

Acker, J., Barry, K. and Esseveld, J. (1991) 'Objectivity and truth: problems in doing feminist research', in M. Fonow and J. Cook (eds) *Beyond Methodology: Feminist Scholarship as Lived Research*, Bloomington: Indiana University Press, pp. 133–52.

Adelman, C. (1993) 'Kurt Lewin and the origins of action research', *Educational Action Research*, 1, 1: 7–14.

Ahmad, B. (1990) *Black Perspectives in Social Work*, Birmingham: Venture Press.

Ahmad, W. and Sheldon, T. (1993) '"Race" and statistics', in M. Hammersley (ed.) *Social Research: Philosophy, Politics and Practice*, London: Sage, pp. 124–30.

Altrichter, H., Posch, P. and Somekh, B. (1993) *Teachers Investigate Their Work: an Introduction to the Methods of Action Research*, London: Routledge.

Aspden, P. (1994) 'Carp pool reflections on the art of doubt', *Times Higher Education Supplement* (Management Education Section), 22 April, p. 21.

Ayer, S. (1994) 'A proper process of scrutiny', *Professional Nurse*, 9, 9: 595–9.

Bartholomew, J. (1972) 'The teacher as researcher: a key to innovation and change', *Hard Cheese*, London: Goldsmiths College, Vol. 1, pp. 12–22.

Barton-Wright, P. (1998) 'Information for users – the plain English campaign', *Q-Net: the Mental Health Quality Assurance Network Bulletin*, 7: 4.

Batteson, R. (1997) 'Before, I asked a second opinion, but now I know I can do it myself: a strategy for improving nurse/occupational therapist communication for managing patients with splints', *Educational Action Research*, 5, 3: 435–48.

Belenky, M., Clinchy, B., Goldberger, N. and Tarule, J. (1986) *Women's Ways of Knowing*, New York: Basic Books.

Bennett, C., Chapman, A., Cliff, D., Garside, M., Hampton, W., Hardwick, R., Higgins, G. and Linton-Beresford, J. (1997) 'Hearing ourselves learn: the development of a critical friendship group for professional development', *Educational Action Research*, 5, 3: 282–402.

Beresford, P. (1992) 'Researching citizen-involvement: a collaborative or colonising experience?', in Barnes, M. and Wistow, G. (eds) *Researching User Involvement* (Nuffield Institute for Health Services Studies), Leeds: University of Leeds Press, pp. 16–32.

Beresford, P. (1999) 'Making participation possible: movements of disabled people and psychiatric survivors', in T. Jordan and A. Lent (eds) *Storming the Millennium: the New Politics of Change*, London: Lawrence and Wishart, pp. 35–50.

Bhaskar, R. (1986) *Scientific Realism and Human Emancipation*, London: Verso.

Bhaskar, R. (1989) *Reclaiming Reality*, London: Verso.

Bhaskar, R. (1993) *Dialectics: the Pulse of Freedom*, London: Verso.

Billingsley, A. (1973) 'Black families and white social science', in J. Ladner (ed.) *The Death of White Sociology*, New York: Vintage Books, pp. 431–50.

Bishop, L. (1995) 'An Approach to Managing Changing Professional Roles Through Exploring "What Is Inspection?"', Msc Dissertation, Chelmsford: Anglia Polytechnic University.

Blair, M. (1998) 'The myth of neutrality in educational research', in P. Connolly and B. Troyna (eds) *Researching Racism in Education*, Buckingham: Open University Press, pp. 12–20.

Bliss, J. (1983) *Qualitative Data Analysis for Educational Research*, Beckenham: Croom Helm.

Bond, M., For Mothers By Mothers Group and Walton, P. (1998) 'Knowing mothers: from practitioner research to self-help and organisational change', *Educational Action Research*, 6, 1: 111–29.

Borkman, T. (1999) *Understanding Self-help/Mutual Aid Groups: Experiential Learning in the Commons*, New Jersey: Rutgers University Press.

Bridges, D. (1999) 'Educational research: pursuit of truth or flight into fancy?', *British Educational Research Journal*, 25, 5: 597–616.

British Sociological Association (1992) 'BSA statement of ethical practice', *Sociology*, 26, 4: 704–6.

Brown, L., Henry, C., Henry J. and McTaggart, R. (1982) 'Action research: notes on the national seminar', in J. Elliott and D. Whitehead (eds) *Action Research for Professional Development and the Improvement of Schooling*, Cambridge: Institute of Education (available from the Centre for Applied Research in Education, University of East Anglia, Norwich), pp. 1–16.

Brown Lee, J. (1997) 'A convergent experience', pp. 231–5, in R. Winter, J. Brown Lee, L. Bishop, M. Maisch, C. McMillan and P. Sobiechowska, 'The ambiguities of educational reform: action research and competence specification in social work education', in S. Hollingsworth (ed.) *International Action Research*, London: Falmer Press, pp. 226–37.

Carr, W. and Kemmis, S. (1986) *Becoming Critical: Education, Knowledge and Action Research*, Lewes: Falmer Press and Deakin University Press.

Central Council for Education and Training in Social Work (1992) *The Requirements for Post Qualifying Education and Training in the Personal Social Services: a Framework for Continuing Professional Development ('Paper 31')*, London: CCETSW.

Chein, I., Cook, S. and Harding, J. (1948) 'The field of action research', *American Psychologist*, 3: 43–50.

Chisholm, R. and Elden, M. (1993) 'Features of emerging action research', *Human Relations*, 46, 2: 275–98.

Chomsky, N. (1993) *Year 501: the Conquest Continues*, London: Verso.

Cohen, L. and Manion, L. (1994) *Research Methods in Education*, 4th edn, London: Routledge.

Collier, A. (1994) *Critical Realism: an Introduction to Roy Bhaskar's Philosophy*, London: Verso.

Collier, J. (1945) 'United States Indian administration as a laboratory of ethnic relations', *Social Research*, 12, 2: 266–303.

Comte, A. (1974 [1830–42]) *The Essential Comte* (selections from the *Course of Positive Philosophy*), ed. S. Andreski, London: Croom Helm.

Cooper, A. (1997) 'Thinking the unthinkable: "white liberal" defences against understanding in anti-racist training', *Journal of Social Work Practice*, 11, 2: 127–37.

Dalal, F. (1997) 'The colour question in psychoanalysis', *Journal of Social Work Practice*, 11, 2: 103–14.

Dartington Social Research Unit (1997) *Newsposter: Research in Practice*, Dartington: Social Research Unit.

Deming, W.E. (1986) *Out of the Crisis*, Cambridge: Cambridge University Press.

Department of Health (1992) *Local Research Ethics Committees*, London: HMSO.

Department of Health (1995) *Child Protection: Messages from Research*, London: HMSO.

Department of Health (1997) *The New NHS*, London: DOH/HMSO.

Dixon, N. (1994) *The Organisational Learning Cycle*, Maidenhead: McGraw-Hill.

Dorney, J. and Flood, C. (1997) 'Breaking gender silences in the curriculum: a retreat intervention with middle school educators', *Educational Action Research*, 5, 1: 71–86.

Elden, M. (1981) 'Sharing the research work: participative research and its role demands', in P. Reason and J. Rowan (eds) *Human Inquiry: a Sourcebook for New Paradigm Research*, Chichester: John Wiley, pp. 253–66.

Elliott, D. and Phipson, S. (1987) *Manual of the Law of Evidence*, 12th edn, London: Sweet and Maxwell.

Elliott, J. (1976) *Developing Hypotheses about Classrooms from Teachers' Practical Constructs: an Account of the Work of the Ford Teaching Project*, Cambridge: Institute of Education (obtainable from the Centre for Applied Research in Education, University of East Anglia, Norwich).

Elliott, J. (1991) *Action Research for Educational Change*, Buckingham: Open University Press.

Elliott, J. (1995) 'What is good action research?', *Action Researcher*, 2: 10–11.

Elliott, J. and Adelman, C. (1975) *Classroom Action Research*, Ford Teaching Practice Documents, Norwich: Centre for Applied Research in Education, University of East Anglia.

Elliott, J. and Adelman, C. (1996) 'Reflecting where the action is: the design of the Ford Teaching Project', in C. O'Hanlon (ed.) *Professional Development Through Action Research in Educational Settings*, London: Falmer Press, pp. 7–18.

English National Board for Nursing, Midwifery and Health Visiting (1990) *A New Structure for Professional Development*, London: ENB.

Essex County Council Social Services (1997) *People First – the Way Ahead: Five Year Development Strategy for Learning Disability Services in Essex, 1997–2002*, Chelmsford: Essex County Council Social Services.

Evidence-Based Medicine Working Group (1992) 'Evidence-based medicine: a new approach to teaching the practice of medicine', *Journal of the American Medical Association*, 268: 2420–5.

Fals-Borda, O. and Rahman, M. (eds) (1991) *Action and Knowledge: Breaking The Monopoly With Participatory Action Research*, London: Intermediate Technology Publications.

Faulkner, A (1997) *Knowing Our Own Minds*, London: Mental Health Foundation.

Fay, B. (1975) *Social Theory and Political Practice*, London: George Allen & Unwin.

Fisher, M. (ed.) (1983) *Speaking of Clients* (Social Services Monographs in Practice) Sheffield: University of Sheffield Joint Unit for Social Services Research.

Fisk, M. (1979) 'Dialectic and ontology', in J. Mepham and D.-H. Ruben (eds) *Issues in Marxist Philosophy, Vol. 1: Dialectics and Method*, Brighton: Harvester Press, pp. 117–44.

Foster, M. (1972) 'An introduction to the theory and practice of action research in work organisations', *Human Relations*, 25, 6: 529–56.

Fox, A. (1974) *Beyond Contract: Work, Power and Trust Relations*, London: Faber.

Freire, P. (1972) *Cultural Action for Freedom*, Harmondsworth: Penguin.

Fuller, R. (1996) 'Evaluating social work effectiveness – a pragmatic approach', in Barnardo's, *What Works? Effective Social Interventions in Child Welfare*, Ilford: Barnardo's, pp. 55–67.

Fuller, R. and Petch, A. (1995) *Practitioner Research: the Reflexive Social Worker*, Buckingham: Open University Press.

Gahan, C. and Hannibal, M. (1998) *Doing Qualitative Research Using QSR NUD*IST*, London: Sage.

Gerrish, K., Husband, C. and Mackenzie, J. (1996) *Nursing for a Multi-Ethnic Society*, Buckingham: Open University Press.

Gibbons, M., Limoges, C., Nowotny, H., Schwartzman, S., Scott, P. and Trow, M. (1994) *The New Production of Knowledge*, London: Sage.

Giddens, A. (1976) *New Rules of Sociological Method*, London: Hutchinson.

Goleman, D. (1996) *Emotional Intelligence*, London: Bloomsbury.

Gorman, H. (1999) 'Practitioner research in community care – personalising the political', in B. Broad (ed.) *The Politics of Social Work Research and Evaluation*, Birmingham: Venture Press, pp. 171–82.

Gouldner, A. (1962) 'Anti-Minotaur: the myth of a value-free sociology', *Social Problems*, 9: 199–213.

Griffiths, M. (1994) 'Autobiography, feminism and the practice of action research', *Educational Action Research*, 2, 1: 71–82.

Guba, E. and Lincoln, Y. (1981) *Effective Evaluation*, San Francisco: Jossey Bass.

Guba, E. and Lincoln, Y. (1989) *Fourth Generation Evaluation*, London: Sage.

Habermas, J. (1974) 'Rationalism divided in two', in A. Giddens (ed.) *Positivism and Sociology*, London: Heinemann.

Habermas, J. (1976) *Legitimation Crisis*, London: Heinemann.

Habermas, J. (1978) *Knowledge and Human Interests*, 2nd edn, London: Heinemann.

Hakes, C. (1991) *Total Quality Management*, London: Chapman and Hall.

Hammersley, M. (1992) 'On feminist methodology', *Sociology*, 26, 2: 187–206.

Harding, S. (1990) 'Feminism and theories of scientific knowledge', *Women – a Cultural Review*, 1, 1: 87–97.

Hart, E. and Bond, M. (1995) *Action Research for Health and Social Care*, Buckingham: Open University Press.

Hart, S. (1995) 'Action-in-reflection', *Educational Action Research*, 3, 2: 211–32.

Hart, S. (2000) *Thinking Through Teaching: a Framework for Enhancing Participation and Learning*, London: David Fulton.

Healy, P. (1995) 'Racism: fact or fiction', *Nursing Standard*, 10, 9: 18–19.

Heasman, P. and Adams, A. (1998) 'Reflecting well on social work practice: Professional competence, reflection and research', *Educational Action Research*, 6, 2: 337–42.

Heckscher, C. (1994) 'Defining the post-bureaucratic type', in C. Heckscher and A. Donnellon (eds) *The Post-Bureaucratic Organisation*, London: Sage.

Heron, J. (1996) *Co-operative Inquiry: Research into the Human Condition*, London: Sage.

Hollingsworth, S. (1994) 'Feminst pedagogy in the research class: an example of teacher research', *Educational Action Research*, 2, 1: 49–70.

Holman, B. (1987) 'Research from the underside', *British Journal of Social Work*, 17: 669–83.

Hugman, R. (1991) *Power in Caring Professions*, Basingstoke: Macmillan.

Hutchins, D. (1988) *Just in Time*, Aldershot: Gower.

Huws, U. (1999) 'Material world: the myth of the weightless economy', in L. Panitch and C. Leys (eds) *Global Capitalism Versus Democracy*, Woodbridge: Merlin Press, pp. 29–55.

Investors in People (1994) *Investing in People*, Sheffield: Investors in People UK.

Israel, J. (1979) *The Language of Dialectics and the Dialectics of Language*, Brighton: Harvester Press.

Jackson, D., Brady, W. and Stein, I. (1999) 'Towards (re)conciliation: (re)constructing relationships between indigenous health works and nurses', *Journal of Advanced Nursing*, 29, 1: 97–103.

Kemmis, S. and McTaggart, R. (1988) *The Action Research Planner*, 3rd edn, Victoria: Deakin University Press.

Kemp, P. (1997) 'Supporting the supporters', *Educational Action Research*, 5, 2.

Kline, N. (1993) *Women and Power*, London: BBC Publications.

Kropotkin, P. (1987 [1902]) *Mutual Aid: a Factor of Evolution*, London: Freedom Press.

Kuhn, T. (1970) *The Structure of Scientific Revolutions*, 2nd edn, Chicago: University of Chicago Press.

Ladner, J. (ed.) (1973) *The Death of White Sociology*, New York: Vintage Books.

Lather, P. (1988) 'Feminist perspectives and empowering research methodologies', *Women's Studies International Forum*, II, 6: 569–81.

Lees, R. (1975) 'The action-research relationship', in R. Lees and G. Smith (eds) *Action Research in Community Development*, London: Routledge and Kegan Paul, pp. 59–66.

Lees, R. and Smith, G. (eds) (1975) *Action Research in Community Development*, London: Routledge and Kegan Paul.

Lewin, K. (1946) 'Action research and minority problems', *Journal of Social Issues*, 2: 34–46.

Lincoln, Y. and Guba, E. (1985) *Naturalistic Inquiry*, Beverly Hills, Calif.: Sage.

Losito, B. and Pozzo, G. (1997) 'The double track: the dichotomy of roles in action research', in S. Hollingsworth (ed.) *International Action Research*, London: Falmer Press, pp. 288–99.

Losito, B., Pozzo, G. and Somekh, B. (1998) 'Exploring the labyrinth of first and second order inquiry in action research', *Educational Action Research*, 6, 2: 219–39.

Loveland, B. (1998) 'The care programme approach – whose is it? Empowering users in the care programme process', *Educational Action Research*, 6, 2: 321–35.

Lyotard, J.-F. (1984) *The Postmodern Condition: a Report on Knowledge*, Manchester: Manchester University Press.

MacDonald, B. (1977) 'A political classification of evaluation studies', in D. Hamilton, B. MacDonald, C. King, D. Jenkins and M. Parlett (eds) *Beyond the Numbers Game: a Reader in Educational Evaluation*, London: Macmillan, pp. 224–7.

MacDonald, G. (1999) 'Evidence-based social care: wheels off the runway?', *Public Money and Management*, January–March: 25–32.

MacFarlane, J. (1998) 'Quality from the users' perspective – a QA framework', *Q-Net: the Mental Health Quality Assurance Network Bulletin*, 7: 4.

McKernan, J. (1996) *Curriculum Action Research*, 2nd edn, London: Kogan Page.

McLellan, D. (1995) *Ideology*, 2nd edn, Buckingham: Open University Press.

McNiff, J. (1988) *Action Research: Principles and Practice*, London: Macmillan.

MacVicar, C. (1995) 'Increasing choice? The evaluation of Linburn Road Respite Care Unit, Dunfermline', in R. Fuller and A. Petch (1995) *Practitioner Research: the Reflexive Social Worker*, Buckingham: Open University Press, pp. 151–70.

Markovic, M. (1984) *Dialectical Theory of Meaning*, Dordrecht: Reidel.

Marks-Maran, D. and Rose, P. (eds) (1997) *Reconstructing Nursing: Beyond Art and Science*, London: Baillère-Tindall.

Marshall, J. (1992) 'Research women in management as a way of life', *Management Education and Development*, 23, 3: 281–9.

Mason, T. (1995) 'Seclusion in special hospitals – a developmental study', unpublished PhD thesis, Cambridge: Anglia Polytechnic University.

Mayer, J. E. and Timms, N. (1970) *The Client Speaks*, London: Routledge and Kegan Paul.

Messner, E. and Rauch, F. (1995) 'Dilemmas of facilitating action research', *Educational Action Research*, 3, 1: 41–53.

Meyer, J. (1993) 'New paradigm research in practice: the trials and tribulations of action research', *Journal of Advanced Nursing*, 18: 1066–72.

Mirza, M. (1998) '"Same voices, same lives?": revisiting black feminist standpoint epistemology', in P. Connolly and B. Troyna (eds) *Researching Racism in Education*, Buckingham: Open University Press, pp. 79–94.

Morgan, D. (1997) *Focus Groups as Qualitative Research*, London: Sage.

Morgan, G. (1986) *Images of Organisation*, London: Sage.

Mullender, A., Everitt, A., Hardiker, P. and Littlewood, J. (1993/4) 'Value issues in research', *Social Action*, 1, 4: 11–18.

Munn-Giddings, C. (1993) '"A different way of knowing": social care values, practitioner research and action research', *Educational Action Research*, 1, 2: 275–85.

Munn-Giddings, C (1998) 'Self-help/mutual aid, gender and citizenship', in V. Ferreira, T. Tavares and S. Portugal (eds) *Shifting Bonds, Shifting Bounds; Women, Mobility and Citizenship in Europe*, Oeiras (Portugal): Celta Editora, pp. 85–104.

Murphy, J. (1990) *Pragmatism: from Peirce to Davidson*, Oxford: Westview Press.

National Health Service Executive [UK] (1998) *Racial Harassment in the National Health Service*, Wetherby: Department of Health.

Neuberger, J. (1992) *Ethics and Health Care: the Role of Research Ethics Committees in the UK*, London: King's Fund.

New Economics Foundation (1997) *Participation Works! 21 Techniques of Community Participation for the Twenty-First Century*, London: New Economics Foundation.

Norris, C. (1996) *Reclaiming Truth*, London: Lawrence & Wishart.

Oakley, A. (1981) 'Interviewing women: a contradiction in terms', in H. Roberts (ed.) *Doing Feminist Research*, London: Routledge and Kegan Paul, pp. 30–61.

Oakley, A. (1996) 'Who's afraid of the randomised controlled trial? The challenge of evaluating the potential of social interventions', in Barnardo's, *What Works? Effective Social Interventions in Child Welfare*, Ilford: Barnardo's, pp. 33–47.

Oliver, M. (1990) *The Politics of Disablement*, London: Macmillan.

Oliver, M. (1996) *Understanding Disability: from Theory to Practice*, Basingstoke: Macmillan.

Omerod, P. (1994) *The Death of Economics*, London: Faber and Faber.

Ovretveit, J. (1986) *Improving Social Work Records and Practice*, Birmingham: British Association of Social Workers.

Palmer, A., Burns, S. and Bulman, C. (1994) *Reflective Practice in Nursing*, Oxford: Blackwell Scientific.

Parlett, M. and Hamilton, D. (1977) 'Evaluation as illumination: a new approach to the study of innovatory programmes', in D. Hamilton, B. McDonald, C. King, D. Jenkins and M. Parlett (eds) *Beyond the Numbers Game: a Reader in Educational Evaluation*, London: Macmillan, pp. 6–22.

Pedler, M., Burgoyne, J. and Boydell, T. (1991) *The Learning Company*, London: McGraw Hill.

Peirce, C. (1992) *The Essential Peirce – Selected Philosophical Writings, Vol. 1 (1867–1893)*, ed. N. Houser and C. Kloesel, Bloomington: Indiana University Press.

Peters, T. (1987) *Thriving on Chaos*, London: Macmillan.

Peters, T. and Waterman, R. (1982) *In Search of Excellence*, New York: Harper & Row.

Popper, K. (1959) *The Logic of Scientific Discovery*, London: Hutchinson.

Popper, K. (1963) *Conjectures and Refutations*, London: Routledge and Kegan Paul.

Posch, P. (1993) 'Action research in environmental education', *Educational Action Research*, 1, 3: 447–55.

Prendergast, S. (1997) *Ethics Guidelines for Research*, Cambridge: Anglia Polytechnic University.

Putnam, H. (1987) *The Many Faces of Realism*, LaSalle, Ill.: Open Court.

Ramberg, B. (1989) *Donald Davidson's Philosophy of Language – an Introduction*, Oxford: Blackwell.

Ramon, S. (1997) 'Assessing innovation as part of individual workers' input: focus on user/carer participation in care management', in S. Baldwin and P. Barker (eds) *International Handbook on Community Care*, London: Routledge.

Rapoport, R. (1970) 'Three dilemmas in action research with special reference to the Tavistock experience', *Human Relations*, 23, 6: 499–513.

Reason, P. (ed.) (1988) *Human Inquiry in Action: Development in New Paradigm Research*, London: Sage.

Reason, P. (1994) *Participation In Human Inquiry*, London: Sage.

Reason, P. and Rowan, J. (eds) (1981) *Human Inquiry: a Sourcebook for New Paradigm Research*, Chichester: John Wiley.

Ricoeur, P. (1981) 'Science and ideology', in *Hermeneutics and the Social Science*, Cambridge: Cambridge University Press, pp. 222–46.

Rorty, R. (1979) *Philosophy and the Mirror of Nature*, Princeton, N.J.: Princeton University Press.

Rose, D. (1999) 'Do it yourselves', *Mental Health Care*, 2, 5: 174–7.

Rose, H. (1994) *Love, Power and Knowledge: Towards a Feminist Transformation of the Sciences*, Cambridge: Polity Press.

Royal College of Nursing (1990) *RCN Standards of Care Project: the Dynamic Standard Setting System*, London: Royal College of Nursing.

Sanford, N. (1970) 'Whatever happened to action research?', *Journal of Social Issues*, 26, 4; reprinted in A. Clarke (ed.) (1976) *Experimenting with Organisational Life – the Action Research Approach*, London: Plenum Press, pp. 19–32.

Schindler, G. (1993) 'The conflict', *Educational Action Research*, I, 3: 457–68.

Schon, D. (1983) *The Reflective Practitioner*, New York: Basic Books.

Schon, D. (1987) *Educating the Reflective Practitioner*, San Francisco: Jossey-Bass.

Schutz, A. (1964) 'The stranger: an essay in social psychology', in A. Broderson (ed.) *Studies in Social Theory*, The Hague: Martinus Nijhoff, pp. 91–105.

Selznick, P. (1964) 'An approach to a theory of bureaucracy', in L. Coser and B. Rosenberg (eds) *Sociological Theory*, 2nd edn, New York: Macmillan, pp. 477–88.

Senge, P. (1990) *The Fifth Discipline – the Art and Practice of the Learning Organisation*, London: Century Business.

Simons, H. (1982a) 'Process evaluation in schools', in R. McCormick (ed.) *Calling Education to Account*, London: Heinemann, pp. 119–32.

Simons, H. (1982b) 'Suggestions for a school self-evaluation based on democratic principles', in R. McCormick (ed.) *Calling Education to Account*, London: Heinemann, pp. 286–95.

Singh, G. (1994) 'Anti-racist social work: political correctness or political action!', *Social Work Education*, 13, 1: 26–31.

Smith, G. (1975) 'Action-research: experimental social administration?', in R. Lees and G. Smith (eds) *Action Research in Community Development*, London: Routledge and Kegan Paul, pp. 188–99.

Somekh, B. (1994) 'Inhabiting each other's castles: towards knowledge and mutual growth through collaboration', *Educational Action Research*, 2, 3: 357–81.

Stacey, R. (1996) *Strategic Management and Organisational Dynamics*, 2nd edn, London: Pitman.

Stake, R. (1967) 'The countenance of educational evaluation', *Teachers College Record*, 68, 7: 523–40.

Stake, R. (1980) 'The case study method in social inquiry', in H. Simons (ed.) *Towards a Science of the Singular*, Norwich: Centre for Applied Research in Education, University of East Anglia.

Stansell, B. (1997) 'How Can I Improve Staff Morale?' (unpublished action research report), Cambridge: Anglia Polytechnic University School of Community Health and Social Studies.

Stenhouse, L. (1975) *An Introduction to Curriculum Research and Development*, London: Heinemann.

Stenhouse, L. (1985a) 'What counts as research?', in J. Ruddock and D. Hopkins (eds) *Research as a Basis for Teaching*, London: Heinemann, pp. 8–19.

Stenhouse, L. (1985b) 'The illuminative research tradition', in J. Ruddock and D. Hopkins (eds) *Research as a Basis for Teaching*, London: Heinemann, pp. 31–2.

Stevenson, M. (1992) 'Columbus and the war on indigenous peoples', *Race and Class*, 33, 3 (*The Curse of Columbus*): 27–45.

Stewart, J. and Sutherland, M. (1992) *The Learning Local Authority*, Luton: Local Government Management Board.

Stringer, E. (1996) *Action Research: a Handbook for Practitioners*, London: Sage.

Tannen, B. (1992) *You Just Don't Understand: Women and Men in Conversation*, London: Virago.

Tavistock Institute (1993) *Human Relations* (special action research issue), 46, 2.

Taylor, R. and Thornicroft, G. (1996) 'Uses and limits of randomised control trials in mental health service research', in G. Thornicroft and M. Tansella (eds) *Mental Health Outcome Measures*, Berlin: Springer, pp. 143–51.

Thompson, N. (1993) *Anti-discriminatory Practice*, London: Macmillan.

Titchen, A. (2000) 'Critical companionship: a conceptual framework for facilitating expertise', in J. Higgs and A. Titchen (eds) *Practice, Knowledge and Expertise in the Health Professions*, Oxford: Butterworth Heinemann.

Towell, D. and Harries, C. (eds) (1979) *Innovation in Patient Care*, London: Croom Helm.

Troyna, B. (1998) '"The whites of my eyes, nose, ears . . .": a reflexive account of "whiteness" in race-related research', in P. Connolly and B. Troyna (eds) *Researching Racism in Education*, Buckingham: Open University Press, pp. 95–108.

Turney, D. (1997) 'Hearing voices, talking difference: a dialogic approach to anti-oppressive practice', *Journal of Social Work Practice*, 11, 2: 115–25.

Twining, W. (1990) *Rethinking Evidence*, Oxford: Blackwell.

Ungerson, C. (1987) *Policy Is Personal: Sex, Gender and Informal Care*, London: Tavistock.

Valla, V. (1994) 'Popular education and knowledge: popular surveillance of health and education services in Brasilian metropolitan areas', *Educational Action Research*, 2, 3: 403–14.

Wadsworth, Y and Hargreaves, K (1993) *What Is Feminist Research?*, Melbourne: Action Research Issues Association.

Ward, H. (1996) 'The looking after children project: asking practitioners to assess outcomes in child care', in Barnardo's, *What Works? Effective Social Interventions in Child Welfare*, Ilford: Barnardo's, pp. 77–89.

Webb, C. (1991) 'Action research', in D. Cormack (ed.) *The Research Process in Nursing*, 2nd edn, Oxford: Blackwell, pp. 155–65.

Weber, M. (1947) 'Legal authority with a bureaucratic administrative staff', in *The Theory of Social and Economic Organisation*, New York: The Free Press, pp. 329–41.

Weber, R. (1985) *Basic Content Analysis*, Beverly Hills, Calif.: Sage.

Whitehead, J. (1989) 'Creating a living educational theory from questions of the kind, "How do I improve my practice?"', *Cambridge Journal of Education*, 19, 1: 41–52.

Whyte, W.F. (ed.) (1991) *Participatory Action Research*, Newbury Park, Calif.: Sage.

Winter, R. (1982) '"Dilemma analysis" – a contribution to methodology for action research', *Cambridge Journal of Education*, 12, 3: 166–74.

Winter, R. (1987) *Action Research and the Nature of Social Inquiry*, Aldershot: Avebury/Gower.

Winter, R. (1989) *Learning from Experience: Principles and Practice in Action Research*, Lewes: Falmer Press.

Winter, R. (1994) 'The relevance for action research of feminist theories of educational development', *Educational Action Research*, 2, 3: 423–6.

Winter, R. (1996) 'Some principles and procedures for the conduct of action research', in O. Zuber-Skerritt (ed.) *New Directions in Action Research*, London: Falmer Press.

Winter, R. (1998) 'Managers, spectators and citizens: where does "theory" come from in action research?', *Educational Action Research*, 6, 3: 361–76.

Winter, R. and Maisch, M. (1996) *Professional Competence and Higher Education: the ASSET Programme*, London: Falmer Press.

Wittgenstein, L. (1968) *Philosophical Investigations*, 3rd edn, Oxford: Blackwell.

Yelloly, M. and Henkel, M. (1995) *Learning and Teaching in Social Work: Towards Reflective Practice*, London: Jessica Kingsley.

Yunus, M. (1998) *Banker to the Poor: the Autobiography of Muhammad Yunus, Founder of the Grameen Bank*, London: Aurum.

Index

1212